AAOS
Comprehensive
Orthopaedic
Review

Study Questions

AAOS
AMERICAN ACADEMY OF
ORTHOPAEDIC SURGEONS

AAOS
Comprehensive
Orthopaedic
Review

Study Questions

Editor

Jay R. Lieberman, MD

Director, New England Musculoskeletal Institute
Professor and Chairman, Department of Orthopaedic Surgery
University of Connecticut Health Center
Farmington, Connecticut

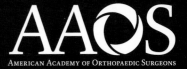

AMERICAN ACADEMY OF ORTHOPAEDIC SURGEONS

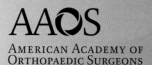

AMERICAN ACADEMY OF ORTHOPAEDIC SURGEONS

The material presented in the **AAOS Comprehensive Orthopaedic Review: Study Questions** has been made available by the American Academy of Orthopaedic Surgeons for educational purposes only. This material is not intended to present the only, or necessarily best, methods or procedures for the medical situations discussed, but rather is intended to represent an approach, view, statement, or opinion of the author(s) or producer(s), which may be helpful to others who face similar situations.

Some drugs or medical devices demonstrated in Academy courses or described in Academy print or electronic publications have not been cleared by the Food and Drug Administration (FDA) or have been cleared for specific uses only. The FDA has stated that it is the responsibility of the physician to determine the FDA clearance status of each drug or device he or she wishes to use in clinical practice.

Furthermore, any statements about commercial products are solely the opinion(s) of the author(s) and do not represent an Academy endorsement or evaluation of these products. These statements may not be used in advertising or for any commercial purpose.

Published 2009 by the
American Academy of Orthopaedic Surgeons
6300 North River Road
Rosemont, IL 60018

Copyright 2009
by the American Academy of Orthopaedic Surgeons

ISBN 978-0-89203-597-7

Printed in the USA

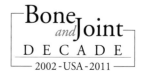

Acknowledgments

Editorial Board
AAOS Comprehensive Orthopaedic Review
Study Questions

Jay R. Lieberman, MD *(Editor)*
Director, New England Musculoskeletal Institute
Professor and Chairman, Department of Orthopaedic
  Surgery
University of Connecticut Health Center
Farmington, Connecticut

Martin I. Boyer, MD, MSc, FRCSC *(Hand and Wrist)*
Associate Professor
Department of Orthopaedic Surgery
Washington University School of Medicine
St. Louis, Missouri

Brian G. Donley, MD *(Foot and Ankle)*
Director, Center for Foot and Ankle
Orthopaedic and Rheumatologic Institute
Cleveland Clinic
Cleveland, Ohio

Leesa M. Galatz, MD *(Shoulder and Elbow)*
Associate Professor, Shoulder and Elbow Service
Department of Orthopaedic Surgery
Washington University
Barnes-Jewish Hospital
St. Louis, Missouri

Jonathan N. Grauer, MD *(Basic Science)*
Associate Professor
Department of Orthopaedics and Rehabilitation
Yale University School of Medicine
New Haven, Connecticut

Robert M. Kay, MD *(Pediatrics)*
Associate Professor
Department of Orthopaedic Surgery
Keck School of Medicine
University of Southern California
Children's Orthopaedic Center
Children's Hospital Los Angeles
Los Angeles, California

Kenneth J. Koval, MD *(Trauma)*
Professor of Orthopaedics
Dartmouth-Hitchcock Medical Center
Lebanon, New Hampshire

Kurt P. Spindler, MD *(Sports Medicine, Knee)*
Kenneth D. Schermerhorn Professor
Vice-Chairman, Department of Orthopaedics
Director, Vanderbilt Sports Medicine Center
Nashville, Tennessee

Thomas Parker Vail, MD *(Total Joint Arthroplasty/*
  Joint Salvage)
Professor and Chairman
Department of Orthopaedic Surgery
University of California, San Francisco
San Francisco, California

Jeffrey C. Wang, MD *(Spine)*
Chief, Orthopaedic Spine Service
Professor, Orthopaedic Surgery and Neurosurgery
UCLA Spine Center
UCLA School of Medicine
Los Angeles, California

Kristy Weber, MD *(Orthopaedic Oncology and Systemic*
  Disease)
Associate Professor of Orthopaedics and Oncology
Department of Orthopaedics
Johns Hopkins University
Baltimore, Maryland

Many of the questions in this book were originally prepared for inclusion in the following AAOS examinations:

1996 Anatomy-Imaging Self-Assessment Examination

1997 Orthopaedic Basic Science Self-Assessment Examination

1997 Musculoskeletal Trauma Self-Assessment Examination

1998 Pediatric Orthopaedic Self-Assessment Examination

1999 Anatomy-Imaging Self-Assessment Examination

2000 Orthopaedic Basic Science Self-Assessment Examination

2000 Musculoskeletal Trauma Self-Assessment Examination

2001 Pediatric Orthopaedic Self-Assessment Examination

2002 Orthopaedic Self-Assessment Examination

2002 Anatomy-Imaging Self-Assessment Examination

2002 Musculoskeletal Tumors and Diseases Self-Assessment Examination

2002 Shoulder and Elbow Self-Assessment Examination

2003 Adult Spine Self-Assessment Examination

2003 Foot and Ankle Self-Assessment Examination

2003 Musculoskeletal Trauma Self-Assessment Examination

2004 Adult Reconstructive Surgery of the Hip and Knee
      Self-Assessment Examination

2004 Pediatric Orthopaedic Self-Assessment Examination

2004 Sports Medicine Self-Assessment Examination

2005 Musculoskeletal Tumors and Diseases Self-Assessment Examination

Preface

Self-assessment is an integral part of preparing for critical orthopaedic examinations. The time-pressed resident or practicing orthopaedic surgeon who has limited hours available for examination preparation can find the prospect of reviewing the entire field of orthopaedics a nearly impossible task. This set of study questions is provided to help focus the reader's efforts. By self-assessing, the reader can identify areas of relative strength and weakness and chart a course of study for areas needing attention, by a close reading of the appropriate section of the *AAOS Comprehensive Orthopaedic Review* and by exploring the additional reading provided in the references listed for each study question as well as other home study programs.

To facilitate this focused study, the questions are organized into 10 content domains: *Basic Science, Pediatric Orthopaedics, Orthopaedic Oncology and Systemic Disease, Sports Medicine, Trauma, Spine, Shoulder and Elbow, Hand and Wrist, Total Joint Arthroplasty/Joint Salvage,* and *Foot and Ankle.* Various aspects of the knee are covered in the sports medicine, trauma, and total joint sections.

Many of the study questions in this book are taken from *Orthopaedic Self-Assessment Examinations* (OSAEs) published by the American Academy of Orthopaedic Surgeons (AAOS). In addition, new questions were written specifically for this publication. All questions were reviewed in 2008 and 2009 to make sure the material included is accurate and reflects current knowledge. I am grateful to the following section editors who, in addition to their considerable duties in editing the review book, read

many hundreds of potential questions, reviewing them for accuracy of content and selecting those they judged most important to include in this volume: Martin Boyer, MD (Hand and Wrist); Brian Donley, MD (Foot and Ankle); Leesa Galatz, MD (Shoulder and Elbow); Jonathan Grauer, MD (Basic Science); Robert Kay, MD (Pediatric Orthopaedics); Ken Koval, MD (Trauma); Kurt Spindler, MD (Sports Medicine); Thomas Vail, MD (Total Joint Arthroplasty/Joint Salvage); Jeff Wang, MD (Spine); and Kristy Weber, MD (Orthopaedic Oncology and Systemic Disease). I also want to thank Marilyn Fox, PhD, and the Department of Publications at the AAOS for their support. This book would not have been possible without the cooperation of the following people in the Department of Electronic Media, Evaluation Programs, Course Operations, and Practice Management Group, who made the study questions available: Howard Mevis, Director; Marcie Lampert, Senior Examinations Coordinator; and Irene Bogdal, Administrative Assistant.

Our goal was to provide the reader with a truly comprehensive review of the field of orthopaedics. We hope that you agree that we have accomplished this objective.

Jay R. Lieberman, MD
Director, New England Musculoskeletal Institute
Professor and Chairman,
Department of Orthopaedic Surgery
University of Connecticut Health Center
Farmington, Connecticut

Table of Contents

Basic Science

Section Editor

Jonathan N. Grauer, MD

Q-1: Titanium, an extremely reactive metal, is one of the most biocompatible implant materials because

1. nothing in the biologic environment reacts with titanium.
2. physiologic conditions inhibit titanium reactions.
3. proteins coat the titanium and "insulate" it from the body.
4. titanium spontaneously forms a stable oxide coating.
5. titanium alloys are less reactive than pure metal.

Q-2: Which of the following cell membrane proteins convey chemotherapeutic resistance to tumor cells?

1. CD44 glycoproteins
2. P-glycoproteins
3. Paracrine peptides
4. Matrix metalloproteinases (MMPs)
5. Stromelysins

Q-3: Bone destruction as a result of multiple myeloma is primarily caused by which of the following cell types?

1. Myeloma cells
2. Macrophages
3. Osteoclasts
4. Plasma cells
5. Pericytes

Q-4: Which of the following antibiotics is bacteriostatic at therapeutic serum concentrations?

1. Penicillin
2. Cefoxitin
3. Clindamycin
4. Vancomycin
5. Bacitracin

Q-5: The administration of ciprofloxacin is contraindicated in which of the following patient populations?

1. Diabetics
2. Alcoholics
3. Intravenous drug abusers
4. Patients with renal failure
5. Children

Q-6: What antibiotic works by inhibiting peptidoglycan synthesis?

1. Penicillin
2. Gentamicin
3. Rifampin
4. Tetracycline
5. Clindamycin

Q-7: Which of the following organisms is (are) most likely to cause hematogenous osteomyelitis in hemodialysis patients?

1. *Escherichia coli* and *Klebsiella pneumoniae*
2. *Staphylococci*
3. *Candida* species
4. Anaerobic oral organisms
5. Anaerobic enteric organisms

Q-8: The pharmacologic effect of warfarin is caused by what mechanism?

1. Inhibition of platelet aggregation
2. Inhibition of hepatic enzymes that activate vitamin K
3. Binding to vitamin K-dependent clotting factors II, VII, IX, and X
4. Binding to antithrombin III, which increases its affinity for activated Factor X and thrombin
5. Direct binding to vitamin K

Q-9: A brittle material such as a ceramic femoral head prosthesis undergoes what type(s) of deformation when loaded to failure?

1. Elastic and plastic
2. Elastic
3. Plastic
4. Viscoelastic
5. Viscoelastic and plastic

Q-10: The risk of human immunodeficiency virus (HIV) transmission via a processed musculoskeletal allograft obtained from an American Association of Tissue Banks (AATB) certified bone bank is estimated to be

1. 1 in 50,000.
2. 1 in 100,000.
3. 1 in 500,000.
4. 1 in 1.5 million.
5. 1 in 5 million.

Q-11: Which of the following methods or parameters would best determine the percentage of aneuploid cells in a malignant tumor?

1. Immunohistochemistry
2. Histiologic mapping
3. Degree of necrosis
4. Presence of dedifferentiation
5. Flow cytometry

Q-12: Which of the following variables most influences the volumetric wear of polyethylene occurring on secondary surfaces (backside wear) in modular total hip and total knee components?

1. Total contact area
2. Roughness of the metal surface
3. Composition of the metal surface
4. Magnitude of the load
5. Relative motion

Q-13: What factor is most likely to decrease the rigidity of an external fixation system?

1. Increased pin diameter
2. Increased pin number
3. Decreased pin separation
4. Decreased pin group separation
5. Increased distance of the side bar to the bone

Q-14: Which of the following functions primarily as an osteoconductive as opposed to an osteoinductive material?

1. Autogenous cortical bone
2. Demineralized bone matrix
3. Freeze-dried cortical allogeneic bone
4. Autogenous cancellous bone
5. Bone morphogenetic protein

Q-15: What antibiotic works by inhibiting DNA gyrase?

1. Penicillin
2. Gentamicin
3. Vancomycin
4. Ciprofloxacin
5. Clindamycin

Q-16: In some cases of osteopetrosis, bone resorption and remodeling are impaired because of a defect in carbonic anhydrase. The function of this enzyme in bone is to

1. promote maturation of mononuclear phagocytes into osteoclasts.
2. degrade osteoid.
3. generate hydrogen ions at the ruffled border.
4. promote coupling between osteoblasts and osteoclasts.
5. initiate stress-related remodeling.

Q-17: The structure of cartilage proteoglycans can be described as

1. multiple hyaluronate molecules bound to core protein, which is subsequently bound to a glycosaminoglycan chain.
2. multiple glycosaminoglycan chains bound to hyaluronate, which is subsequently bound to core protein.
3. multiple glycosaminoglycans bound to core protein, which is subsequently bound to hyaluronate via a link protein.
4. multiple link proteins bound to core protein, which is subsequently bound to glycosaminoglycan.
5. multiple hyaluronate chains bound to link protein, which is subsequently bound to glycosaminoglycan.

Q-18: A newly discovered gene (retinoblastoma gene) is expressed in normal cells. Loss of this gene results in a malignant phenotype. What type of gene is being described?

1. Dominant oncogene
2. Recessive oncogene
3. Proto-oncogene
4. Suppressor gene
5. Transgene

Q-19: What component of frozen allograft bone has the least amount of immunogenicity?

1. Bone marrow cells
2. Proteoglycans
3. Hydroxyapatite
4. Cytokines
5. Cell surface proteins

Q-20: What portion of the knee meniscus has the greatest concentration of mechanoreceptors?

1. Peripheral one third
2. Central one third
3. Inner two thirds
4. Anterior horn
5. Posterior horn

Q-21: Figure 1 shows the radiograph of a 6-year-old girl who has a right thoracic scoliosis that measures 60°. Examination shows multiple café-au-lait spots, and family history reveals that the child's mother has the same disorder. The gene responsible for this disorder codes for

1. dystrophin.
2. frataxin.
3. neurofibromin.
4. peripheral myelin protein.
5. sulfate transport protein.

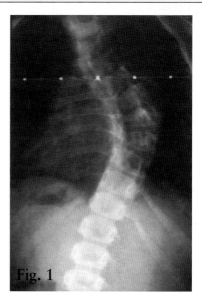

Fig. 1

Q-22: In children, scurvy has the greatest effect on bone formation in the

1. physis.
2. diaphysis.
3. epiphysis.
4. metaphysis.
5. articular surface.

Q-23: Warfarin limits the risk of deep venous thrombosis (DVT) by which of the following actions?

1. Competitive inhibition of vitamin K-dependent clotting factors
2. Inhibition of the posttranslational modification of vitamin K-dependent clotting factors
3. Reversible inhibition of platelet function
4. Irreversible inhibition of platelet function
5. Potentiation of antithrombin III

Q-24: What is the most common bacterium found in an infection caused by a human bite?

1. *Eikenella*
2. *Pasturella multocida*
3. *Borrelia burgdorferi*
4. *Salmonella typhosa*
5. Methicillin-resistant *Staphylococcus aureus*

Q-25: The rate of chondrocyte maturation in the growth plate is directly regulated by an interaction between systemic hormones and

1. electric fields.
2. local growth factors.
3. oxygen tension.
4. mechanical forces.
5. calcium concentrations.

Q-26: A genetic defect in type X collagen is most likely to result in which of the following conditions?

1. Multiple early fractures
2. Osteoporosis
3. Chondrodysplasia
4. Joint laxity
5. Inflammatory arthritis

Q-27: Most natural biologic materials are anisotropic, meaning that their stress-strain curve exhibits

1. different moduli for compressive and tensile tests.
2. a high degree of nonlinearity.
3. a high sensitivity to the size of the test specimen.
4. dependence on the rate of loading.
5. dependence on the direction of load application.

Q-28: Which of the following factors is most commonly associated with late aseptic loosening of cemented acetabular components?

1. Increased frictional torque
2. Recurrent neck-socket impingement
3. Fatigue failure of cement
4. Poor initial component fixation
5. Polyethylene wear

Q-29: Which of the following processes will most greatly increase the wear damage to an ultrahigh molecular weight polyethylene articulating surface?

1. Ethanol sterilization
2. Third body inclusion
3. Cold flow deformation
4. Gamma radiation sterilization
5. Ion implantation on the mating metallic surface

Q-30: What is the function of a transcription factor?

1. Bind to DNA and influence gene expression
2. Bind to cell membrane receptors and induce phosphorylation
3. Package DNA
4. Unwind DNA
5. Dehydrate cellular proteins

Q-31: What is the most common bacterium found in an infection caused by a tick bite?

1. *Eikenella*
2. *Vibrio vulnificus*
3. *Borrelia burgdorferi*
4. *Clostridium perfringens*
5. Methicillin-resistant *Streptococcus*

Q-32: Methicillin-resistant *Staphylococcus aureus* can be treated effectively with an oral quinolone and which of the following antibiotics to achieve synergy?

1. Penicillin
2. Probenecid
3. Rifampin
4. Cefoxitin
5. Amoxicillin

Q-33: A fully differentiated osteoclast has receptors for which of the following proteins?

1. Parathyroid hormone (PTH)
2. Calcitonin
3. Cholecalciferol
4. Bone morphogenetic protein (BMP)
5. Interleukin-2 (IL-2)

Q-34: Cephalosporins are effective antibiotic agents because of their action on what aspect of bacterial metabolism?

1. DNA gyrase
2. Cell wall
3. mRNA
4. Cell membrane
5. Protein

Q-35: Repair of the peripheral one third of the meniscus is sometimes possible because it has which of the following characteristics?

1. Increased blood supply
2. Appropriate viscoelasticity
3. High glycoprotein concentration
4. High type II collagen concentration
5. Large size

Q-36: During the first 2 years of life, which of the following actions is most responsible for increasing structural stability of the physis?

1. The change from a flat to an undulating physis
2. The growth of the zone of Ranvier
3. Increased strength of the points of insertion of muscles onto bone
4. Increased penetration of proprioceptive nerve endings about the physis
5. Increased capillary penetration about the physis

Q-37: Virtually all biological materials are viscoelastic, which means that their mechanical behavior is dependent on what factor?

1. Load applied
2. Cross-sectional area
3. Rate of loading
4. Mode of loading
5. Direction of loading

Q-38: When a long bone is subjected to a bending moment, the greatest tensile stresses are located

1. within the cortex.
2. at the neutral axis.
3. at a periosteal surface.
4. at an endosteal surface.
5. along the bending axis.

Q-39: What is the dominant component of articular cartilage extracellular matrix by weight?

1. Water
2. Collagen
3. Keratan sulfate
4. Chondroitin sulfate
5. Nerve and lymphatic tissue

A-1: Titanium, an extremely reactive metal, is one of the most biocompatible implant materials because

1. nothing in the biologic environment reacts with titanium.
2. physiologic conditions inhibit titanium reactions.
3. proteins coat the titanium and "insulate" it from the body.
4. titanium spontaneously forms a stable oxide coating.
5. titanium alloys are less reactive than pure metal.

PREFERRED RESPONSE: 4

DISCUSSION: Titanium rapidly forms an adherent oxide, TiO_2, when exposed to oxygen. This process of self-passivation effectively covers the surface of titanium and titanium alloys with a nonreactive ceramic coating and makes these materials extremely biocompatible.

REFERENCES: Black J: *Orthopaedic Biomaterials in Research and Practice.* New York, NY, Churchill Livingstone, 1988, pp 57-81.
Simon SR (ed): *Orthopaedic Basic Science.* Rosemont, IL, American Academy of Orthopaedic Surgeons, 1994, pp 467-474.

A-2: Which of the following cell membrane proteins convey chemotherapeutic resistance to tumor cells?

1. CD44 glycoproteins
2. P-glycoproteins
3. Paracrine peptides
4. Matrix metalloproteinases (MMPs)
5. Stromelysins

PREFERRED RESPONSE: 2

DISCUSSION: One of the mechanisms of chemotherapeutic resistance of cancer cells is through the expression of the multidrug resistance gene 1 (MDR1). MDR1 codes for a membrane phosphoglycoprotein (p-glycoprotein). P-glycoprotein is an energy-dependent efflux pump that is associated with resistance to hydrophobic agents. The presence of p-glycoprotein in chondrosarcoma has been hypothesized to contribute to its chemotherapeutic resistance. CD44 glycoprotein is a cell surface cytokine found on metastatic tumor cells that binds to subendothelial basement membranes. Paracrine peptides are growth factors found in the local tissue environment, rather than tumor cell-produced growth factors (autocrine peptides) that promote metastatic tumor growth. MMPs are proteases produced by malignant cells that degrade tissue basement membranes to assist in metastasis. Stromelysins are MMPs that degrade proteoglycan core protein, laminin, fibronectin, and nonhelical portions of basement membrane collagens.

REFERENCES: Terek RM, Schwartz GK, Devaney K, et al: Chemotherapy and p-glycoprotein expression in chondrosarcoma. *J Orthop Res* 1998;16:585-590.
Pastan I, Gottesman M: Multiple-drug resistance in human cancer. *N Engl J Med* 1987;316:1388-1393.

A-3: Bone destruction as a result of multiple myeloma is primarily caused by which of the following cell types?

1. Myeloma cells
2. Macrophages
3. Osteoclasts
4. Plasma cells
5. Pericytes

PREFERRED RESPONSE: 3

DISCUSSION: Myeloma is commonly associated with bone destruction. Osteoclasts appear to be the major cell type involved in bone osteolysis. Osteoclasts have been reported to cluster on bone-resorbing surfaces adjacent to collections of myeloma cells. In addition, cultures of human myeloma cells in vitro produce several osteoclast activating factors, including lymphotoxin, interleukin-l, and interleukin-6. Myeloma cells have not been reported to directly destroy bone. Osteoblast function is inhibited by the presence of myeloma cells. Pericytes derive from the vascular endothelium and are hypothesized to function as osteoblast progenitor cells.

REFERENCES: Mundy GR, Yoneda T: Facilitation and suppression of bone metastasis. *Clin Orthop Relat Res* 1995;312:34-44.
Mundy GR: Mechanisms of osteolytic bone destruction. *Bone* 1991;12(suppl 1):S1-6.

A-4: Which of the following antibiotics is bacteriostatic at therapeutic serum concentrations?

1. Penicillin
2. Cefoxitin
3. Clindamycin
4. Vancomycin
5. Bacitracin

PREFERRED RESPONSE: 3

DISCUSSION: Penicillin and cephalosporins such as cefoxitin, vancomycin, and bacitracin are all bactericidal by causing loss of bacterial cell wall viability, either by activating enzymes that disrupt cell walls or by inhibiting synthesis of cell walls. Clindamycin is bacteriostatic and acts by inhibiting protein synthesis.

REFERENCES: Sande MA, Kapusnik-Uner JE, Mandell GL: Antimicrobial agents, in Gilman AG (ed): *Goodman and Gilman's The Pharmacological Basis of Therapeutics,* ed 8. New York, NY, McGraw, 1990, p 1019.
Pruitt BA, McManus WF, McManus AT, et al: Infections: Bacteriology, antibiotics and chemotherapy, in Jupiter JB (ed): *Flynn's Hand Surgery, ed 4*. Baltimore, MD, Williams & Wilkins, 1991, p 713.

Answers: Basic Science

A-5: The administration of ciprofloxacin is contraindicated in which of the following patient populations?

1. Diabetics

2. Alcoholics

3. Intravenous drug abusers

4. Patients with renal failure

5. Children

PREFERRED RESPONSE: 5

DISCUSSION: Quinolone antibiotics such as ciprofloxacin have produced arthropathy in immature mammals and, although these lesions have not been reported in humans, these drugs are not recommended for use in children. The two major drug interactions to be aware of with ciprofloxacin are the significant decrease in absorption of the drug when taken orally with magnesium or aluminum-containing antacids, and the increase in serum concentration when theophylline is administered with ciprofloxacin.

REFERENCES: Frymoyer JW (ed): *Orthopaedic Knowledge Update 4: Home Study Syllabus.* Rosemont, IL, American Academy of Orthopaedic Surgeons, 1993, p 157.
Sande MA, Kapusnik-Uner JE, Mandell GL: Antimicrobial agents, in Gilman AG (ed): *Goodman and Gilman's The Pharmacological Basis of Therapeutics,* ed 8. New York, NY, McGraw, 1990, p 1059.

A-6: What antibiotic works by inhibiting peptidoglycan synthesis?

1. Penicillin

2. Gentamicin

3. Rifampin

4. Tetracycline

5. Clindamycin

PREFERRED RESPONSE: 1

DISCUSSION: The beta-lactam antibiotics such as penicillin are thought to work by inhibiting peptidoglycan synthesis by binding to the bacterial cell membrane surface penicillin-binding proteins. Rifampin inhibits bacterial RNA synthesis. Gentamicin, clindamycin, and tetracycline act via different mechanisms to interfere with bacterial RNA function.

REFERENCES: Simon SR (ed): *Orthopaedic Basic Science.* Rosemont, IL, American Academy of Orthopaedic Surgeons, 1994, p 505.
Saude MA, Kapusnik-Uner JE, Mandell GL: Antimicrobial agents, in Gilman AG (ed): *Goodman and Gilman's The Pharmacological Basis of Therapeutics,* ed 8. New York, NY, McGraw, 1990, p 1019.

A-7: Which of the following organisms is (are) most likely to cause hematogenous osteomyelitis in hemodialysis patients?

1. *Escherichia coli* and *Klebsiella pneumoniae*
2. *Staphylococci*
3. *Candida* species
4. Anaerobic oral organisms
5. Anaerobic enteric organisms

PREFERRED RESPONSE: 2

DISCUSSION: Hemodialysis patients are at increased risk for hematogenous osteomyelitis because indwelling intravenous catheters used over the long term serve as a source of infection. *Staphylococcus aureus* and *S epidermidis* are the organisms most commonly isolated. The ribs and thoracic vertebrae are the most frequently affected bones.

REFERENCE: Gupta M, Frenkel LD: Acute osteomyelitis, in Jauregui LE (ed): *Diagnosis and Management of Bone Infections.* New York, NY, Marcel Dekker, 1995, p 15.

A-8: The pharmacologic effect of warfarin is caused by what mechanism?

1. Inhibition of platelet aggregation
2. Inhibition of hepatic enzymes that activate vitamin K
3. Binding to vitamin K-dependent clotting factors II, VII, IX, and X
4. Binding to antithrombin III, which increases its affinity for activated Factor X and thrombin
5. Direct binding to vitamin K

PREFERRED RESPONSE: 2

DISCUSSION: Warfarin acts by inhibiting hepatic enzymes, vitamin K epoxide, and possibly vitamin K reductase. This inhibition leads to reduced carboxylation of vitamin K-dependent proteins (prothrombin and factors VII, IX, and X). The therapeutic effect of warfarin on the clotting cascade is delayed by the time necessary for normal clotting factors to be turned over and replaced by decarboxylated factors. Factor VII, with a half-life of 6 to 7 hours, is the first to be affected. The early onset of therapeutic anticoagulation may be limited by the simultaneous suppression of the antithrombogenic factor, Protein C, which is also a carboxylated vitamin K-dependent protein. Warfarin does not act by binding directly to vitamin K or to clotting factors.

REFERENCES: Zimlich RH, Fulbright BM, Friedman RJ: Current status of anticoagulation therapy after total hip and total knee arthroplasty. *J Am Acad Orthop Surg* 1996;4:54-62.
Colwell CW, Spiro TE, Trowbridge AA, et al: Use of enoxaparin, a low-molecular-weight heparin, and unfractionated heparin for the prevention of deep vein thrombosis after elective hip replacement: A clinical trial comparing efficacy and safety. *J Bone Joint Surg Am* 1994;76:3-14.
RD Heparin Arthroplasty Group: RD heparin compared with warfarin for prevention of venous thromboembolic disease following total hip or knee arthroplasty. *J Bone Joint Surg Am* 1994;76:1174-1185.

A-9: A brittle material such as a ceramic femoral head prosthesis undergoes what type(s) of deformation when loaded to failure?

1. Elastic and plastic
2. Elastic
3. Plastic
4. Viscoelastic
5. Viscoelastic and plastic

PREFERRED RESPONSE: 2

DISCUSSION: Brittle materials undergo only fully recoverable (elastic) deformation prior to fracture. Brittle materials have little or no capacity to undergo permanent (plastic) deformation prior to fracture. The properties of brittle materials are neither temperature nor rate dependent (viscoelastic).

REFERENCES: Burstein AH, Wright TM: *Fundamentals of Orthopaedic Biomechanics.* Baltimore, MD, Williams & Wilkins, 1994, pp 95-129.
Simon SR (ed): *Orthopaedic Basic Science.* Rosemont, IL, American Academy of Orthopaedic Surgeons, 1994, pp 449-452.

A-10: The risk of human immunodeficiency virus (HIV) transmission via a processed musculoskeletal allograft obtained from an American Association of Tissue Banks (AATB) certified bone bank is estimated to be

1. 1 in 50,000.
2. 1 in 100,000.
3. 1 in 500,000.
4. 1 in 1.5 million.
5. 1 in 5 million.

PREFERRED RESPONSE: 4

DISCUSSION: In a recent review, the risk of HIV transmission in patients receiving processed musculoskeletal allografts from reputable bone banks was estimated to be 1 in 1.5 million. The following precautions are important: Bone banks certified by the AATB screen all donors by taking a social and medical history and performing serology for hepatitis B surface antigen, hepatitis B core antibody, hepatitis C antibody, syphilis, human T cell leukemia virus antibody, HIV-I and -II antibody and HIV-I antigen (P24). Some banks examine donor tissues for HIV using polymerase chain reaction technology. Using this technology, one infected cell can be reliably detected in a population of 10^6 uninfected cells. Additionally, the interval between inoculation of a person with the virus and detection of the virus is shorter than with antibody tests. When the tissue or bone is processed (debrided, washed, soaked in ethanol or antibiotics), the risk is further reduced. To date there has been no documented case of disease transmission by processed musculoskeletal allografts.

REFERENCE: Tomford WW: Transmission of disease through transplantation of musculoskeletal allografts. *J Bone Joint Surg Am* 1995;77:1742-1754.

Answers: Basic Science

A-11: Which of the following methods or parameters would best determine the percentage of aneuploid cells in a malignant tumor?

1. Immunohistochemistry

2. Histiologic mapping

3. Degree of necrosis

4. Presence of dedifferentiation

5. Flow cytometry

PREFERRED RESPONSE: 5

DISCUSSION: Flow cytometry is a method by which the amount of DNA in cells is quantified. Thousands of cell nuclei, normal and neoplastic, are passed through a machine that uses a fluorescent dye as a marker of the DNA content. The pattern generated can be characterized as either normal or abnormal based on the cell ploidy. By convention, the amount of DNA in an ovum or sperm is haploid, and normal cells are diploid (euploid) in the G_0 phase of the cell cycle, twice the amount of DNA (tetraploid) is seen during cell division. Normal flow cytometry patterns demonstrate a large diploid spike with a much smaller tetraploid spike representing those few cells undergoing division. Abnormal amounts of DNA (aneuploid) show patterns outside of these two spikes. Immunohistochemical analysis can assist in histiologic classification of tumors but does not measure aneuploidy. The degree of necrosis and presence of dedifferentiation may signify a high-grade lesion, but does not relate to the aneuploid nature of malignant cells.

REFERENCES: Simon SR (ed): *Orthopaedic Basic Science*. Rosemont, IL, American Academy of Orthopaedic Surgeons, 1994, pp 219-276.
Mankin HJ, Conner JF, Schiller AL, et al: Grading of bone tumors by analysis of nuclear DNA content using flow cytometry. *J Bone Joint Surg Am* 1985;67:404-413.

A-12: Which of the following variables most influences the volumetric wear of polyethylene occurring on secondary surfaces (backside wear) in modular total hip and total knee components?

1. Total contact area

2. Roughness of the metal surface

3. Composition of the metal surface

4. Magnitude of the load

5. Relative motion

PREFERRED RESPONSE: 5

DISCUSSION: Wear is the removal of material that occurs as the result of relative motion between two opposed surfaces. All of these factors can influence the volume of backside polyethylene wear; however, the most important factor is relative motion. Surfaces in contact without relative motion do not wear.

REFERENCE: McKellop HA, Campbell P, Park SH, et al: The origin of submicron polyethylene wear debris in total hip arthroplasty. *Clin Orthop Relat Res* 1995;311:3-20.

A-13: What factor is most likely to decrease the rigidity of an external fixation system?

1. Increased pin diameter
2. Increased pin number
3. Decreased pin separation
4. Decreased pin group separation
5. Increased distance of the side bar to the bone

PREFERRED RESPONSE: 5

DISCUSSION: An increase in pin length (bone surface to frame) significantly increases the deformability to load, and reduces the construct rigidity. The longer the length of a rod or pin, the greater the deformation under a given load. As the point of attachment of the sidebar is moved further from the bone surface, the effective pin length is increased.

REFERENCES: Chao EYS, Aru HT: Biomechanics of fracture fixation, in Mow VC, Hayes WC (eds): *Basic Orthopaedic Biomechanics*. New York, NY, Raven Press, 1991, pp 309-315.
Chao EYS, Kasman RA, An KN: Rigidity and stress analysis of external fracture fixation devices: A theoretical approach. *J Biomech* 1982;15:971-983.

A-14: Which of the following functions primarily as an osteoconductive as opposed to an osteoinductive material?

1. Autogenous cortical bone
2. Demineralized bone matrix
3. Freeze-dried cortical allogeneic bone
4. Autogenous cancellous bone
5. Bone morphogenetic protein

PREFERRED RESPONSE: 3

DISCUSSION: Freeze-dried cortical allografts are almost exclusively osteoconductive. All of the above materials have been used to augment bone repair. Osteoconduction is a property of bone graft materials, which provide a three-dimensional trellis for the ingrowth of host capillaries and osteoprogenitor cells. Osteoinduction involves the recruitment and differentiation of undifferentiated mesenchymal stem cells from the surrounding host tissues to osteoblasts. Osteoinductive substances can promote bone formation in ectopic sites. Autogenous bone grafts are osteogenic, which means they possess the intrinsic potential to form new bone. They also are osteoconductive. Allografts are not considered osteoinductive because this property is lost through processing to eliminate immunologic barriers. Bone morphogenetic proteins are purely osteoinductive.

REFERENCES: Burchardt H: The biology of bone graft repair. *Clin Orthop Relat Res* 1983;174:28-42.
Goldberg VM, Stevenson S: The biology of bone grafts. *Semin Arthroplasty* 1993;4:58-63.
Damien CJ, Parsons JR: Bone graft and bone graft substitutes: A review of current technology and applications. *J Appl Biomater* 1991;2:187-208.

Answers: Basic Science

A-15: What antibiotic works by inhibiting DNA gyrase?

1. Penicillin
2. Gentamicin
3. Vancomycin
4. Ciprofloxacin
5. Clindamycin

PREFERRED RESPONSE: 4

DISCUSSION: The quinolone antibiotics such as ciprofloxacin function by inhibiting DNA gyrase. Gentamicin and clindamycin act via different mechanisms to interfere with bacterial RNA function. Penicillin binds to bacterial surface membrane proteins. inhibiting peptidoglycan synthesis. Vancomycin interferes with the insertion of glycan subunits into the cell wall.

REFERENCES: Simon SR (ed): *Orthopaedic Basic Science.* Rosemont, IL, American Academy of Orthopaedic Surgeons, 1994, p 505.
Frymoyer JW (ed): *Orthopaedic Knowledge Update 4: Home Study Syllabus.* Rosemont, IL, American Academy of Orthopaedic Surgeons, 1993, p 157.

A-16: In some cases of osteopetrosis, bone resorption and remodeling are impaired because of a defect in carbonic anhydrase. The function of this enzyme in bone is to

1. promote maturation of mononuclear phagocytes into osteoclasts.
2. degrade osteoid.
3. generate hydrogen ions at the ruffled border.
4. promote coupling between osteoblasts and osteoclasts.
5. initiate stress-related remodeling.

PREFERRED RESPONSE: 3

DISCUSSION: Osteoclasts are attached to underlying bone via integrin receptors in the clear zone. This effectively seals the space below the osteoclasts. Hydrogen ions produced by carbonic anhydrase are pumped into the space across the ruffled border of the osteoclasts. In the ruffled border space, the underlying hydroxyapatite is solubilized in the low pH and calcium ions are released. Patients who are deficient in carbonic anhydrase cannot resorb bone by this mechanism.

REFERENCES: Simon SR (ed): *Orthopaedic Basic Science.* Rosemont, IL, American Academy of Orthopaedic Surgeons, 1994, pp 185-217.
Poss R (ed): *Orthopaedic Knowledge Update 3: Home Study Syllabus.* Park Ridge, IL, American Academy of Orthopaedic Surgeons, 1990, pp 29-45.

A-17: The structure of cartilage proteoglycans can be described as

1. multiple hyaluronate molecules bound to core protein, which is subsequently bound to a glycosaminoglycan chain.

2. multiple glycosaminoglycan chains bound to hyaluronate, which is subsequently bound to core protein.

3. multiple glycosaminoglycans bound to core protein, which is subsequently bound to hyaluronate via a link protein.

4. multiple link proteins bound to core protein, which is subsequently bound to glycosaminoglycan.

5. multiple hyaluronate chains bound to link protein, which is subsequently bound to glycosaminoglycan.

PREFERRED RESPONSE: 3

DISCUSSION: Cartilage proteoglycans are large negatively charged molecules with a molecular weight of several million and a spatial configuration reminiscent of a test tube brush. The core of the brush is the hyaluronate (a complex sugar), to which are attached many proteoglycan core proteins through an interaction with link protein. On each core protein are many glycosaminoglycan chains.

REFERENCES: Bullough PO, Vigorita VJ: *Atlas of Orthopaedic Pathology.* Baltimore, MD, University Press, 1984, p 34.
Simon SR (ed): *Orthopaedic Basic Science.* Rosemont, IL, American Academy of Orthopaedic Surgeons, 1994, pp 9-11.

A-18: A newly discovered gene (retinoblastoma gene) is expressed in normal cells. Loss of this gene results in a malignant phenotype. What type of gene is being described?

1. Dominant oncogene

2. Recessive oncogene

3. Proto-oncogene

4. Suppressor gene

5. Transgene

PREFERRED RESPONSE: 4

DISCUSSION: The retinoblastoma (RB) gene encodes for a protein that regulates a specific oncogene that, if absent, results in oncogene expression. The RB gene is termed a tumor suppressor gene. Oncogenes, when expressed, result in a malignant phenotype. A proto-oncogene is a normal gene. A transgene is not normally found in an organism, but it can be artificially placed into the single-celled embryo and therefore will be present in all cells of that organism.

REFERENCES: Simon SR (ed): *Orthopaedic Basic Science.* Rosemont, IL, American Academy of Orthopaedic Surgeons, 1994, pp 219-276.
Lewin B: *Genes,* ed 3. New York, NY, John Wiley & Sons, 1987, pp 698-715.

Answers: Basic Science

A-19: What component of frozen allograft bone has the least amount of immunogenicity?

1. Bone marrow cells
2. Proteoglycans
3. Hydroxyapatite
4. Cytokines
5. Cell surface proteins

PREFERRED RESPONSE: 3

DISCUSSION: Large frozen allografts are composite materials and contain a variety of potential antigens. Allografts are primarily subjected to cellular mechanisms, as opposed to humoral rejection mechanisms. Class I and class II cellular antigens, which are encoded by the major histocompatibility complex (MHC) contained within the allograft, are the major alloantigens that are recognized by host T-lymphocytes. Cellular populations that contribute to this antigen pool include marrow adipose tissue, microvascular endothelium, and retinacular activating cells, with those of granulocytic origin being the most inflammatory. The extracellular matrix in the graft elicits a measurable antigenic response, but this response is greatly diminished when compared with the cellular components. Type I collagen, which represents nearly 90% of the organic matrix of bone, has been shown to stimulate both humoral and cell-mediated responses in vivo. The noncollagenous portion of organic bone matrix, consisting of large proteoglycan molecules as well as osteocalcin, osteopontin, and other glycoproteins, has been reported to stimulate immune responsiveness. Hydroxyapatite, the mineral component of bone, has not been shown to elicit an immune response. The failure of allograft incorporation is associated with the degree of allograft cellularity, as well as the MHC incompatibility between allografts and host tissues.

REFERENCES: Horowitz MC, Friedlaender GE: Induction of specific T-cell responsiveness to allogeneic bone. *J Bone Joint Surg Am* 1991;73:1157-1168.
Muscolo DL, Caletti E, Schajowicz F, Araujo ES, Makino A: Tissue-typing in human massive allografts of frozen bone. *J Bone Joint Surg Am* 1987;69:583-595.
Trentham DE, Townes AS, Kang AH, David JR: Humoral and cellular sensitivity to collagen and type II collagen induced arthritis in rats. *J Clin Invest* 1978;61:89-96.

A-20: What portion of the knee meniscus has the greatest concentration of mechanoreceptors?

1. Peripheral one third
2. Central one third
3. Inner two thirds
4. Anterior horn
5. Posterior horn

PREFERRED RESPONSE: 5

DISCUSSION: The neural elements are found in greatest concentration in the horns of the meniscus, and particularly in the posterior horns. The presence of these mechanoreceptors may play a role in sensory feedback of the knee.

REFERENCES: Buckwalter JA, Einhorn TA, Simon SR (eds): *Orthopaedic Basic Science: Biology and Biomechanics of the Musculoskeletal System,* ed 2. Rosemont, IL, American Academy of Orthopaedic Surgeons, 2000, pp 532-545.
O'Connor BL: The mechanoreceptor innervation of the posterior attachments of the lateral meniscus of the dog knee joint. *J Anat* 1984;138:15-26.

A-21: Figure 1 shows the radiograph of a 6-year-old girl who has a right thoracic scoliosis that measures 60°. Examination shows multiple café-au-lait spots, and family history reveals that the child's mother has the same disorder. The gene responsible for this disorder codes for

1. dystrophin.
2. frataxin.
3. neurofibromin.
4. peripheral myelin protein.
5. sulfate transport protein.

PREFERRED RESPONSE: 3

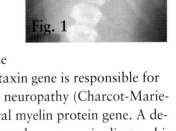
Fig. 1

DISCUSSION: The patient has the dystrophic type of scoliosis seen in patients with neurofibromatosis type I (NF-1). The NF-1 gene is located on chromosome 17 and codes for neurofibromin, believed to be a tumor-suppresser gene. Abnormalities in the dystrophin gene are seen in Duchenne muscular dystrophy and Becker muscular dystrophy. A mutation in the frataxin gene is responsible for Friedreich ataxia. The most common type of hereditary motor and sensory neuropathy (Charcot-Marie-Tooth), HMSN type IA is caused by a complete duplication of the peripheral myelin protein gene. A defect in the cellular sulfate transport protein results in undersulfation of proteoglycans seen in diastrophic dysplasia.

REFERENCE: Beaty JH: *Orthopaedic Knowledge Update 6.* Rosemont, IL, American Academy of Orthopaedic Surgeons, 1999, pp 225-234.

Answers: Basic Science

A-22: In children, scurvy has the greatest effect on bone formation in the

1. physis.
2. diaphysis.
3. epiphysis.
4. metaphysis.
5. articular surface.

PREFERRED RESPONSE: 4

DISCUSSION: Deficiency of vitamin C produces a decrease in chondroitin sulfate synthesis, and a deficiency in collagen cross-linking is seen in the metaphysis. The microscopic appearance of the cartilaginous portion of the growth plate is normal but the metaphysis is quite abnormal. It appears that the deficiency in the metaphysis is related to the large amount of type I collagen normally found in this region. Radiographic findings may include the accumulation of calcified cartilage at the metaphysis-growth plate junction that results in a white line on the radiograph (white line of Fraenkel). The trabeculae are sparse and there is a generalized osteoporosis. The metaphyseal bone is weakened with microfractures and marginal spurs (Pelkin sign). Displacement of the growth plate may occur. The epiphyseal nucleus is also markedly radiolucent, but the calcified cartilage is unaffected, producing an appearance of ringed epiphyses (Wimberger sign).

REFERENCES: Simon SR (ed): *Orthopaedic Basic Science*. Rosemont, IL, American Academy of Orthopaedic Surgeons, 1994, pp 185-217.
Ramar S, Sivaramakrishnan V, Manoharan K: Scurvy: A forgotten disease. *Arch Phys Med Rehabil* 1993;74:92-95.

A-23: Warfarin limits the risk of deep venous thrombosis (DVT) by which of the following actions?

1. Competitive inhibition of vitamin K-dependent clotting factors
2. Inhibition of the posttranslational modification of vitamin K-dependent clotting factors
3. Reversible inhibition of platelet function
4. Irreversible inhibition of platelet function
5. Potentiation of antithrombin III

PREFERRED RESPONSE: 2

DISCUSSION: Warfarin is an oral anticoagulant that inhibits the posttranslational carboxylation of clotting factors II, VII, IX, and X (the so-called "vitamin K-dependent clotting factors") in the liver. When these factors are not carboxylated, they cannot bind calcium or function in the clotting cascade. Therefore, warfarin does not competitively inhibit the factors, but rather reduces their active concentration. Aspirin and its analogues inhibit platelet function. The potentiation of antithrombin III is the mechanism by which heparin functions as an anticoagulant.

REFERENCE: Gilman AG, et al: *The Pharmacological Basis of Therapeutics*. New York, NY, MacMillan Publishing.

A-24: What is the most common bacterium found in an infection caused by a human bite?

1. *Eikenella*
2. *Pasturella multocida*
3. *Borrelia burgdorferi*
4. *Salmonella typhosa*
5. Methicillin-resistant *Staphylococcus aureus*

PREFERRED RESPONSE: 1

DISCUSSION: The human bite is the most common source for *Eikenella*, and a cat bite is a source of *Pasturella multocida*. Lyme disease is caused by a tick bite (either Ixodes dammini or Io pacificus) that carries the bacteria *Borrelia burgdorferi*. *Staphylococcus* and *Streptococcus* remain the most common bacteria that cause orthopaedic infections and must always be assumed present until cultures or response (or lack of response) prove otherwise.

REFERENCES: Beaty JH (ed): *Orthopaedic Knowledge Update 6*. Rosemont, IL, American Academy of Orthopaedic Surgeons, 1999, pp 191-203.
Kasser JR (ed): *Orthopaedic Knowledge Update 5*. Rosemont, IL, American Academy of Orthopaedic Surgeons, 1996, pp 149-161, 295-309.
Buckwalter JA, Einhorn TA, Simon SR (eds): *Orthopaedic Basic Science: Biology and Biomechanics of the Musculoskeletal System,* ed 2. Rosemont, IL, American Academy of Orthopaedic Surgeons, 2000, pp 240-259.

A-25: The rate of chondrocyte maturation in the growth plate is directly regulated by an interaction between systemic hormones and

1. electric fields.
2. local growth factors.
3. oxygen tension.
4. mechanical forces.
5. calcium concentrations.

PREFERRED RESPONSE: 2

DISCUSSION: Local growth factors directly regulate the rate of chondrocyte maturation in the growth plate. A signaling loop involving parathyroid-related peptide (PTHrP), which is a potent inhibitor of chondrocyte maturation, and indian hedgehog has been well described. Indian hedgehog is produced by growth plate chondrocytes and regulates the expression of PTHrP. Systemic factors, such as vitamin D and growth hormone, also have important effects on chondrocyte differentiation, but indirectly regulate this process. While electric fields may influence fracture healing, a role in physeal chondrocyte maturation has not been identified. Mechanical forces are important for normal growth, but the nature of their effects is not known. Calcification of the cartilaginous matrix is essential for primary bone formation, but external calcium concentrations do not affect differentiation. In the past, a low oxygen tension was

(continued on next page)

Answers: Basic Science

(A-25: *continued*)

considered responsible for chondrocyte hypertrophy and differentiation, but that is now known to be incorrect.

REFERENCES: Grimsrud CD, Romano PR, D'Souza M, et al: BMP-6 is an autocrine stimulator of chondrocyte differentiation. *J Bone Miner Res* 1999;14:475-482.

Erickson DM, Harris SE, Dean DD, et al: Recombinant bone morphogenetic protein (BMP)-2 regulates costochondral growth plate chondrocytes and induces expression of BMP-2 and BMP-4 in a cell maturation-dependent manner. *J Orthop Res* 1997;15:371-380.

A-26: A genetic defect in type X collagen is most likely to result in which of the following conditions?

1. Multiple early fractures
2. Osteoporosis
3. Chondrodysplasia
4. Joint laxity
5. Inflammatory arthritis

PREFERRED RESPONSE: 3

DISCUSSION: Type X collagen is a short-chain, nonfibrillar collagen that is produced only by hypertrophic chondrocytes during the process of endochondral ossification. This collagen is found in the matrix in association with hypertrophic chondrocytes in all areas of endochondral bone formation, including growth plate, fracture callus, and heterotopic bone formation. Although a specific role for type X collagen has not been identified in endochondral bone formation, a genetic defect in this collagen is associated with Schmid metaphyseal chondrodysplasia, which is characterized by short limbs and bowing of the legs that is aggravated by walking. Similar to defects in type I collagen, which give rise to osteogenesis imperfecta, multiple separate mutations have been identified in patients with Schmid metaphyseal chondrodysplasia. More than 10 separate mutations have been identified thus far and all involve the noncollagenous globular region of the type X collagen molecule. Multiple early fractures are associated with osteogenesis imperfecta, a genetic defect in type I collagen. Joint laxity is associated with diseases such as Ehlers-Danlos syndrome, which results from a genetic defect in lysyl oxidase, an enzyme involved in collagen cross-linking and which also leads to hyperdistensible skin. Inflammatory arthritis is not associated with collagen disorders. Osteoporosis results from a decrease in bone density, and whereas most cases are idiopathic, some individuals with osteoporosis have been identified as having mild and previously unrecognized disorders of type I collagen consistent with osteogenesis imperfecta.

REFERENCE: Warman ML, Abbott M, Apte SS, et al: A type X collagen mutation causes Schmid metaphyseal chondrodysplasia. *Nat Genet* 1993;5:79-82.

Answers: Basic Science

A-27: Most natural biologic materials are anisotropic, meaning that their stress-strain curve exhibits

1. different moduli for compressive and tensile tests.

2. a high degree of nonlinearity.

3. a high sensitivity to the size of the test specimen.

4. dependence on the rate of loading.

5. dependence on the direction of load application.

PREFERRED RESPONSE: 5

DISCUSSION: Isotropic materials have the same elastic properties in three orthogonal directions; anisotropy means that the properties are different when loading in at least one direction. A ligament that is very stiff in the direction of the collagen fibers, but much more compliant in the two transverse directions, is a simple example. Knowing and reporting the direction of load on a test sample is extremely important in measuring the properties of anisotropic materials. The tensile and compressive properties of ligaments are also very different, but this is not anisotropy; isotropic materials can also behave in this manner (eg, cement). Stress-strain curves that vary with the test rate are a hallmark of viscoelastic materials; those sensitive to sample size indicate heterogeneity. Nonlinearity can result from many compositional and structural features.

REFERENCES: Ratner B, Hoffman AS, Schoen FJ, et al: *Biomaterials Science*. San Diego, CA, Academic Press, 1996, pp 16-17.
Buckwalter JA, Einhorn TA, Simon SR (eds): *Orthopaedic Basic Science: Biology and Biomechanics of the Musculoskeletal System*, ed 2. Rosemont, IL, American Academy of Orthopaedic Surgeons, 2000, pp 182-215.

A-28: Which of the following factors is most commonly associated with late aseptic loosening of cemented acetabular components?

1. Increased frictional torque

2. Recurrent neck-socket impingement

3. Fatigue failure of cement

4. Poor initial component fixation

5. Polyethylene wear

PREFERRED RESPONSE: 5

DISCUSSION: Surgical and autopsy specimens consistently document the presence of macrophages containing many submicron polyethylene wear particles in cement-bone interfacial tissue. Progressive disruption of the cement-bone interface by this inflammatory process results in late component loosening.

REFERENCE: Schmalzried TP, Kwong LM, Jasty M, et al: The mechanism of loosening of cemented acetabular components in total hip arthroplasty: Analysis of specimens retrieved at autopsy. *Clin Orthop Relat Res* 1992;274:60-78.

A-29: Which of the following processes will most greatly increase the wear damage to an ultrahigh molecular weight polyethylene articulating surface?

1. Ethanol sterilization

2. Third body inclusion

3. Cold flow deformation

4. Gamma radiation sterilization

5. Ion implantation on the mating metallic surface

PREFERRED RESPONSE: 2

DISCUSSION: While recent data suggest that both storage and sterilization techniques affect the wear properties of ultrahigh molecular weight polyethylene, the most dramatic increase in wear is associated with third body inclusion on the articular surface.

REFERENCES: Simon SR (ed): *Orthopaedic Basic Science*. Rosemont, IL, American Academy of Orthopaedic Surgeons, 1994, pp 449-486.

McKellop HA, Campbell P, Park SH, et al: The origin of submicron polyethylene wear debris in total hip arthroplasty. *Clin Orthop Relat Res* 1995;311:3-20.

A-30: What is the function of a transcription factor?

1. Bind to DNA and influence gene expression

2. Bind to cell membrane receptors and induce phosphorylation

3. Package DNA

4. Unwind DNA

5. Dehydrate cellular proteins

PREFERRED RESPONSE: 1

DISCUSSION: Transcription factors bind to DNA and initiate gene transcription. A variety of transcription factors have been identified and some have a specific role in bone and cartilage physiology. Many transcription factors are present in the cell in an inactive form, but are activated by a series of phosphorylation reactions that follow the binding of a growth factor or other ligand to a specific cellular receptor. Cancers are frequently associated with the abnormal activation of transcription factors. Histones are molecules that bind and package DNA, but are not involved in transcription. Helicases unwind DNA and are involved in DNA synthesis, while metalloproteinases are enzymes that are involved in tissue catabolism and are involved in the pathogenesis of arthritis.

REFERENCES: Schmitt JM, Hwang K, Winn SR, Hollinger JO: Bone morphogenetic proteins: An update on basic biology an clinical relevance. *J Orthop Res* 1999;17:269-278.

Reddi AH: Initiation of fracture repair by bone morphogenetic proteins. *Clin Orthop Relat Res* 1998;355:S66-S72.

Buckwalter JA, Einhorn TA, Simon SR (eds): *Orthopaedic Basic Science: Biology and Biomechanics of the Musculoskeletal System,* ed 2. Rosemont, IL, American Academy of Orthopaedic Surgeons, 2000, pp 20-76.

A-31: What is the most common bacterium found in an infection caused by a tick bite?

1. *Eikenella*
2. *Vibrio vulnificus*
3. *Borrelia burgdorferi*
4. *Clostridium perfringens*
5. Methicillin-resistant *Streptococcus*

PREFERRED RESPONSE: 3

DISCUSSION: Lyme disease is caused by a tick bite (either Ixodes dammini or Io pacificus) that carries the bacterium *Borrelia* burgdorferi. The human bite is the most common source for *Eikenella*, and a cat bite is a source of *Pasturella multocida*. Brackish water can cause a devastating infection of *Vibrio vulnificus*. *Staphylococcus* and *Streptococcus* remain the most common bacteria that cause orthopaedic infections and must always be assumed present until cultures or response (or lack of response) prove otherwise.

REFERENCES: Beaty JH (ed): *Orthopaedic Knowledge Update 6*. Rosemont, IL, American Academy of Orthopaedic Surgeons, 1999, pp 191-203.
Kasser JR (ed): *Orthopaedic Knowledge Update 5*. Rosemont, IL, American Academy of Orthopaedic Surgeons, 1996, pp 149-161, 295-309.
Buckwalter JA, Einhorn TA, Simon SR (eds): *Orthopaedic Basic Science: Biology and Biomechanics of the Musculoskeletal System*, ed 2. Rosemont, IL, American Academy of Orthopaedic Surgeons, 2000, pp 240-259.

A-32: Methicillin-resistant *Staphylococcus aureus* can be treated effectively with an oral quinolone and which of the following antibiotics to achieve synergy?

1. Penicillin
2. Probenecid
3. Rifampin
4. Cefoxitin
5. Amoxicillin

PREFERRED RESPONSE: 3

DISCUSSION: Rifampin has been shown to have synergy with quinolones in the treatment of methicillin-resistant *Staphylococcus aureus* and methicillin-resistant *Staphylococcus epidermidis*. Each of the two antibiotics lessens the development of resistant mutants.

REFERENCES: Chambers HF: Methicillin resistance in staphylococci: Molecular and biochemical basis and clinical implications. *Clin Microbiol Rev* 1997;10:781-791.
Drancourt M, Stein A, Argenson JN, et al: Oral rifampin plus ofloxacin for treatment of Staphylococcus-infected orthopaedic implants. *Antimicrob Agents Chemother* 1993;37:1214-1218.

Answers: Basic Science

A-33: A fully differentiated osteoclast has receptors for which of the following proteins?

1. Parathyroid hormone (PTH)
2. Calcitonin
3. Cholecalciferol
4. Bone morphogenetic protein (BMP)
5. Interleukin-2 (IL-2)

PREFERRED RESPONSE: 2

DISCUSSION: Osteoclasts resorb bone in response to specific systemic and intracellular signals. Regulation of osteoclastic bone resorption depends on the way its physiologic function is regulated through receptor mediated pathways. Calcitonin is a peptide hormone that directly binds to a cell surface receptor on osteoclasts to inhibit osteoclast function. Although PTH is frequently regarded as an agent that stimulates bone resorption, osteoclasts do not possess receptors for this hormone; instead, they are signaled to resorb bone by osteoblasts, the cells that possess receptors to PTH. IL-2 is an immuno-modulatory cytokine that does not directly influence osteoclast function. BMP is the name for a family of osteoinductive proteins, many of which have receptors in osteoblast progenitor cells, but not in fully differentiated osteoclasts. Although osteoclast precursors do directly respond to 1,25 dihydroxychole-calciferol, they do not have a receptor for cholecalciferol itself (vitamin D).

REFERENCES: Suda T, Udagawa N, Takahashi N: Cells of bone: Osteoclast generation, in Bilezikian JP, Raisz LG, Rodan GA (eds): *Principles of Bone Biology.* San Diego, CA, Academic Press, 1996, pp 87-102.
Mundy GR: Bone resorbing cells, in *Primer on the Metabolic Bone Diseases and Disorders of Mineral Metabolism,* ed 3. Philadelphia, PA, Lippincot-Raven, 1996, pp 16-24.

A-34: Cephalosporins are effective antibiotic agents because of their action on what aspect of bacterial metabolism?

1. DNA gyrase
2. Cell wall
3. mRNA
4. Cell membrane
5. Protein

PREFERRED RESPONSE: 2

DISCUSSION: The mechanism of action has been defined for seven antibiotic classes. The cephalosporin action is to inhibit cell wall synthesis. Quinolones inhibit DNA gyrase. Beta-lactam antibiotics bind to the surface of the cell membrane. Aminoglycosides inhibit protein synthesis by binding to ribosomal RNA. Rifampin inhibits RNA synthesis in bacteria.

REFERENCE: Simon SR (ed): *Orthopaedic Basic Science.* Rosemont, IL, American Academy of Orthopaedic Surgeons, 1994, pp 489-517.

A-35: Repair of the peripheral one third of the meniscus is sometimes possible because it has which of the following characteristics?

1. Increased blood supply

2. Appropriate viscoelasticity

3. High glycoprotein concentration

4. High type II collagen concentration

5. Large size

PREFERRED RESPONSE: 1

DISCUSSION: The outer one third of the meniscus is well vascularized, and this characteristic allows for an excellent healing potential.

REFERENCES: Buckwalter JA, Einhorn TA, Simon SR (eds): *Orthopaedic Basic Science: Biology and Biomechanics of the Musculoskeletal System,* ed 2. Rosemont, IL, American Academy of Orthopaedic Surgeons, pp 2000, 532-545.
Arnozczky SP: Gross and vascular anatomy of the meniscus and its role in meniscal healing, regeneration and remodeling, in Mow VC, Arnozczky SP, Jackson DW (eds): *Knee Meniscus Basic and Clinical Foundations.* New York, NY, Raven Press, 1992, pp 1-14.

A-36: During the first 2 years of life, which of the following actions is most responsible for increasing structural stability of the physis?

1. The change from a flat to an undulating physis

2. The growth of the zone of Ranvier

3. Increased strength of the points of insertion of muscles onto bone

4. Increased penetration of proprioceptive nerve endings about the physis

5. Increased capillary penetration about the physis

PREFERRED RESPONSE: 2

DISCUSSION: The zone of Ranvier provides the earliest increase in strength of the physis. During the first year of life, the zone spreads over the adjacent metaphysis to form a fibrous circumferential ring bridging from the epiphysis to the diaphysis. This ring increases the mechanical strength of the physis. The zone also helps the physis grow latitudinally. In turn, the increased width of the physis helps the physis further resist mechanical forces. The change in shape of the physis to its progressively more undulating form is also a factor in increasing physeal strength, but this occurs over a longer period of time, as the child's activity level increases. The undulations of the physis seen in some growth plates also add to stability but to a lesser extent. The other changes contribute little toward increasing physeal strength.

REFERENCES: Burkus JK, Ogden JA: Development of the distal femoral epiphysis: A microscopic morphological investigation of the zone of Ranvier. *J Pediatr Orthop* 1984;4:661-668.
Shapiro F, Holtrop ME, Glimcher MJ: Organization and cellular biology of the perichondrial ossification groove of Ranvier: A morphological study in rabbits. *J Bone Joint Surg Am* 1977;59:703-723.

Answers: Basic Science

A-37: Virtually all biological materials are viscoelastic, which means that their mechanical behavior is dependent on what factor?

1. Load applied
2. Cross-sectional area
3. Rate of loading
4. Mode of loading
5. Direction of loading

PREFERRED RESPONSE: 3

DISCUSSION: Viscoelastic materials exhibit both viscous and elastic behavior. Elastic materials have the same stress-strain relationship regardless of the rate at which the load is applied. Viscoelastic behavior is dependent upon the strain rate; the modulus increases as the strain rate increases. The faster a load is applied to such materials the more elastic they behave. Many materials, both elastic and viscoelastic (including bone), have different properties in tension and compression. Ligaments are an excellent example, stiff in tension but not in compression. Materials that have different mechanical properties in different directions are called anisotropic.

REFERENCES: Black J: *Orthopaedic Biomaterials in Research and Practice.* New York, NY, Churchill Livingstone, 1988, pp 57-81.
Simon SR (ed): *Orthopaedic Basic Science.* Rosemont, IL, American Academy of Orthopaedic Surgeons, 1994, p 456.

A-38: When a long bone is subjected to a bending moment, the greatest tensile stresses are located

1. within the cortex.
2. at the neutral axis.
3. at a periosteal surface.
4. at an endosteal surface.
5. along the bending axis.

PREFERRED RESPONSE: 3

DISCUSSION: The greatest tensile stresses are on the convex outer surface of the bone. In bending, the neutral axis is where the transition occurs from tension to compressive stress, and stresses are at a minimum. In a symmetrical structure, the neutral axis and the benign axis align, but in an asymmetric structure such as a long bone, the axes do not align.

REFERENCES: Timoshenko S, Young DH: *Elements of Strength of Materials,* ed 5. New York, NY, Van Nostrand Reinhold, 1968, pp 70-74.
Burstein AH, Wright TM: *Fundamentals of Orthopaedic Biomechanics.* Baltimore, MD, Williams and Wilkins, 1994.

A-39: What is the dominant component of articular cartilage extracellular matrix by weight?

1. Water

2. Collagen

3. Keratan sulfate

4. Chondroitin sulfate

5. Nerve and lymphatic tissue

PREFERRED RESPONSE: 1

DISCUSSION: Articular cartilage is a highly organized viscoelastic material, and load transmission depends on the specific composition of the extracellular matrix. Articular cartilage is devoid of neural, lymphatic, and blood vessel tissue. The extracellular matrix consists of water, proteoglycans, and collagen. Water comprises most of the wet weight (65% to 80%). Type II collagen comprises 95% of the collagen. The collagen and proteoglycan (keratan sulfate and chondroitin sulfate) matrix and its high water content are responsible for the mechanical properties of the articular cartilage.

REFERENCES: Buckwalter JA, Mankin HJ: Articular cartilage: Degeneration and osteoarthritis, repair, regeneration, and transplantation. *Instr Course Lect* 1998;47:487-504.
Koval KJ (ed): *Orthopaedic Knowledge Update 7*. Rosemont, IL, American Academy of Orthopaedic Surgeons, 2002, pp 3-18.

Pediatric Orthopaedics

Section Editor

Robert M. Kay, MD

Q-1: Figure 1 shows the radiograph of a 7-year-old patient who has a bilateral Trendelenburg limp and limited range of hip motion but no pain. His work-up should include

1. a skeletal survey.
2. genetic evaluation.
3. cardiac evaluation.
4. coagulation studies.
5. an MRI scan of the hips.

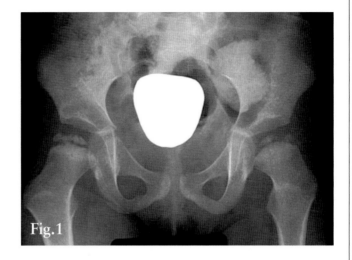

Fig.1

Q-2: A 2-week-old infant has been referred for evaluation of nonmovement of the left hip. History reveals that the patient was delivered 6 weeks premature by cesarean section. Examination reveals no fever, and there is mild swelling of the thigh. Passive movement of the hip appears to elicit tenderness and very limited hip motion. A radiograph of the pelvis shows mild subluxation of the left hip. The next step in evaluation should consist of

1. aspiration of the left hip.
2. application of a Pavlik harness.
3. a gallium scan.
4. an MRI scan of the spine.
5. modified Bryant traction.

Q-3: A 9-year-old boy who is small for his age has a painful limp and limited hip motion. Radiographs of the pelvis are shown in Figures 2A and 2B. In addition to managing the problem with the hip, what laboratory studies should be obtained?

1. Serum protein electrophoresis
2. Serum glucose and hemoglobin A1C
3. WBC and differential blood cell count

(continued on next page)

(Q-3 continued)

4. Thyroxin and thyroid-stimulating hormone

5. Transferrin and total iron-binding capacity

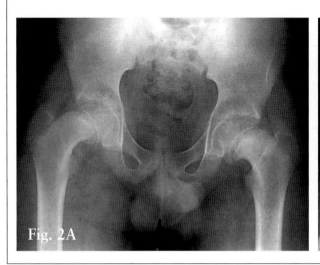

Fig. 2A

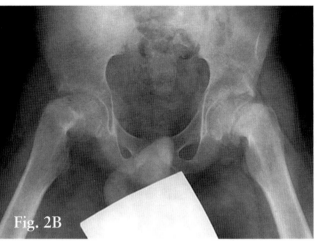

Fig. 2B

Q-4: Figure 3 shows the current radiographs of a 13-year-old boy who was treated for an elbow fracture 1 year ago. He is neurovascularly intact. What is the most important component of treatment if reconstruction is being considered?

1. Construction of the annular ligament

2. Restoration of the radioulnar articulation

3. Restoration and maintenance of ulnar length and alignment

4. Adequate immobilization postoperatively in 120° of flexion

5. Placement of a Kirschner wire from the radial head to the capitellum

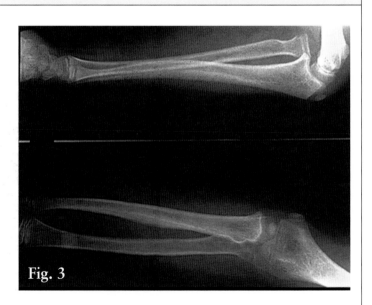

Fig. 3

Q-5: A 12-year-old girl has had lower back pain for the past 6 months that interferes with her ability to participate in sports. She denies any history of radicular symptoms, sensory changes, or bowel or bladder dysfunction. Examination reveals a shuffling gait, restriction of forward bending, and tight hamstrings. Radiographs show a grade III spondylolisthesis of L5 on S1, with a slip angle of 20°. Management should consist of

1. brace treatment.
2. laminectomy, nerve root decompression, and in situ fusion of L4 to the sacrum.
3. in situ fusion of L4 to the sacrum.
4. excision of the L5 lamina.
5. physical therapy.

Q-6: Marfan syndrome is most likely associated with defects in which of the following structural proteins?

1. Elastin
2. Fibrillin
3. Fibronectin
4. Type II collagen
5. Type III collagen

Q-7: The inheritance of the deformity shown in Figure 4 is most commonly

1. autosomal-recessive.
2. autosomal-dominant.
3. X-linked dominant.
4. mitochondrial.
5. sporadic.

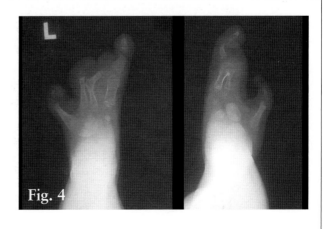

Fig. 4

Q-8: A 7-year-old boy with a closed supracondylar fracture of the distal humerus is unable to flex the distal interphalangeal (DIP) joint of his index finger and the interphalangeal (IP) joint of his thumb. These findings are most likely due to a deficit involving fibers of which of the following nerves?

1. Ulnar
2. Radial
3. Musculocutaneous
4. Anterior interosseous
5. Posterior interosseous

Q-9: A 14-year-old girl with polyarticular juvenile rheumatoid arthritis (JRA) has severe neck pain and reports the onset of urinary incontinence. A lateral radiograph and lateral tomogram of the cervical spine are shown in Figures 5A and 5B. An MRI scan of the upper cervical spine is shown in Figure 5C. Management should consist of

1. a rigid cervical orthosis.
2. a soft cervical collar.
3. posterior C1-2 fusion with halo immobilization.
4. administration of methotrexate.
5. activity restrictions.

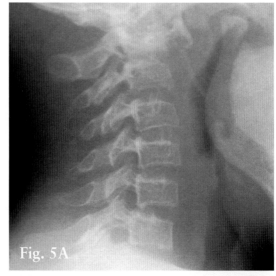

Fig. 5A

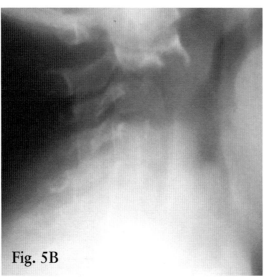

Fig. 5B

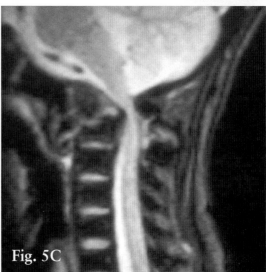

Fig. 5C

Q-10: Figure 6 shows the radiograph of a 13-year-old boy who has low back pain and tight hamstrings. There are no sensory or motor deficits. What is the recommended treatment for this condition?

1. Gill procedure
2. Thoracolumbosacral orthosis
3. Direct repair of the pars defect
4. Posterolateral fusion from L4 to the sacrum
5. Combined anteroposterior fusion from L5 to the sacrum

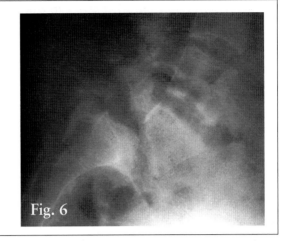

Fig. 6

Q-11: A 12-year-old girl has progressive development of cavus feet. Examination reveals slightly diminished vibratory sensation on the bottom of the foot. Reflexes are 1+ at the knees and ankles. Motor examination shows that all muscles are 5/5 in the foot, except the peroneal and anterior tibial muscles are rated as 4+/5. Which of the following studies is considered most diagnostic?

1. Nerve conduction velocity studies
2. Biopsy of the quadriceps femoris muscle
3. Biopsy of the sural nerve
4. DNA testing
5. Chromosomal analysis

Q-12: Figure 7 shows the lateral cervical radiograph of a 2-year-old girl who was an unrestrained passenger in a motor vehicle accident. She is able to move her neck freely without pain, and her neurologic examination is normal. Management should include

1. observation.
2. anterior decompression.
3. upper cervical arthrodesis.
4. application of a soft collar.
5. immobilization in a halo vest.

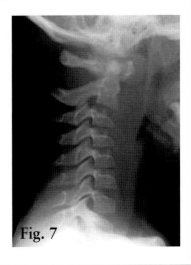

Fig. 7

Q-13: An 11-year-old boy has had a fever and pain and swelling over the lateral aspect of his right ankle for the past 3 days. Examination reveals warmth, swelling, and tenderness over the lateral malleolus, and he has a temperature of 103.2° F (39.5° C). Laboratory studies show a WBC count of 13,200/mm³ with 61% neutrophils, an erythocyte sedimentation rate of 112 mm/h, and a C-reactive protein of 15.7. Radiographs and a T2-weighted MRI scan are shown in Figures 8A through 8C. Aspiration yields 1 mL of purulent fluid. Management should now consist of

1. oral antibiotics and a follow-up office appointment the next day.
2. incision and drainage of the distal fibular metaphysis.
3. indium-labeled WBC scan.
4. antituberculous medication for 6 months.
5. three-phase technetium Tc 99m bone scan.

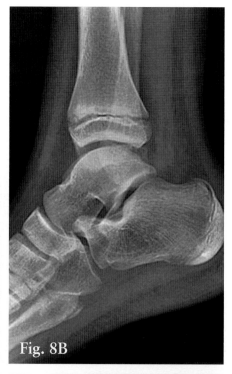

Fig. 8B

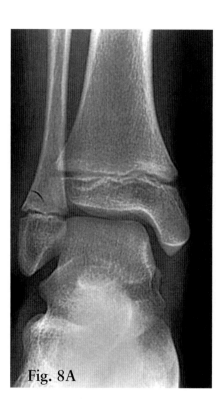

Fig. 8A

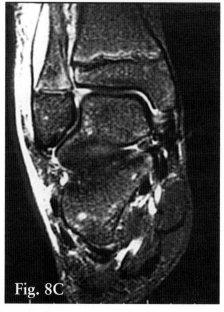

Fig. 8C

Q-14: A newborn has a flail right upper extremity after a difficult right occiput anterior vaginal delivery. Examination shows an obvious fracture of the right clavicle. Following stimulation, there is no movement of the arm or hand and there appears to be no sensation in the hand. Management should include

1. a CT scan arteriogram.
2. an MRI scan of the brachial plexus.
3. nerve conduction velocity studies and an electromyogram.
4. surgical exploration and repair of the brachial plexus.
5. observation for 60 days before obtaining further tests.

Q-15: The most severe and rapidly progressive form of congenital scoliosis is

1. block vertebra.
2. semisegmented hemivertebra.
3. fully segmented hemivertebra.
4. unilateral unsegmented bar.
5. unilateral unsegmented bar with contralateral hemivertebra.

Q-16: Figures 9A and 9B show the radiographs of an 11-year-old boy who felt a pop and immediate pain in his right knee as he was driving off his right leg to jam a basketball. Examination reveals that the knee is flexed, and the patient is unable to actively extend it or bear weight on that side. There is also a large effusion. Management should include

1. ice and elevation, followed by graduated range-of-motion exercises.
2. a long leg cast.
3. excision of the fragment.
4. open reduction and internal fixation.
5. observation until maturity, followed by anterior cruciate ligament repair.

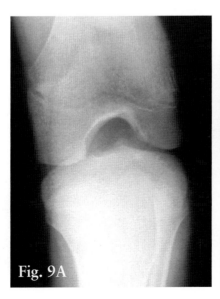

Fig. 9A

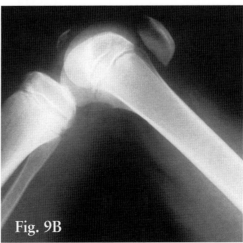

Fig. 9B

Q-17: Posterior spinal fusion for scoliosis should be performed on a patient with Duchenne muscular dystrophy when

1. he patient is still ambulatory.
2. lordotic posture is present.
3. the forced vital capacity (FVC) is less than 30% of the predicted value.
4. curve magnitude measures 25° or greater.
5. orthotic management fails.

Q-18: Which of the following deformities is most likely associated with slight valgus of the femur, dimpling over the tibia, mild leg-length deficiency, increased heel valgus, and tarsal coalition?

1. Type 1 fibular hemimelia
2. Type 2 tibial hemimelia
3. Type 4 proximal femoral focal deficiency (PFFD)
4. Posterior medial bowing of the tibia
5. Congenital pseudarthrosis of the tibia

Q-19: A 4-year-old boy is seen in the emergency department with a 2-day history of left groin pain and a limp. His parents deny any history of injury. Examination of the hip shows a 5° hip flexion position, 20° of abduction, internal rotation to 15°, and external rotation to 30°. His temperature is 100.9°F (38.3°C). Blood studies show a normal WBC count, and the erythrocyte sedimentation rate is 18 mm/h. The C-reactive protein is pending. A radiograph is shown in Figure 10. What is the most likely diagnosis?

1. Perthes disease
2. Transient synovitis
3. Slipped capital femoral epiphysis (SCFE)
4. Septic arthritis
5. Juvenile arthritis

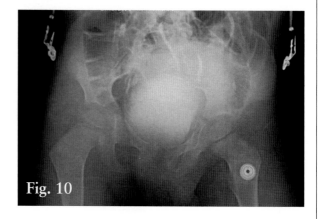
Fig. 10

Q-20: A 7-year-old patient has had a painless limp for several months. Examination reveals pain and spasm with internal rotation, and abduction is limited to 10° on the involved side. Management consists of 1 week of bed rest and traction, followed by an arthrogram. A maximum abduction/internal rotation view is shown in Figure 11A, and abduction and adduction views are shown in Figures 11B and 11C. The studies are most consistent with

1. Catterall II involvement.
2. tubercular synovitis.
3. Herring type A involvement.
4. hinge abduction.
5. osteochondritis dissecans.

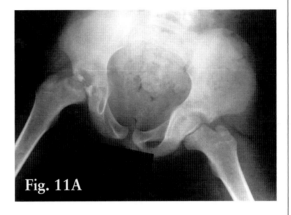

Fig. 11A

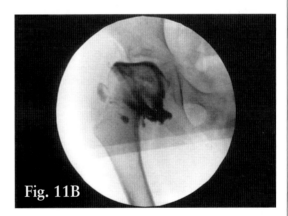

Fig. 11B

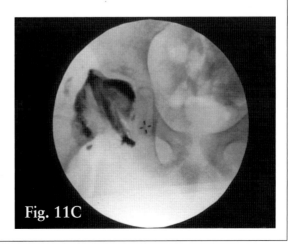

Fig. 11C

Q-21: Figure 12 shows the radiograph of a 3-year-old child with progressive bowlegs. Laboratory studies show a calcium level of 9.5 mg/dL (normal 9.0 to 11.0 mg/dL), a phosphorus level of 4.2 mg/dL (normal 3 to 5.7 mg/dL), and an alkaline phosphatase level of 305 IU/L (normal 104 to 345 IU/L). What is the most likely diagnosis?

1. Blount disease
2. Hypophosphatemic rickets
3. Nutritional rickets
4. Schmid metaphyseal dysostosis
5. Jansen metaphyseal dysostosis

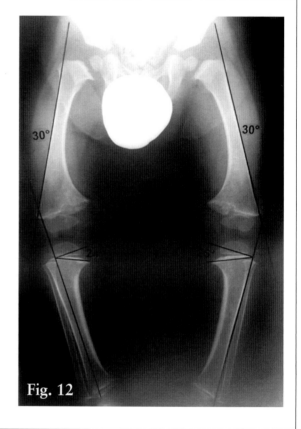

Fig. 12

Q-22: Which of the following clinical scenarios represents an appropriate indication for convex hemiepiphysiodesis/hemiarthrodesis in the treatment of a child with a congenital spinal deformity?

1. A 3-year-old child with a hemivertebra opposite a contralateral bar and thoracic scoliosis that measures 53°
2. A 4-year-old child with a fully segmented L1 hemivertebra and scoliosis that measures 80°
3. A 4-year-old child with a fully segmented T10 hemivertebra and scoliosis that measures 50°
4. A 4-year-old child with a posterolateral hemivertebra at the thoracolumbar junction and a kyphoscoliotic deformity that measures 45°
5. A 10-year-old child with a hemivertebra and scoliosis that measures 50°

Q-23: Which of the following types of iliac osteotomy provides the greatest potential for increased coverage?

1. Ganz periacetabular
2. Pemberton innominate
3. Salter innominate
4. Sutherland double innominate
5. Steele triple innominate

Q-24: Figure 13 shows the radiograph of an 18-year-old patient who has severe knee pain. Treatment consisting of osteotomy should be performed

1. above the tibial tubercle.
2. at or just below the tibial tubercle.
3. in the tibial diaphysis.
4. on both the femur and tibia.
5. on the femur alone.

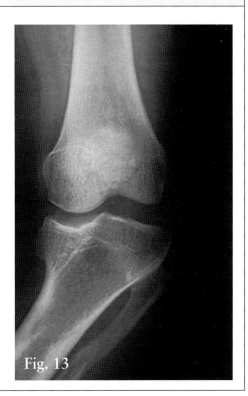

Fig. 13

Q-25: Examination of a 6-year-old boy who sustained a displaced Salter-Harris type II fracture of the distal radius reveals 35° of volar angulation. A satisfactory reduction is obtained with the aid of a hematoma block. At the 10-day follow-up examination, radiographs show loss of reduction and 35° of volar angulation. Management should now consist of

1. acceptance of the malalignment and continued cast immobilization.
2. repeat closed reduction with the aid of IV morphine and midazolam.
3. repeat closed reduction with the aid of IV ketamine.
4. repeat closed reduction with the patient under general anesthesia.
5. gentle open reduction with smooth cross-pin fixation.

Q-26: Figure 14 shows the radiograph of a 13-year-old girl who has scoliosis. She has long, slender fingers, and when she grasps her left wrist with her right hand, the index finger and thumb overlap by 3 cm. She wears glasses for myopia. A preoperative work-up should include

1. an echocardiogram.
2. neurofibromin testing.
3. a serum fibrillin level.
4. an MRI scan of the spine.
5. a urine mucopolysaccharide screen.

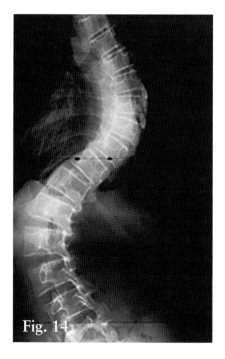

Fig. 14

Q-27: Figure 15 shows the radiograph of an 11-year-old boy with Duchenne muscular dystrophy who has been nonambulatory for the past 2 years. Management of the spinal deformity should consist of

1. wheelchair modifications and custom-molded inserts.
2. posterior fusion with instrumentation.
3. anterior and posterior fusion.
4. observation and reexamination in 6 months.
5. thoracolumbosacral orthosis bracing.

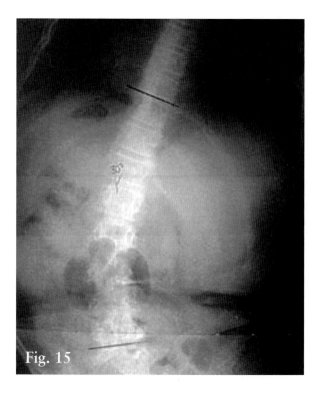

Fig. 15

Q-28: Which of the following patients is considered the most appropriate candidate for selective dorsal rhizotomy?

1. Nonambulatory 2-year-old with spastic diplegia
2. Nonambulatory 2-year-old with spastic quadriplegia
3. Nonambulatory 12-year-old with spastic quadriplegia
4. Ambulatory 4-year-old with spastic diplegia
5. Ambulatory 9-year-old with hemiplegia and athetosis

Q-29: A 2-day-old infant has the hyperextended knee deformity shown in Figure 16. No other deformities are found on examination. A radiograph shows that the ossified portion of the proximal tibia is slightly anterior to that of the distal femur. Management should consist of

1. gentle stretching and serial casting.
2. Bryant traction for 1 to 2 weeks, followed by closed reduction.
3. percutaneous quadriceps recession, followed by serial casting.
4. delayed open reduction at age 6 months to avoid iatrogenic damage to either the distal femoral or proximal tibial physes.
5. a renal ultrasound.

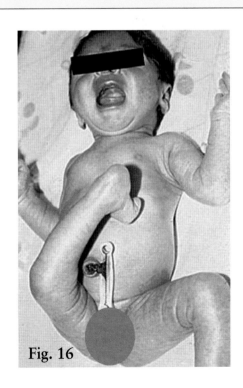

Fig. 16

Q-30: A 10-year-old boy has activity-related knee pain that is poorly localized. He denies locking, swelling, or giving way. Examination shows mild tenderness at the medial femoral condyle and painless full range of motion without ligamentous instability. Radiographs are shown in Figures 17A through 17C. What is the best course of action?

1. Knee arthroscopy with drilling of the lesion
2. Limited activity for 6 to 12 weeks
3. Removal of the loose body
4. Biopsy of the lesion
5. Open reduction and internal fixation

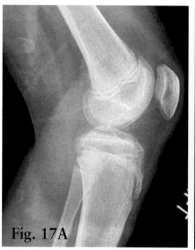 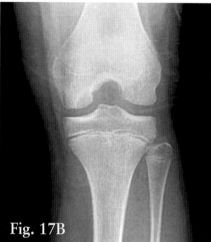 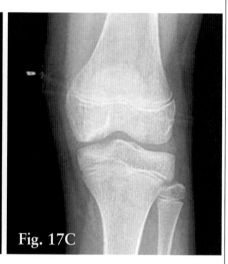

Fig. 17A   Fig. 17B   Fig. 17C

Q-31: A 3-year-old boy has a rigid 40° lumbar scoliosis that is the result of a fully segmented L5 hemivertebra. All other examination findings are normal. Management should consist of

1. in situ posterior fusion.
2. hemivertebral resection and fusion.
3. convex hemiepiphyseodesis.
4. observation with follow-up in 6 months.
5. thoracolumbosacral orthosis bracing.

Q-32: Examination of a 7-year-old boy reveals 20° of valgus following a lawn mower injury to the lateral femoral epiphysis. Treatment consists of total distal femoral epiphyseodesis and varus osteotomy. Following surgery, he has a limb-length discrepancy of 3 cm and 5° of genu valgum. Assuming that he undergoes no further treatment, the patient's predicted limb-length discrepancy at maturity would be how many centimeters?

1. Less than 7
2. 7 to 10
3. 11 to 13
4. 14 to 17
5. Greater than 17

Q-33: Figure 18 shows the hand deformities of a 3-year-old girl who has short stature. The most likely diagnosis is

1. achondroplasia.
2. pseudoachondroplasia.
3. diastrophic dysplasia.
4. metaphyseal chondrodysplasia.
5. multiple epiphyseal dysplasia.

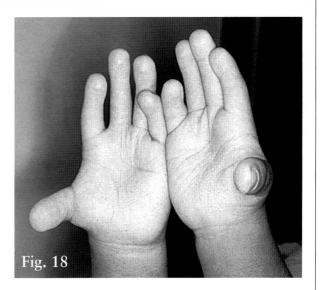

Fig. 18

Q-34: A 4-year-old child sustains a spiral fracture to the tibia in an unwitnessed fall. History reveals three other fractures to long bones, and the parents are vague about the etiology of each. There is no family history of bone disease. The parents ask if the child has osteogenesis imperfecta (OI); however, there are no clinical or radiographic indications of this diagnosis. In addition to fracture care, management should include

1. notification of child protective services and hospital admission.
2. a punch biopsy of skin for collagen analysis.
3. DNA testing for OI.
4. calcium, phosphate, and alkaline phosphatase studies.
5. placement of intramedullary rods to prevent further fractures.

Q-35: Figure 19 shows the clinical photograph of a 3-month-old infant with a foot deformity that has been nonprogressive since birth. Examination reveals that the deformity corrects actively and with passive manipulation. There is no associated equinus. Management should consist of

1. serial casting.
2. UCBL orthoses.
3. abductor hallucis lengthening.
4. observation and parental reassurance.
5. corrective shoes.

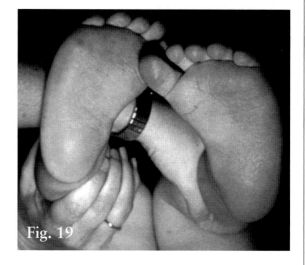

Fig. 19

Q-36: Figure 20 shows the radiograph of a 7-year-old girl with a low thoracic-level myelomeningocele. She has a history of skin ulcers over the apex of the deformity, but her current skin condition is good. Management of the spinal deformity should consist of

1. physical therapy for hip stretching exercises.
2. kyphectomy and posterior fusion with instrumentation.
3. anterior release and fusion using a rib strut graft.
4. anterior release and strut grafting and posterior fusion with instrumentation.
5. bracing.

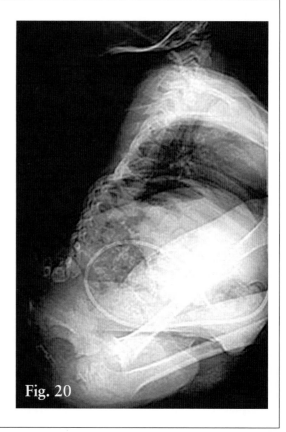

Fig. 20

Q-37: Development of a valgus deformity in children after a fracture of the proximal tibial metaphysis most likely results from

1. lateral physeal arrest.
2. tethering by the fibula.
3. periosteal interposition.
4. asymmetric physeal growth.
5. anterior tibial artery stenosis.

Q-38: The preferred surgical approach to the elbow of a child with an irreducible type III supracondylar distal humerus fracture and pulseless extremity is through which of the following muscle intervals?

1. Pronator teres and the brachialis
2. Pronator teres and the triceps
3. Pronator teres and the biceps
4. Brachioradialis and the biceps
5. Brachioradialis and the brachialis

Q-39: A 2-year-old girl has had lethargy, fever, and abdominal pain for the past 6 months. In addition to multiple lytic lesions in the long bones and calvaria shown on the skeletal survey, the radiograph of the spine shown in Figure 21A reveals a vertebral lesion. A biopsy specimen is shown in Figure 21B. The most likely diagnosis is

1. leukemia.
2. tuberculosis.
3. Langerhans cell histiocytosis.
4. metastatic neuroblastoma.
5. multifocal osteomyelitis.

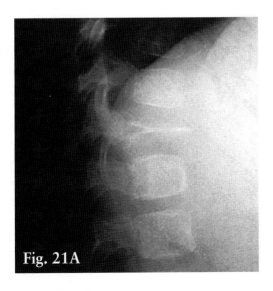

Fig. 21A

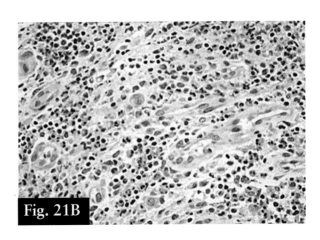

Fig. 21B

Q-40: Progressive paralysis is most likely to be seen in association with what type of congenital vertebral abnormality?

1. Anterior failure of formation
2. Anterior failure of segmentation
3. Posterior failure of formation
4. Posterior failure of segmentation
5. Lateral failure of segmentation

Q-41: Figure 22 shows the radiograph of a girl who has had a 3-month history of activity-related foot pain. She has had two previous ankle sprains on this side. Examination reveals that subtalar motion is limited and there is mild heel valgus. Which of the following studies will best confirm your diagnosis?

1. Comparison radiograph of the contralateral foot
2. Calcaneal radiograph
3. Electromyography (EMG) and a nerve conduction velocity study
4. CT scan
5. Rheumatoid factor

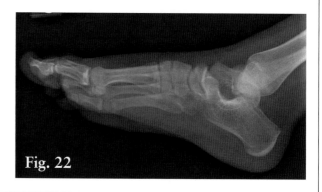

Fig. 22

Q-42: Figure 23 shows a newborn who has severe multiple symmetric joint contractures, including adduction/internal rotation of the shoulders, extended elbows, flexion-ulnar deviation of the wrists, thumbs in the palm of the hands, dislocated hips, knee flexion deformity, and clubfeet. The most likely diagnosis is

1. amyoplasia multiplex congenital.
2. Friedreich ataxia.
3. distal arthrogryposis.
4. spinal muscle atrophy.
5. thoracic-level myelomeningocele.

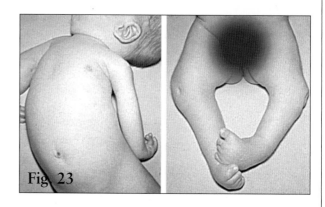

Fig. 23

Q-43: Figure 24A shows the clinical photograph of a 2-year-old boy who has a deformity of the left leg. Examination reveals eight cutaneous markings similar to those shown in Figure 24B. Radiographs are shown in Figure 24C. Management should consist of

1. fragmentation, realignment, and intramedullary nailing of the tibia.
2. resection of the dysplastic region of the tibia and insertion of a vascularized fibula.
3. supplemental vitamin D and phosphate.
4. a clamshell orthosis.
5. observation for spontaneous remodeling.

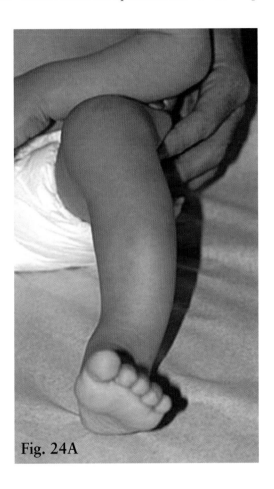

Fig. 24A

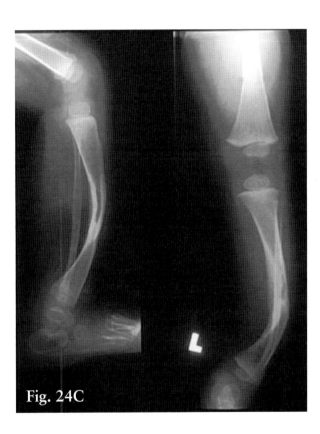

Fig. 24C

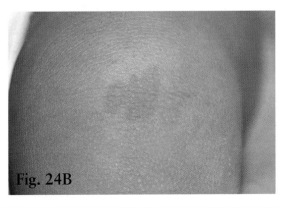

Fig. 24B

Q-44: A 10-year-old girl has had a painful 40° left thoracic scoliosis for the past 16 months. A bone scan shows a localized area of uptake in the T10 vertebra, and a CT scan of this area is shown in Figure 25. Treatment for the lesion should include

1. observation.
2. surgical excision.
3. a thoracolumbosacral orthosis.
4. posterior spinal fusion and instrumentation of T5-L3.
5. administration of nonsteroidal anti-inflammatory medication for a prolonged period.

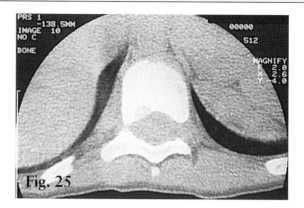

Fig. 25

Q-45: A 6-year-old boy with spastic diplegic cerebral palsy has a crouched gait. Examination reveals hip flexion contractures of 15° and popliteal angles of 70°. Equinus contractures measure 10° with the knees extended. Which of the following surgical procedures, if performed alone, will worsen the crouching?

1. Iliopsoas release from the lesser trochanter
2. Iliopsoas release at the pelvic brim
3. Hamstring lengthening
4. Heel cord lengthening
5. Split posterior tibial tendon transfer

Q-46: Figure 26 shows the pedigree of a family with an unusual type of muscular dystrophy. This pedigree is most consistent with what type of inheritance pattern?

1. Autosomal dominant
2. Autosomal recessive
3. X-linked dominant
4. X-linked recessive
5. Mitochondrial inheritance

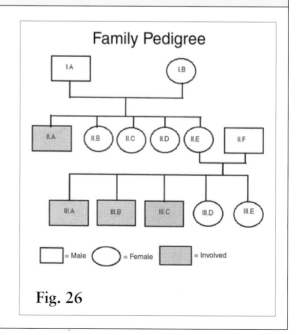

Fig. 26

Q-47: A 13-year-old boy sustains a closed injury to his knee after a fall. A radiograph is shown in Figure 27. Treatment should consist of which of the following?

1. Long leg cast in extension
2. Long leg cast in 45° of flexion
3. Percutaneous pinning with smooth wires and a cylinder cast
4. Anterior cruciate ligament reconstruction and early motion
5. Open reduction and internal fixation with lag screws and a cylinder cast

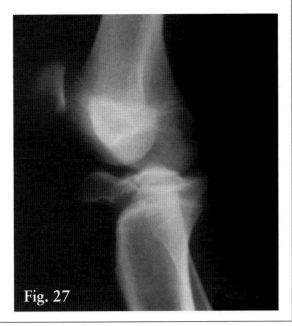

Fig. 27

Q-48: An obese 4-year-old boy has infantile Blount disease. Radiographs reveal a metaphyseal-diaphyseal angle of 18° and a depression of the medial proximal tibial physis. Management should consist of

1. observation.
2. varus prevention orthoses.
3. physeal bar resection.
4. proximal tibial osteotomy that produces a neutral mechanical axis.
5. proximal tibial osteotomy that produces 10° of valgus.

Q-49: In girls with idiopathic scoliosis, peak height velocity (PHV) typically occurs at what point?

1. Before Risser 1 and menarche
2. After Risser 1 and menarche
3. Between Risser 1 and menarche
4. After menarche but before Risser 1
5. At Risser 2

Q-50: Which of the following pathogens are most commonly associated with neonatal septic arthritis and osteomyelitis?

1. *Staphylococcus aureus* and *Escherichia coli*
2. *Staphylococcus aureus* and group A streptococci
3. *Staphylococcus aureus* and group B streptococci
4. *Haemophilus influenzae* and *Escherichia coli*
5. *Haemophilus influenzae* and group A streptococci

Q-51: Figure 28 shows the radiograph of a 10-year-old girl who reports chronic shoulder pain after her gymnastics classes. Examination reveals pain on internal and external rotation but no instability. What is the most likely diagnosis?

1. Acromial fracture
2. Humeral stress fracture
3. Acromioclavicular joint separation
4. Fracture of the surgical neck of the scapula
5. Triceps avulsion fracture

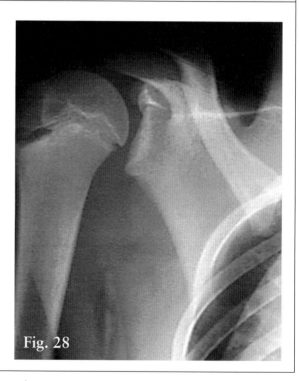

Fig. 28

Q-52: When counseling a patient with hypophosphatemic rickets, which of the following scenarios will always result in a child with the same disorder?

1. Female patient who has a female child
2. Female patient who has a male child
3. Male patient who has a female child
4. Male patient who has a male child
5. Disorder not inherited

Q-53: A 3-year-old patient with L3 myelomeningocele has bilateral dislocated hips. Management should consist of

1. observation.
2. bilateral open reduction.
3. bilateral open reduction and psoas transfers.
4. bilateral open reduction and external oblique transfers.
5. bilateral valgus osteotomies.

Q-54: During soft-tissue release for an idiopathic clubfoot, it is noted that the peroneus longus tendon has been transected in the midfoot. Failure to repair this structure may lead to

1. cavus.
2. claw toes.
3. a dorsal bunion.
4. hindfoot valgus.
5. forefoot pronation.

Q-55: A newborn with bilateral talipes equinovarus undergoes serial manipulation and casting. What is the primary goal of manipulation?

1. Rotation of the foot laterally around the fixed talus
2. Simultaneous abduction of the metatarsals and dorsiflexion of the talus
3. Lateral translation of the calcaneus
4. Anterolateral translation of the navicular
5. Dorsiflexion of the calcaneus with forefoot eversion

Q-56: In patients with neurofibromatosis, what is the most important sign of impending rapid progression of a spinal deformity?

1. Apical curve rotation
2. Anterior vertebral body erosions
3. Cervical spine involvement
4. Penciling of three or more ribs
5. Curve magnitude of greater than 50°

A-1: Figure 1 shows the radiograph of a 7-year-old patient who has a bilateral Trendelenburg limp and limited range of hip motion but no pain. His work-up should include

1. a skeletal survey.
2. genetic evaluation.
3. cardiac evaluation.
4. coagulation studies.
5. an MRI scan of the hips.

PREFERRED RESPONSE: 1

DISCUSSION: The radiograph shows bilateral flattening of the femoral heads with mottling and "fragmentation" suggestive of Legg-Calvé-Perthes disease. However, when these changes occur bilaterally and are symmetric, multiple epiphyseal dysplasia or spondyloepiphyseal dysplasia should be suspected. Skeletal survey will show irregularity of the secondary ossification centers. With these conditions, there is no true osteonecrosis and no evidence that orthotic or surgical "containment" will alter the outcome of progressive degenerative arthritis. Cardiac anomalies and coagulopathies are not associated with the epiphyseal dysplasias.

REFERENCES: Crossan JF, Wynne-Davies R, Fulford GE: Bilateral failure of the capital femoral epiphysis: Bilateral Perthes disease, multiple epiphyseal dysplasia, pseudoachondroplasia, and spondyloepiphyseal dysplasia congenita and tarda. *J Pediatr Orthop* 1983;3:297-301.
Sponseller PD: The skeletal dysplasias, in Morrissy RT, Weinstein SL (eds): *Lovell and Winter's Pediatric Orthopaedics*, ed 5. Philadelphia, PA, Lippincott Williams & Wilkins, 2001, pp 269-270.

A-2: A 2-week-old infant has been referred for evaluation of nonmovement of the left hip. History reveals that the patient was delivered 6 weeks premature by cesarean section. Examination reveals no fever, and there is mild swelling of the thigh. Passive movement of the hip appears to elicit tenderness and very limited hip motion. A radiograph of the pelvis shows mild subluxation of the left hip. The next step in evaluation should consist of

1. aspiration of the left hip.
2. application of a Pavlik harness.
3. a gallium scan.
4. an MRI scan of the spine.
5. modified Bryant traction.

PREFERRED RESPONSE: 1

DISCUSSION: The diagnosis of bone and joint sepsis in a newborn is difficult because of the relative lack of obvious signs and symptoms. Fever is usually absent. A study of 34 newborns with osteomyelitis identified prematurity and delivery by cesarean section as predisposing factors. In that study, the most common clinical findings were pseudoparalysis, local swelling, and pain on passive movement. Because

(continued on next page)

(A-2 continued)

early diagnosis is so important, any infant who exhibits these findings should be suspected as having bone or joint sepsis. Once the area of involvement is identified, aspiration is mandatory. In newborns who have an infection about the hip, radiographs may reveal subluxation. In this patient, septic arthritis must be ruled out by aspiration of the hip. Developmental dysplasia of the hip is not painful and is not accompanied by localized swelling. If no purulent material is obtained at the time of hip aspiration, an arthrogram should be obtained to rule out epiphysiolysis of the proximal femur. Because the area of involvement has been identified by clinical examination, a gallium scan or MRI scan of the spine is not indicated.

REFERENCES: Knudsen CJ, Hoffman EB: Neonatal osteomyelitis. *J Bone Joint Surg Br* 1990; 72:846-851.

Morrissy RT: Bone and joint sepsis, in Morrissy RT, Weinstein SL (eds): *Lovell and Winter's Pediatric Orthopaedics*, ed 4. Philadelphia, Pa, Lippincott-Raven, 1996, pp 579-624.

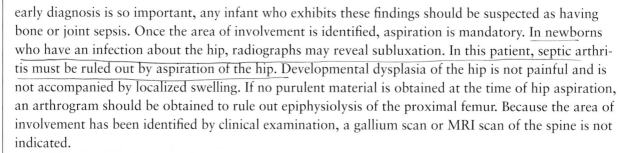

A-3: A 9-year-old boy who is small for his age has a painful limp and limited hip motion. Radiographs of the pelvis are shown in Figures 2A and 2B. In addition to managing the problem with the hip, what laboratory studies should be obtained?

1. Serum protein electrophoresis
2. Serum glucose and hemoglobin A1C
3. WBC and differential blood cell count
4. Thyroxin and thyroid-stimulating hormone
5. Transferrin and total iron-binding capacity

PREFERRED RESPONSE: 4

DISCUSSION: The child has bilateral slipped capital femoral epiphyses (SCFE). SCFE usually develops in early adolescence, but can occur in younger children with endocrine disorders such as panhypopituitarism and hypothyroidism. Any child younger than age 10 years or older than age 16 years who has SCFE should be carefully evaluated for an underlying endocrine problem. Unrecognized endocrine disorders can increase the risks of anesthesia.

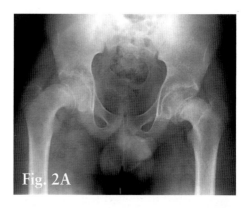

Fig. 2A

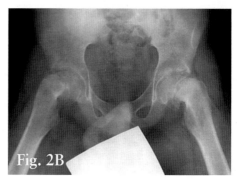

Fig. 2B

REFERENCES: Loder RT, Wittenberg B, DeSilva G: Slipped capital femoral epiphysis associated with endocrine disorders. *J Pediatr Orthop* 1995;15:349-356.

Wells D, King JD, Roe TF, et al: Review of slipped capital femoral epiphysis associated with endocrine disease. *J Pediatr Orthop* 1993;13:610-614.

A-4: Figure 3 shows the current radiographs of a 13-year-old boy who was treated for an elbow fracture 1 year ago. He is neurovascularly intact. What is the most important component of treatment if reconstruction is being considered?

1. Construction of the annular ligament
2. Restoration of the radioulnar articulation
3. Restoration and maintenance of ulnar length and alignment
4. Adequate immobilization postoperatively in 120° of flexion
5. Placement of a Kirschner wire from the radial head to the capitellum

PREFERRED RESPONSE: 3

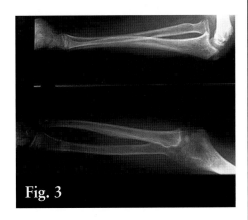

Fig. 3

DISCUSSION: Restoration of ulnar length and alignment is usually sufficient to allow complete reduction of the radial head. Reconstruction of the annular ligament may be unnecessary, and while immobilization in 100° to 110° of flexion is helpful in maintaining reduction, 120° is excessive and risks vascular compromise. Pins across the radiocapitellar joint frequently break and should be avoided. Pinning from the proximal radius to the ulna is safer and can stabilize the radiocapitellar joint just as well.

REFERENCES: Beaty JH, Kasser JR: Fractures about the elbow. *Instr Course Lect* 1995;44:199-215. Mehta SD: Flexion osteotomy of ulna for untreated Monteggia fracture in children. *Indian J Surg* 1985;47:15-19.

A-5: A 12-year-old girl has had lower back pain for the past 6 months that interferes with her ability to participate in sports. She denies any history of radicular symptoms, sensory changes, or bowel or bladder dysfunction. Examination reveals a shuffling gait, restriction of forward bending, and tight hamstrings. Radiographs show a grade III spondylolisthesis of L5 on S1, with a slip angle of 20°. Management should consist of

1. brace treatment.
2. laminectomy, nerve root decompression, and in situ fusion of L4 to the sacrum.
3. in situ fusion of L4 to the sacrum.
4. excision of the L5 lamina.
5. physical therapy.

PREFERRED RESPONSE: 3

(continued on next page)

(A-5 continued)

DISCUSSION: Indications for surgical treatment of spondylolisthesis include pain and/or progression of deformity. Specifically, surgery is necessary when there is persistent pain or a neurologic deficit that fails to respond to nonsurgical therapy, there is significant slip progression, or the slip is greater than 50%. For patients with mild spondylolisthesis, in situ posterolateral L5-S1 fusion is adequate. In patients with more severe slips (greater than 50%), extension of the fusion to L4 offers better mechanical advantage. Postoperative immobilization may be achieved with instrumentation, casting, or both. In patients with a slip angle of greater than 45°, reduction of the lumbosacral kyphosis with instrumentation or casting is desirable to prevent slip progression. Laminectomy alone is contraindicated in a child. Nerve root decompression is indicated if radiculopathy is present clinically.

REFERENCES: Seitsalo S, Osterman K, Hyvarinen H, Tallroth K, Schlenzka D, Poussa M: Progression of spondylolisthesis in children and adolescents: A long-term follow-up of 272 patients. *Spine* 1991;16:417-421.

Newton PO, Johnston CE II: Analysis and treatment of poor outcomes following in situ arthrodesis in adolescent spondylolisthesis. *J Pediatr Orthop* 1997;17:754-761.

A-6: Marfan syndrome is most likely associated with defects in which of the following structural proteins?

1. Elastin
2. Fibrillin
3. Fibronectin
4. Type II collagen
5. Type III collagen

Type I -
Ligaments & bone
Type II -
Cartilage

PREFERRED RESPONSE: 2

DISCUSSION: Most patients with Marfan syndrome have abnormalities in fibrillin, a structural protein found in ligaments. Marfan syndrome has been linked to a fibrillin gene on chromosome 15, as has ectopia lentis. Congenital contractural arachnodactyly has been linked to a fibrillin gene on chromosome 5. A few patients with a marfanoid habitus have an anomaly of type I collagen, the major collagen component of bone and ligaments. Type II collagen is the main collagen found in articular cartilage. A type II collagen anomaly is associated with spondyloepiphyseal dysplasia and Kneist syndrome. A type III collagen anomaly has been seen in one form of Ehlers-Danlos syndrome. Fibronectin and elastin anomalies have not yet been shown to be associated with specific diseases.

REFERENCES: Tsipouras P, Del Mastro R, Sarfarazi M, et al: Genetic linkage of the Marfan syndrome, ectopia lentis, and congenital contractural arachnodactyly to the fibrillin genes on chromosomes 15 and 5: The International Marfan Syndrome Collaborative Study. *N Engl J Med* 1992;326:905-909.

Zaleske DJ: Metabolic and endocrine abnormalities, in Morrissy RT, Weinstein SL (eds): *Lovell and Winter's Pediatric Orthopaedics*, ed 4. Philadelphia, PA, Lippincott-Raven, 1996, vol 1, pp 137-201.

A-7: The inheritance of the deformity shown in Figure 4 is most commonly

1. autosomal recessive.
2. autosomal dominant.
3. X-linked dominant.
4. mitochondrial.
5. sporadic.

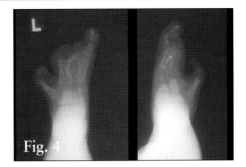

Fig. 4

PREFERRED RESPONSE: 2

DISCUSSION: Cleft hand and cleft foot malformations are commonly inherited as autosomal-dominant traits and are associated with a number of syndromes. An autosomal-recessive and an X-linked inheritance pattern have also been described, but these are much less common and are usually atypical. In the common autosomal-dominant condition, nearly one third of the known carriers of the gene show no hand or foot abnormalities. This is known as reduced penetrance. The disorder may be variably expressed; affected family members often exhibit a range from mild abnormalities in one limb only to severe anomalies in four limbs. Variable expressivity and reduced penetrance can cause difficulty in counseling families regarding future offspring in an affected family. Many patients have a cleft hand that may be caused by the split-hand, split-foot gene (SHFM1) localized on chromosome 7q21.

REFERENCE: Kay SPJ: Cleft hand, in Green DP (ed): *Green's Operative Hand Surgery*. Philadelphia, PA, Churchill Livingstone, 1999, pp 402-414.

A-8: A 7-year-old boy with a closed supracondylar fracture of the distal humerus is unable to flex the distal interphalangeal (DIP) joint of his index finger and the interphalangeal (IP) joint of his thumb. These findings are most likely due to a deficit involving fibers of which of the following nerves?

1. Ulnar
2. Radial
3. Musculocutaneous
4. Anterior interosseous
5. Posterior interosseous

PREFERRED RESPONSE: 4

DISCUSSION: Inability to flex the DIP joint of the index finger and IP joint of the thumb indicates a motor deficit to the anterior interosseous nerve. The posterior interosseous, radial, ulnar, and musculocutaneous nerves do not innervate the profundus to the index finger nor the flexor pollicis longus.

REFERENCES: Kasser JR (ed): *Orthopaedic Knowledge Update 5*. Rosemont, IL, American Academy of Orthopaedic Surgeons, 1996, pp 259-267.
Cramer KE, Green NE, Devito DP: Incidence of anterior interosseous nerve palsy in supracondylar humerus fractures in children. *J Pediatr Orthop* 1993;13:502-505.

A-9: A 14-year-old girl with polyarticular juvenile rheumatoid arthritis (JRA) has severe neck pain and reports the onset of urinary incontinence. A lateral radiograph and lateral tomogram of the cervical spine are shown in Figures 5A and 5B. An MRI scan of the upper cervical spine is shown in Figure 5C. Management should consist of

1. a rigid cervical orthosis.

2. a soft cervical collar.

3. posterior C1-2 fusion with halo immobilization.

4. administration of methotrexate.

5. activity restrictions.

PREFERRED RESPONSE: 3

DISCUSSION: The plain radiograph and tomogram show an abnormality of the upper cervical spine, with erosion of the dens. The MRI scan shows evidence of cord impingement. The cervical spine is frequently involved in polyarticular JRA. Stiffness and autofusion are commonly seen, but C1-2 instability can also occur secondary to synovitis and bony erosion. Basilar invagination is rare in JRA. There is no consensus regarding fusion in the asymptomatic patient. In patients with symptoms and neurologic signs, posterior C1-2 fusion is indicated.

REFERENCES: Fried JA, Athreya B, Gregg JR, Das M, Doughty R: The cervical spine in juvenile rheumatoid arthritis. *Clin Orthop Relat Res* 1983;179:102-106.
Hensinger RN, DeVito PD, Ragsdale CG: Changes in the cervical spine in juvenile rheumatoid arthritis. *J Bone Joint Surg Am* 1986;68:189-198.

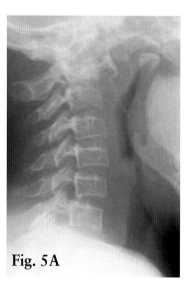

Fig. 5A

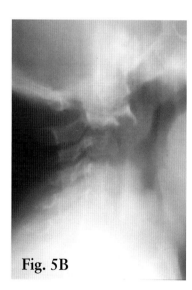

Fig. 5B

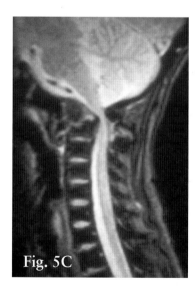

Fig. 5C

A-10: Figure 6 shows the radiograph of a 13-year-old boy who has low back pain and tight hamstrings. There are no sensory or motor deficits. What is the recommended treatment for this condition?

1. Gill procedure
2. Thoracolumbosacral orthosis
3. Direct repair of the pars defect
4. Posterolateral fusion from L4 to the sacrum
5. Combined anteroposterior fusion from L5 to the sacrum

PREFERRED RESPONSE: 4

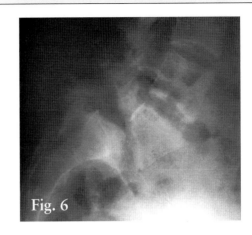

Fig. 6

DISCUSSION: The standard treatment of spondylolisthesis in skeletally immature patients with greater than 50% slippage is a posterolateral fusion from L4 to the sacrum. An orthosis will not prevent progression of the slip. Isolated decompression (Gill procedure) is contraindicated in adolescents as it increases the likelihood of progressive slippage. Direct repair of pars defects is appropriate for L3 or L4 spondylolysis without spondylolisthesis. Anterior procedures are not generally indicated in adolescents with grade III spondylolistheses.

REFERENCES: Bradford DS, Iza J: Repair of the defect in spondylolysis or minimal degrees of spondylolisthesis by segmental wire fixation and bone grafting. *Spine* 1985;10:673-679.
Harris IE, Weinstein SL: Long-term follow-up of patients with grade-III and IV spondylolisthesis: Treatment with and without posterior fusion. *J Bone Joint Surg Am* 1987;69:960-969.
Pizzutillo PD, Mirenda W, MacEwen GD: Posterolateral fusion for spondylolisthesis in adolescence. *J Pediatr Orthop* 1986;6:311-316.

A-11: A 12-year-old girl has progressive development of cavus feet. Examination reveals slightly diminished vibratory sensation on the bottom of the foot. Reflexes are 1+ at the knees and ankles. Motor examination shows that all muscles are 5/5 in the foot, except the peroneal and anterior tibial muscles are rated as 4+/5. Which of the following studies is considered most diagnostic?

1. Nerve conduction velocity studies
2. Biopsy of the quadriceps femoris muscle
3. Biopsy of the sural nerve
4. DNA testing
5. Chromosomal analysis

PREFERRED RESPONSE: 4

DISCUSSION: The patient most likely has a form of Charcot-Marie-Tooth disease, or hereditary motor sensory neuropathy (HMSN). The most common varieties can now be diagnosed by DNA testing. Muta-

(continued on next page)

(A-11 continued)

tions have been detected in the peripheral myelin protein-22 (PMP-22) gene in HMSN type IA and in the connexin gene in the X-linked HMSN. Specific DNA diagnosis is useful in genetic counseling. Routine chromosomal testing most likely would not detect these mutations. Nerve conduction velocity study results are normal in some types of HMSN, and delayed nerve conduction, when found, indicates a peripheral neuropathy but does not specify the type or inheritance pattern. Biopsy of the sural nerve or of the quadriceps can be informative in some patients, but is not as specific as DNA testing. These procedures are most often reserved for patients with negative DNA test results.

REFERENCES: Chance PF: Molecular genetics of hereditary neuropathies. *J Child Neurol* 1999;14:43-52.
Bell C, Haites N: Genetic aspects of Charcot-Marie-Tooth disease. *Arch Dis Child* 1998;78:296-300.

A-12: Figure 7 shows the lateral cervical radiograph of a 2-year-old girl who was an unrestrained passenger in a motor vehicle accident. She is able to move her neck freely without pain, and her neurologic examination is normal. Management should include

1. observation.
2. anterior decompression.
3. upper cervical arthrodesis.
4. application of a soft collar.
5. immobilization in a halo vest.

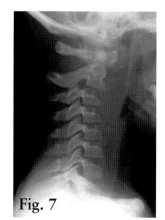

Fig. 7

PREFERRED RESPONSE: 1

DISCUSSION: In children, injuries to the upper cervical spine are more common than injuries to the lower cervical spine. Radiographic findings that would indicate significant trauma in adults, such as anterior soft-tissue widening, may be normal variants in the cervical spine of a child. This child has pseudosubluxation of C2 on C3. Pseudosubluxation occurs because children have less slope to their articular facet joints and increased ligamentous laxity. It is possible to differentiate pseudosubluxation from more serious spinal problems by drawing a line along the front of the posterior elements of C1, C2, and C3, as described by Swischuk. Pseudosubluxation of C2 on C3 is a normal finding, so treatment is not indicated.

REFERENCES: Ehara S, el-Khoury GY, Sato Y: Cervical spine injury in children: Radiologic manifestations. *Am J Roentgenol* 1988;151:1175-1178.
Swischuk LE: Anterior displacement of C2 in children: Physiologic or pathologic. *Radiology* 1977;122:759-763.

A-13: An 11-year-old boy has had a fever and pain and swelling over the lateral aspect of his right ankle for the past 3 days. Examination reveals warmth, swelling, and tenderness over the lateral malleolus, and he has a temperature of 103.2° F (39.5° C). Laboratory studies show a WBC count of 13,200/mm³ with 61% neutrophils, an erythocyte sedimentation rate of 112 mm/h, and a C-reactive protein of 15.7. Radiographs and a T2-weighted MRI scan are shown in Figures 8A through 8C. Aspiration yields 1 mL of purulent fluid. Management should now consist of

1. oral antibiotics and a follow-up office appointment the next day.
2. incision and drainage of the distal fibular metaphysis.
3. indium-labeled WBC scan.
4. antituberculous medication for 6 months.
5. three-phase technetium Tc 99m bone scan.

PREFERRED RESPONSE: 2

DISCUSSION: The initial signs and symptoms of acute hematogenous osteomyelitis vary widely but usually include fever, bone pain, and impaired use of the involved extremity. In lower extremity infections, the child may limp or refuse to walk. Examination often reveals bone tenderness. In more advanced cases, erythema, warmth, and swelling may be present. The WBC and neutrophil counts are not always elevated, but the erythocyte sedimentation rate will be abnormal in more than 90% of patients. When the infection is diagnosed early, before a subperiosteal abscess has formed, antibiotics alone may be adequate to treat the infection. This patient has a more advanced infection, however, with the MRI scan revealing a subperiosteal abscess that was confirmed by aspiration. When an abscess is present, surgical drainage is generally indicated to remove devitalized tissue and to enhance the efficacy of the antibiotics. Further studies, such as bone or indium scans, are not necessary and will delay definitive treatment.

REFERENCES: Scott RJ, Christofersen MR, Robertson WW Jr, et al: Acute osteomyelitis in children: A review of 116 cases. *J Pediatr Orthop* 1990;10:649-652.
Vaughan PA, Newman NM, Rosman MA: Acute hematogenous osteomyelitis. *J Pediatr Orthop* 1987;7:652-655.

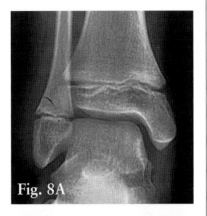

Fig. 8A

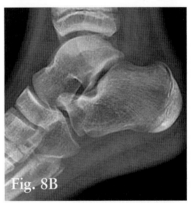

Fig. 8B

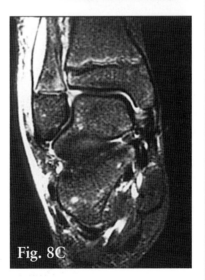

Fig. 8C

A-14: A newborn has a flail right upper extremity after a difficult right occiput anterior vaginal delivery. Examination shows an obvious fracture of the right clavicle. Following stimulation, there is no movement of the arm or hand and there appears to be no sensation in the hand. Management should include

1. a CT scan arteriogram.
2. an MRI scan of the brachial plexus.
3. nerve conduction velocity studies and an electromyogram.
4. surgical exploration and repair of the brachial plexus.
5. observation for 60 days before obtaining further tests.

PREFERRED RESPONSE: 5

DISCUSSION: The patient's signs and symptoms suggest the clinical appearance of a brachial plexus palsy. Fractures of the clavicle can mimic this disorder, and sensory testing in infants can be difficult. Recovery of function in patients with obstetric palsy is common, even if the initial loss of function appears to be severe. Observation for 60 to 90 days frequently reveals substantial functional improvement, obviating the need for surgery or further diagnostic testing. Surgical repair of the lesion is advocated by some authors for severe loss of function that is still present after age 3 months. Early diagnostic studies have not been helpful in planning treatment, although an MRI scan obtained at a later time can assist with surgical planning. There is no indication for an arteriogram.

REFERENCES: Sedel L: The results of surgical repair of brachial plexus injuries. *J Bone Joint Surg Br* 1982;64:54-66.
Jahnke AH Jr, Bovill DF, McCarroll HR Jr, et al: Persistent brachial plexus birth palsies. *J Pediatr Orthop* 1991;11:533-537.

A-15: The most severe and rapidly progressive form of congenital scoliosis is

1. block vertebra.
2. semisegmented hemivertebra.
3. fully segmented hemivertebra.
4. unilateral unsegmented bar.
5. unilateral unsegmented bar with contralateral hemivertebra.

PREFERRED RESPONSE: 5

DISCUSSION: In the various types of congenital scoliosis, the combination of unilateral unsegmented bar with contralateral hemivertebra leads to the most rapid progression. The various types of congenital scoliosis in decreasing order of progression include unilateral unsegmented bar, fully segmented hemivertebra, semisegmented hemivertebra, and block vertebra.

REFERENCES: Kasser JR (ed): *Orthopaedic Knowledge Update 5*. Rosemont, IL, American Academy of Orthopaedic Surgeons, 1996, pp 551-572.
McMaster MJ, David CV: Hemivertebra as a cause of scoliosis: A study of 104 patients. *J Bone Joint Surg Br* 1986;68:588-595.

Answers: Pediatric Orthopaedics

A-16: Figures 9A and 9B show the radiographs of an 11-year-old boy who felt a pop and immediate pain in his right knee as he was driving off his right leg to jam a basketball. Examination reveals that the knee is flexed, and the patient is unable to actively extend it or bear weight on that side. There is also a large effusion. Management should include

1. ice and elevation, followed by graduated range-of-motion exercises.
2. a long leg cast.
3. excision of the fragment.
4. open reduction and internal fixation.
5. observation until maturity, followed by anterior cruciate ligament repair.

PREFERRED RESPONSE: 4

DISCUSSION: Fractures through the cartilage on the inferior pole of the patella, the so-called sleeve fracture, are often difficult to diagnose because of the paucity of ossified bone visible on the radiographs. If the fracture is missed and the fragments are widely displaced, the patella may heal in an elongated configuration that may result in compromise of the extensor mechanism function. The treatment of choice is open reduction and internal fixation using a tension band wire technique to achieve close approximation of the fragments and restore full active knee extension.

REFERENCES: Heckman JD, Alkire CC: Distal patellar pole fractures: A proposed common mechanism of injury. *Am J Sports Med* 1984;12:424-428.
Tolo VT: Fractures and dislocations around the knee, in Green NE, Swiontkowski MF (eds): *Skeletal Trauma in Children*. Philadelphia, Pa, WB Saunders, 1994, vol 3, pp 380-382.

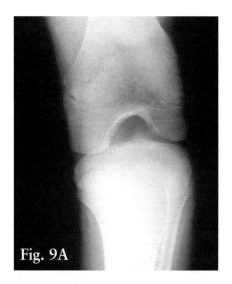
Fig. 9A

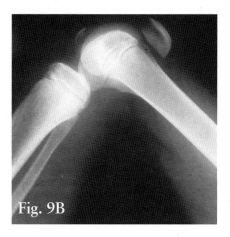
Fig. 9B

A-17: Posterior spinal fusion for scoliosis should be performed on a patient with Duchenne muscular dystrophy when

1. the patient is still ambulatory.
2. lordotic posture is present.
3. the forced vital capacity (FVC) is less than 30% of the predicted value.
4. curve magnitude measures 25° or greater.
5. orthotic management fails.

PREFERRED RESPONSE: 4

DISCUSSION: Progressive scoliosis develops in most patients with Duchenne muscular dystrophy. The onset of spinal deformity typically follows the cessation of walking, and curves can be expected to progress about 10° per year. Posterior spinal fusion with instrumentation should be performed as soon as a curve of 25° or greater is documented and before deterioration of pulmonary function (a FVC of less than 30%) precludes surgery. Patients with kyphotic posture tend to progress more rapidly than those with lordotic posture. Brace treatment is contraindicated because it is not definitive and it may mask curve progression while pulmonary function is concomitantly worsening.

REFERENCES: Beaty JH (ed): *Orthopaedic Knowledge Update 6*. Rosemont, Ill, American Academy of Orthopaedic Surgeons, 1999, pp 635-651.
Mubarak SJ, Morin WD, Leach J: Spinal fusion in Duchenne muscular dystrophy: Fixation and fusion to the sacropelvis? *J Pediatr Orthop* 1993;13:752-757.

A-18: Which of the following deformities is most likely associated with slight valgus of the femur, dimpling over the tibia, mild leg-length deficiency, increased heel valgus, and tarsal coalition?

1. Type 1 fibular hemimelia
2. Type 2 tibial hemimelia
3. Type 4 proximal femoral focal deficiency (PFFD)
4. Posterior medial bowing of the tibia
5. Congenital pseudarthrosis of the tibia

PREFERRED RESPONSE: 1

Anteromedial Bowing

DISCUSSION: Fibular hemimelia can exist in three forms; type 1 represents the milder form with a hypoplastic fibular present. An associated abnormality commonly found with fibular hypoplasia is anteromedial bowing of the tibia, with a skin dimple overlying the deformity. Abnormalities of the ankle joint (such as a ball-and-socket ankle and a valgus position of the hindfoot) are common, and tarsal coalition frequently exists. The patient almost always has some mild shortening of the femur, valgus of the distal

(continued on next page)

(A-18 continued)

femur, and anteroposterior knee instability. While tarsal coalition is present in some forms of PFFD, a type 4 deformity is associated with severe shortening, as is type 2 tibial hemimelia. Posterior medial bowing is associated with mild leg-length deficiency, although it is not associated with tarsal coalition. Congenital pseudarthrosis of the tibia is often seen in association with neurofibromatosis and frequently has a fracture that fails to heal.

REFERENCES: Day HJB: The ISO/ISPO classification of congenital limb deficiency, in Bowker JHG, Michael JW (eds): *Atlas of Limb Prosthetics: Surgical, Prosthetic, and Rehabilitation Principles*, ed 2. St Louis, MO, Mosby-Year Book, 1992, pp 743-748.
Achterman C, Kalamchi A: Congenital deficiency of the fibula. *J Bone Joint Surg Br* 1979;61:133-137.
Grogan DP, Holt GR, Ogden JA: Talocalcaneal coalition in patients who have fibular hemimelia or proximal femoral focal deficiency: A comparison of the radiographic and pathological findings. *J Bone Joint Surg Am* 1994;76:1363-1370.

A-19: A 4-year-old boy is seen in the emergency department with a 2-day history of left groin pain and a limp. His parents deny any history of injury. Examination of the hip shows a 5° hip flexion position, 20° of abduction, internal rotation to 15°, and external rotation to 30°. His temperature is 100.9°F (38.3°C). Blood studies show a normal WBC count, and the erythrocyte sedimentation rate is 18 mm/h. The C-reactive protein is pending. A radiograph is shown in Figure 10. What is the most likely diagnosis?

1. Perthes disease
2. Transient synovitis
3. Slipped capital femoral epiphysis (SCFE)
4. Septic arthritis
5. Juvenile arthritis

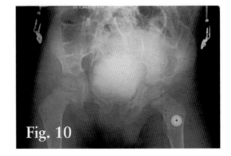
Fig. 10

PREFERRED RESPONSE: 2

DISCUSSION: Transient synovitis is the most common cause of hip pain in children. Males are affected more often than females, and this a typical age for this problem. Normal radiographs rule out SCFE and Perthes disease. The normal WBC count, temperature, ability to walk, and normal ESR make septic arthritis unlikely. Both juvenile arthritis and transient synovitis are diagnoses of exclusion and the subsequent clinical course would differentiate. Transient synovitis usually lasts less than 4 or 5 days. With juvenile arthritis, the ESR usually is elevated.

REFERENCES: Kocher MS, Mandiga R, Zurakowski D, Barnewolt C, Kasser J: Validation of a clinical prediction rule for the differentiation between septic arthritis and transient synovitis of the hip in children. *J Bone Joint Surg Am* 2004;86:1629-1635.
Kocher MS, Zurakowski D, Kasser J: Differentiating between septic arthritis and transient synovitis of the hip in children: An evidence-based clinical prediction algorithm. *J Bone Joint Surg Am* 1999;81:1662-1670.

A-20: A 7-year-old patient has had a painless limp for several months. Examination reveals pain and spasm with internal rotation, and abduction is limited to 10° on the involved side. Management consists of 1 week of bed rest and traction, followed by an arthrogram. A maximum abduction/internal rotation view is shown in Figure 11A, and abduction and adduction views are shown in Figures 11B and 11C. The studies are most consistent with

1. Catterall II involvement.
2. tubercular synovitis.
3. Herring type A involvement.
4. hinge abduction.
5. osteochondritis dissecans.

PREFERRED RESPONSE: 4

DISCUSSION: The radiographs show classic hinge abduction. The diagnostic feature is the failure of the lateral epiphysis to slide under the acetabular edge with abduction, and the abduction view shows medial dye pooling because of distraction of the hip joint. Persistent hinge abduction has been shown to prevent femoral head remodeling by the acetabulum. Radiographic changes are characteristic of severe involvement with Legg-Calve-Perthes disease. The Catterall classification cannot be well applied without a lateral radiograph, but this degree of involvement would likely be considered a grade III or IV. Because the lateral pillar is involved, this condition would be classified as type C using the Herring lateral pillar classification scheme.

REFERENCE: Reinker KA: Early diagnosis and treatment of hinge abduction in Legg-Perthes disease. *J Pediatr Orthop* 1996;16:3-9.

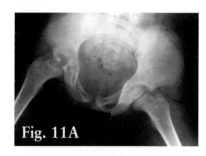
Fig. 11A

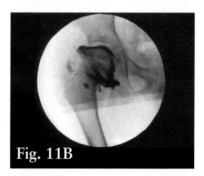
Fig. 11B

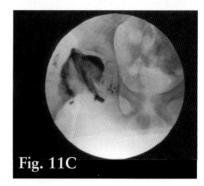
Fig. 11C

A-21: Figure 12 shows the radiograph of a 3-year-old child with progressive bowlegs. Laboratory studies show a calcium level of 9.5 mg/dL (normal 9.0 to 11.0 mg/dL), a phosphorus level of 4.2 mg/dL (normal 3 to 5.7 mg/dL), and an alkaline phosphatase level of 305 IU/L (normal 104 to 345 IU/L). What is the most likely diagnosis?

1. Blount disease
2. Hypophosphatemic rickets
3. Nutritional rickets
4. Schmid metaphyseal dysostosis
5. Jansen metaphyseal dysostosis

widened physes

PREFERRED RESPONSE: 4

DISCUSSION: The patient has bowlegs associated with very wide physes, particularly noted at the hips. The widening of the growth plates is a classic sign of rickets; however, the normal levels of calcium, phosphorus, and alkaline phosphatase rule out both nutritional and hypophosphatemic rickets. Patients with nutritional rickets or hypophosphatemic rickets have hypophosphatemia and increased alkaline phosphatase levels. Jansen metaphyseal dysostosis has very severe radiographic findings that are not found in this patient; however, these radiographic findings are classic for Schmid metaphyseal dysostosis. This disorder is caused by a mutation in the gene for type X collagen, which is found only in the growth plates of growing children.

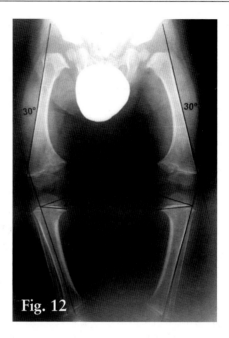

Fig. 12

REFERENCES: Lachman RS, Rimoin DL, Spranger J: Metaphyseal chondrodysplasia, Schmid type: Clinical and radiographic delineation with a review of the literature. *Pediatr Radiol* 1988;18:93-102. Warman ML, Abbot M, Apte SS, et al: A type X collagen mutation causes Schmid metaphyseal chondrodysplasia. *Nat Genet* 1993;5:79-82.

found only in growth plate of children

A-22: Which of the following clinical scenarios represents an appropriate indication for convex hemiepiphysiodesis/hemiarthrodesis in the treatment of a child with a congenital spinal deformity?

1. A 3-year-old child with a hemivertebra opposite a contralateral bar and thoracic scoliosis that measures 53°
2. A 4-year-old child with a fully segmented L1 hemivertebra and scoliosis that measures 80°
3. A 4-year-old child with a fully segmented T10 hemivertebra and scoliosis that measures 50°
4. A 4-year-old child with a posterolateral hemivertebra at the thoracolumbar junction and a kyphoscoliotic deformity that measures 45°
5. A 10-year-old child with a hemivertebra and scoliosis that measures 50°

(continued on next page)

Answers: Pediatric Orthopaedics

(A-22 continued)

PREFERRED RESPONSE: 3

DISCUSSION: Convex hemiarthrodesis and hemiepiphysiodesis are procedures designed to gradually reduce curve magnitude in congenital scoliosis because of hemivertebrae. They are used to surgically create an anterior and posterior bar to arrest growth on the convexity of the existing deformity. Success of the technique is predicated on continued growth on the concave side of the deformity. Prerequisites for this procedure include curves of limited length (less than or equal to five vertebrae), curves of reasonable magnitude (less than 70°), absence of kyphosis, concave growth potential, and appropriate age (younger than age 5 years).

REFERENCE: Winter RB, Lonstein JE, Denis F, Sta-Ana de la Rosa H: Convex growth arrest for progressive congenital scoliosis due to hemivertebrae. *J Pediatr Orthop* 1988;8:633-638.

Correct to less than 40° saphne (flexible)

A-23: Which of the following types of iliac osteotomy provides the greatest potential for increased coverage?

1. Ganz periacetabular
2. Pemberton innominate
3. Salter innominate
4. Sutherland double innominate
5. Steele triple innominate

PREFERRED RESPONSE: 1

DISCUSSION: The degree of acetabular dysplasia and the age of the child are important considerations when choosing what type of osteotomy to perform. The ability to obtain concentric reduction is a prerequisite of all osteotomies that redirect the acetabulum. Procedures that cut all three pelvic bones allow more displacement and, therefore, correction of acetabular dysplasia. The closer the osteotomy is to the acetabulum, the greater the coverage of the femoral head. Compared with the other acetabular osteotomies, the Ganz periacetabular osteotomy provides the greatest potential for correcting acetabular deficiency because there are no bone or ligamentous restraints to limit correction, but it has the disadvantage of being a technically demanding procedure. The amount of coverage provided by the Salter osteotomy is limited.

REFERENCES: Millis MB, Poss R, Murphy SB: Osteotomies of the hip in the prevention and treatment of osteoarthritis. *Instr Course Lect* 1992;41:145-154.
Weinstein SL: Developmental hip dysplasia and dislocation, in Morrissy RT, Weinstein SL (eds): *Lovell and Winter's Pediatric Orthopaedics*, ed 4. Philadelphia, PA, Lippincott-Raven, 1996, pp 903-950.

A-24: Figure 13 shows the radiograph of an 18-year-old patient who has severe knee pain. Treatment consisting of osteotomy should be performed

1. above the tibial tubercle.
2. at or just below the tibial tubercle.
3. in the tibial diaphysis.
4. on both the femur and tibia.
5. on the femur alone.

PREFERRED RESPONSE: 2

DISCUSSION: Very large corrections of tibial deformity can be achieved at or just below the tibial tubercle. This level of osteotomy maintains the relationship between the tubercle and the rest of the joint, does not alter patellofemoral mechanics, and avoids complicating possible future conversion to total knee arthroplasty. High tibial osteotomy is contraindicated for large corrections because of excessive elevation of the tibial tubercle and overhang of the lateral plateau. Correction in the tibial diaphysis creates a zigzag pattern in the tibia by correcting below the deformity and risks nonunion in cortical bone. There is no evidence that the femur is deformed; therefore, femoral osteotomy is not indicated.

REFERENCE: Murphy SB: Tibial osteotomy for genu varum: Indications, preoperative planning, and technique. *Orthop Clin North Am* 1994;25:477-482.

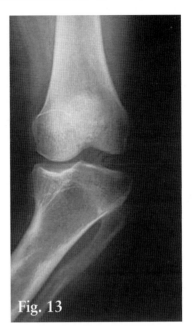
Fig. 13

A-25: Examination of a 6-year-old boy who sustained a displaced Salter-Harris type II fracture of the distal radius reveals 35° of volar angulation. A satisfactory reduction is obtained with the aid of a hematoma block. At the 10-day follow-up examination, radiographs show loss of reduction and 35° of volar angulation. Management should now consist of

1. acceptance of the malalignment and continued cast immobilization.
2. repeat closed reduction with the aid of IV morphine and midazolam.
3. repeat closed reduction with the aid of IV ketamine.
4. repeat closed reduction with the patient under general anesthesia.
5. gentle open reduction with smooth cross-pin fixation.

PREFERRED RESPONSE: 1

DISCUSSION: In a 6-year-old child with a physeal fracture, the healing response 10 days after injury is so advanced that manipulation would have to be very forceful to be successful. A forceful manipulation in a patient this age increases the risk of early growth arrest and a significant disability because 80% of the growth of the radius comes from the distal physis. Because of the large contribution of growth from the distal radial physis and the angulation being in the plane of wrist motion, the potential for remodel-

(continued on next page)

(A-25 continued)

ing of this fracture is great. It is highly probable that this fracture will completely remodel in 1 to 2 years of growth. In this patient, even a "gentle" open reduction would probably require enough force that the physis would be damaged.

REFERENCES: Dimeglio A: Growth in pediatric orthopaedics, in Morrissy RT, Weinstein SL (eds): *Lovell and Winter's Pediatric Orthopaedics*, ed 5. Philadelphia, PA, Lippincott Williams and Wilkins, 2001, pp 33-62.

Waters PM: Forearm and wrist fractures, in Richards BS (ed): *Orthopaedic Knowledge Update: Pediatrics*. Rosemont, IL, American Academy of Orthopaedic Surgeons, 1996, pp 251-258.

A-26: Figure 14 shows the radiograph of a 13-year-old girl who has scoliosis. She has long, slender fingers, and when she grasps her left wrist with her right hand, the index finger and thumb overlap by 3 cm. She wears glasses for myopia. A preoperative work-up should include

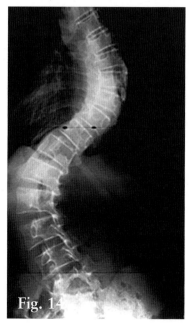

Fig. 14

1. an echocardiogram.
2. neurofibromin testing. — *neroFibromatosis* (handwritten)
3. a serum fibrillin level.
4. an MRI scan of the spine.
5. a urine mucopolysaccharide screen.

PREFERRED RESPONSE: 1

DISCUSSION: The patient has Marfan syndrome. In these patients, aortic dilation can be life-threatening and aortic rupture has been reported as a complication of spinal surgery. An ultrasound measurement of the diameter of the aorta should be done preoperatively and on a yearly basis thereafter, and treatment with beta blockers and avoidance of stressful activities should be prescribed prophylactically if dilation is present. An MRI scan of the spine is not indicated in the work-up of this disease. Urine mucopolysaccharide screening is used to rule out mucopolysaccharidoses, but this patient has no sign of these diseases. While fibrillin levels are abnormal in patients with Marfan syndrome, this is a structural protein and abnormality cannot be determined by serum measurement. Abnormalities of neurofibromin are associated with neurofibromatosis, not Marfan syndrome.

REFERENCES: Birch JG, Herring JA: Spinal deformity in Marfan syndrome. *J Pediatr Orthop* 1987;7:546-552.

Shores J, Berger KR, Murphy EA, et al: Progression of aortic dilation and the benefit of long-term beta-adrenergic blockade in Marfan's syndrome. *N Engl J Med* 1994;330:1335-1341.

Tsipouras P, Del Mastro R, Sarfarazi M, et al: Genetic linkage of the Marfan syndrome, ectopia lentis, and congenital contractural arachnodactyly to the fibrillin genes on chromosomes 15 and 5: The International Marfan Syndrome Collaborative Study. *New Engl J Med* 1992;326:905-909.

A-27: Figure 15 shows the radiograph of an 11-year-old boy with Duchenne muscular dystrophy who has been nonambulatory for the past 2 years. Management of the spinal deformity should consist of

1. wheelchair modifications and custom-molded inserts.
2. posterior fusion with instrumentation.
3. anterior and posterior fusion.
4. observation and reexamination in 6 months.
5. thoracolumbosacral orthosis bracing.

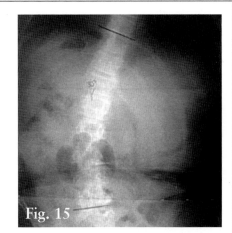

Fig. 15

PREFERRED RESPONSE: 2

DISCUSSION: The presence of any curve greater than 20° in a nonambulatory patient with Duchenne muscular dystrophy is an indication for posterior fusion with instrumentation. Because of progressive cardiomyopathy and pulmonary deficiency, waiting until the curve is larger can increase the risk of pulmonary or cardiac complications during or following surgery. There is some disagreement as to whether all such fusions must extend to the pelvis. Bracing or other nonsurgical management is ineffective and is not indicated in this situation.

REFERENCES: Sussman M: Duchenne muscular dystrophy. *J Am Acad Orthop Surg* 2002;10:138-151. Mubarek SJ, Morin WD, Leach J: Spinal fusion in Duchenne muscular dystrophy: Fixation and fusion to the sacropelvis? *J Pediatr Orthop* 1993;13:752-757.

A-28: Which of the following patients is considered the most appropriate candidate for selective dorsal rhizotomy?

1. Nonambulatory 2-year-old with spastic diplegia
2. Nonambulatory 2-year-old with spastic quadriplegia
3. Nonambulatory 12-year-old with spastic quadriplegia
4. Ambulatory 4-year-old with spastic diplegia
5. Ambulatory 9-year-old with hemiplegia and athetosis

PREFERRED RESPONSE: 4

DISCUSSION: While other surgical and nonsurgical options exist for management of spasticity, the criteria originally laid out by Peacock and associates describe the most appropriate candidate for rhizotomy as a patient with spastic diplegia who is between the ages of 4 to 8 years and has a stable gait pattern that is limited by lower extremity spasticity. Rhizotomy is not recommended in patients with athetosis because of unpredictable results. In addition, rhizotomy should be avoided in nonambulatory patients with spastic quadriplegia because it is associated with significant spinal deformities.

(continued on next page)

(A-28 continued)

REFERENCES: Peacock WJ, Arens LJ, Berman B: Cerebral palsy spasticity: Selective posterior rhizotomy. *Pediatr Neurosci* 1987;13:61-66.

Oppenheim WL: Selective posterior rhizotomy for spastic cerebral palsy: A review. *Clin Orthop Relat Res* 1990;253:20-29.

Mooney JF III, Millis MB: Spinal deformity after selective dorsal rhizotomy in patients with cerebral palsy. *Clin Orthop Relat Res* 1999;364:48-52.

A-29: A 2-day-old infant has the hyperextended knee deformity shown in Figure 16. No other deformities are found on examination. A radiograph shows that the ossified portion of the proximal tibia is slightly anterior to that of the distal femur. Management should consist of

1. gentle stretching and serial casting.
2. Bryant traction for 1 to 2 weeks, followed by closed reduction.
3. percutaneous quadriceps recession, followed by serial casting.
4. delayed open reduction at age 6 months to avoid iatrogenic damage to either the distal femoral or proximal tibial physes.
5. a renal ultrasound.

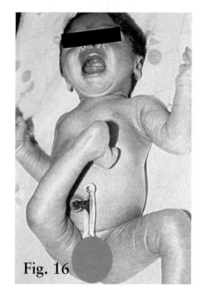

Fig. 16

PREFERRED RESPONSE: 1

DISCUSSION: Congenital dislocation of the knee is an uncommon deformity that varies in presentation from simple hyperextension to complete anterior dislocation of the tibia on the femur. Treatment varies with the age at presentation and the severity of the deformity. Most authors recommend early nonsurgical management. A recent study of 24 congenital knee dislocations in 17 patients found that satisfactory results were obtained in most instances using closed treatment. Based on their findings, the authors concluded that immediate reduction or serial casting should be performed when the patient is seen early after birth. If the patient is seen late and correction cannot be achieved by serial casting, traction followed by closed or open reduction may be necessary. Early percutaneous quadriceps recession has been described for complex congenital knee dislocations associated with underlying disorders, such as arthrogryposis and Ehlers-Danlos syndrome. Ultrasound of the hip is required in all patients with congenital dislocation of the knee because 50% of these patients will have associated developmental dysplasia of the hip.

REFERENCES: Ko JY, Shih CH, Wenger DR: Congenital dislocation of the knee. *J Pediatr Orthop* 1999;19:252-259.

Johnson E, Audell R, Oppenheim WL: Congenital dislocation of the knee. *J Pediatr Orthop* 1987;7:194-200.

Roy DR, Crawford AH: Percutaneous quadriceps recession: A technique for management of congenital hyperextension deformities of the knee in the neonate. *J Pediatr Orthop* 1989;9:717-719.

A-30: A 10-year-old boy has activity-related knee pain that is poorly localized. He denies locking, swelling, or giving way. Examination shows mild tenderness at the medial femoral condyle and painless full range of motion without ligamentous instability. Radiographs are shown in Figures 17A through 17C. What is the best course of action?

1. Knee arthroscopy with drilling of the lesion
2. Limited activity for 6 to 12 weeks
3. Removal of the loose body
4. Biopsy of the lesion
5. Open reduction and internal fixation

PREFERRED RESPONSE: 2

DISCUSSION: The radiographs show an osteochondritis dissecans (OCD) lesion in the medial femoral condyle of a skeletally immature patient. The lesion is not displaced from its bed. Nonsurgical management of a stable OCD lesion in a patient with open physes consists of a period of activity limitation and occasional immobilization. Unstable lesions, loose bodies, and patients with closed physes require more aggressive treatment. Most of the surgical procedures can be done arthroscopically. Because the radiographic appearance is typical, biopsy is unnecessary. The radiographs do not show an osteocartilaginous loose body, and the patient reports no catching or locking; therefore, removal of the loose body is not indicated.

REFERENCES: Linden B: Osteochondritis dissecans of the femoral condyles: A long term follow-up study. *J Bone Joint Surg Am* 1977;59:769-776.
Cahill BR: Osteochondritis dissecans of the knee: Treatment of juvenile and adult forms. *J Am Acad Orthop Surg* 1995;3:237-247.
Cahill BR, Phillips MR, Navarro R: The results of conservative management of juvenile osteochondritis dissecans using joint scintigraphy: A prospective study. *Am J Sports Med* 1989;17:601-606.

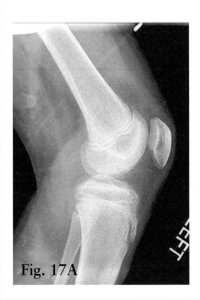

Fig. 17A

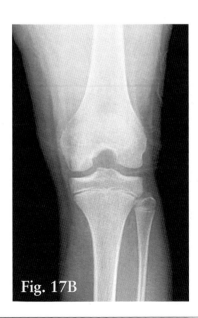

Fig. 17B

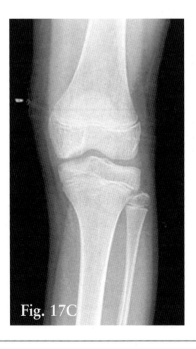

Fig. 17C

A-31: A 3-year-old boy has a rigid 40° lumbar scoliosis that is the result of a fully segmented L5 hemivertebra. All other examination findings are normal. Management should consist of

1. in situ posterior fusion.
2. hemivertebral resection and fusion.
3. convex hemiepiphyseodesis.
4. observation with follow-up in 6 months.
5. thoracolumbosacral orthosis bracing.

PREFERRED RESPONSE: 2

DISCUSSION: Near complete correction and rebalancing of the spine can be achieved by hemivertebral resection that may be done as either a simultaneous or a staged procedure in the young patient. This eliminates the problem of future progression and possible development of compensatory curves. Nonsurgical management is not indicated in congenital scoliosis. Convex hemiepiphyseodesis is best suited for patients younger than age 5 years who have a short curve caused by fully segmented hemivertebrae that correct to less than 40° with the patient supine. Hemiepiphyseodesis and isolated posterior fusion are not indicated.

REFERENCES: Bradford DS, Boachie-Adjei O: One-stage anterior and posterior hemivertebral resection and arthrodesis for congenital scoliosis. *J Bone Joint Surg Am* 1990;72:536-540.
Lazar RD, Hall JE: Simultaneous anterior and posterior hemivertebra excision. *Clin Orthop Relat Res* 1999;364:76-84.

A-32: Examination of a 7-year-old boy reveals 20° of valgus following a lawn mower injury to the lateral femoral epiphysis. Treatment consists of total distal femoral epiphyseodesis and varus osteotomy. Following surgery, he has a limb-length discrepancy of 3 cm and 5° of genu valgum. Assuming that he undergoes no further treatment, the patient's predicted limb-length discrepancy at maturity would be how many centimeters?

1. Less than 7
2. 7 to 10
3. 11 to 13
4. 14 to 17
5. Greater than 17

PREFERRED RESPONSE: 3

DISCUSSION: The distal femoral epiphysis grows approximately 1 cm per year, and in boys growth ceases at approximately age 16 years. Therefore, the patient's limb-length discrepancy at maturity would be 12 cm (9 cm plus the 3-cm discrepancy he has from the previous surgery).

REFERENCES: Little DG, Nigo L, Aiona MD: Deficiencies of current methods for the timing of epiphyseodesis. *J Pediatr Orthop* 1996;16:173-179.
Westh RN, Menelaus MB: A simple calculation for the timing of epiphyseal arrest: A further report. *J Bone Joint Surg Br* 1981;63:117-119.

A-33: Figure 18 shows the hand deformities of a 3-year-old girl who has short stature. The most likely diagnosis is

1. achondroplasia.
2. pseudoachondroplasia.
3. diastrophic dysplasia.
4. metaphyseal chondrodysplasia.
5. multiple epiphyseal dysplasia.

PREFERRED RESPONSE: 3

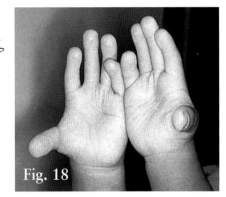

Fig. 18

DISCUSSION: The thumb deformity shown in Figure 18 is termed a "hitchhiker's thumb" and is a distinctive feature of diastrophic dysplasia. Although achondroplasia, pseudoachondroplasia, multiple epiphyseal dysplasia, and metaphyseal chondrodysplasia are all associated with dwarfism, none of these disorders is associated with this distinctive abducted and hypermobile deformity of the thumb. Diastrophic dysplasia was described by Lamy and Maroteaux in 1960 and is inherited as an autosomal-recessive trait. Diastrophic dysplasia is caused by a mutation of a gene coding for a sulfate transport protein located on chromosome 5. The patient is severely dwarfed with the limbs being very short (micromelia) and will reach an eventual adult height of 80 cm to 140 cm. The shortening of the limbs is more severe in the proximal segment than the distal segment and is termed rhizomelic. Diastrophic dysplasia is associated with multiple anomalies including scoliosis, cervical kyphosis, thoracolumbar kyphosis, lumbar lordosis, and flexion contractures of the hips, knees, and elbows. The distinctive feature of diastrophic dysplasia is shortening of the first metacarpal and metatarsal, resulting in the "hitchhiker's thumb" and bilateral clubfoot deformities. Another distinctive feature is a deformity of the external ears termed "cauliflower ears." The ears become thickened and twisted with furrowed lobes and narrowing of the external auditory canal. The patient with diastrophic dysplasia usually has normal intelligence and no abnormalities of the heart or kidney.

REFERENCES: Bethem D, Winter RB, Lutter L: Disorders of the spine in diastrophic dwarfism. *J Bone Joint Surg Am* 1980;62:529-536.
Bassett GS, Scott CI Jr: The osteochondrodysplasias, in Morrissy RT (ed): *Lovell and Winter's Pediatric Orthopaedics*, ed 3. Philadelphia, PA, JB Lippincott, 1990, vol 1, pp 91-142.
Hollister DW, Lachman RS: Diastrophic dwarfism. *Clin Orthop Relat Res* 1976;114:61-69.

A-34: A 4-year-old child sustains a spiral fracture to the tibia in an unwitnessed fall. History reveals three other fractures to long bones, and the parents are vague about the etiology of each. There is no family history of bone disease. The parents ask if the child has osteogenesis imperfecta (OI); however, there are no clinical or radiographic indications of this diagnosis. In addition to fracture care, management should include

1. notification of child protective services and hospital admission.
2. a punch biopsy of skin for collagen analysis.
3. DNA testing for OI.
4. calcium, phosphate, and alkaline phosphatase studies.
5. placement of intramedullary rods to prevent further fractures.

(continued on next page)

(A-34 continued)

PREFERRED RESPONSE: 1

DISCUSSION: Child abuse and OI are frequently both in the differential diagnosis of a child with multiple fractures. If OI is suspected, testing is appropriate to confirm this diagnosis. This may include skull radiographs to look for wormian bones and/or fibroblast culturing and collagen analysis of a punch biopsy. Unfortunately, because of the large number of mutations that can yield the disease, DNA testing is not commercially available for OI. In this patient, however, the physician suspects nonaccidental trauma and is legally obligated in most states to notify child protective services. Because the child may be at considerable risk of further injury, hospitalization is indicated to protect the child until child protective services can complete a home investigation and assess the degree of risk. Work-up for both OI and child abuse can be done during the hospitalization.

REFERENCES: Rockwood CA, Wilkins KE, King RE (eds): *Fractures in Children*. Philadelphia, PA, JB Lippincott, 1984, vol 3, pp 173-175.
Kempe CH, Silverman FN, Stelle BF, Droegemueller W, Silver HK: The battered-child syndrome. *JAMA* 1962;181:17-24.
Akbarnia BA, Akbarnia NO: The role of the orthopedist in child abuse and neglect. *Orthop Clin North Am* 1976;7:733-742.

A-35: Figure 19 shows the clinical photograph of a 3-month-old infant with a foot deformity that has been nonprogressive since birth. Examination reveals that the deformity corrects actively and with passive manipulation. There is no associated equinus. Management should consist of

1. serial casting.
2. UCBL orthoses.
3. abductor hallucis lengthening.
4. observation and parental reassurance.
5. corrective shoes.

PREFERRED RESPONSE: 4

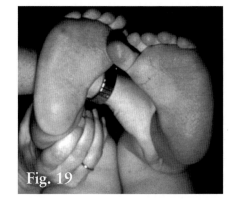
Fig. 19

DISCUSSION: The patient has bilateral metatarsus adductus deformities. In a long-term follow-up study by Farsetti and associates, deformities that were passively correctable spontaneously resolved and no treatment was required. More rigid deformities were successfully treated with serial manipulation, with good results in 90%. There were no poor results. Therefore, observation is the management of choice for passively correctable deformities. In feet that are more rigid, serial manipulation and casting is the management of choice.

REFERENCE: Farsetti P, Weinstein SL, Ponseti IV: The long-term functional and radiographic outcomes of untreated and non-operatively treated metatarsus adductus. *J Bone Joint Surg Am* 1994;76:257-265.

A-36: Figure 20 shows the radiograph of a 7-year-old girl with a low thoracic-level myelomeningocele. She has a history of skin ulcers over the apex of the deformity, but her current skin condition is good. Management of the spinal deformity should consist of

1. physical therapy for hip stretching exercises.
2. kyphectomy and posterior fusion with instrumentation.
3. anterior release and fusion using a rib strut graft.
4. anterior release and strut grafting and posterior fusion with instrumentation.
5. bracing.

PREFERRED RESPONSE: 2

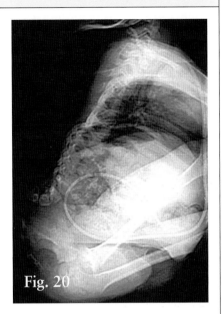

Fig. 20

DISCUSSION: This form of severe kyphosis results in intractable difficulties with sitting position, compression of internal organs, and chronic skin breakdown. Kyphectomy and posterior fusion with instrumentation, while associated with a high rate of complications, provides one of the best solutions to this clinical dilemma. The other choices are either completely ineffective or inadequate in managing this degree of deformity.

REFERENCES: Lindseth RE: Spine deformity in myelomeningocele. *Instr Course Lect* 1991;40:273-279. Sharrard J, Drennan JC: Osteotomy excision of the spine for lumbar kyphosis in older children with myelomeningocele. *J Bone Joint Surg Br* 1972;54:50-60.

A-37: Development of a valgus deformity in children after a fracture of the proximal tibial metaphysis most likely results from

1. lateral physeal arrest.
2. tethering by the fibula.
3. periosteal interposition.
4. asymmetric physeal growth.
5. anterior tibial artery stenosis.

PREFERRED RESPONSE: 4

DISCUSSION: The incidence of proximal tibial metaphyseal fracture in children is estimated at 5 per 1,000 children per year. Of these, approximately 15% develop a valgus deformity. Closure of the physeal plates is rarely seen and typically there is overgrowth at both the proximal and distal ends of the tibia

(continued on next page)

(A-37 continued)

following the fracture. Studies of the "growth arrest lines" and bone scan analysis suggest that there is an asymmetric stimulation of the proximal tibial physeal plate with more medial than lateral growth, resulting in a valgus deformity. Lateral physeal arrest, tethering by the fibula, and periosteal interposition are suggested theories that attempt to explain the deformity, but they have not been proven.

REFERENCES: Skak SV, Jensen TT, Poulsen TD: Fracture of the proximal metaphysis of the tibia in children. *Injury* 1987;18:149-156.

Ogden JA, Ogden DA, Pugh L, et al: Tibia valga after proximal metaphyseal fractures in childhood: A normal biologic response. *J Pediatr Orthop* 1995;15:489-494.

Zionts LE, Harcke HT, Brooks KM, MacEwen GD: Posttraumatic tibia valga: A case demonstrating asymmetric activity at the proximal growth plate on technetium bone scan. *J Pediatr Orthop* 1987;7:458-462.

A-38: The preferred surgical approach to the elbow of a child with an irreducible type III supracondylar distal humerus fracture and pulseless extremity is through which of the following muscle intervals?

1. Pronator teres and the brachialis
2. Pronator teres and the triceps
3. Pronator teres and the biceps
4. Brachioradialis and the biceps
5. Brachioradialis and the brachialis

PREFERRED RESPONSE: 1

DISCUSSION: In a type III supracondylar distal humerus fracture of the elbow, the brachial artery can become incarcerated, yielding a pulseless extremity. In this situation, closed reduction may not be effective; therefore, open management is often necessary. The preferred surgical approach to the brachial artery and to this fracture is the anterior approach to the cubital fossa. The lacertus fibrosis is incised, and the dissection is carried out between the brachialis (musculocutaneous nerve) and the pronator teres (median nerve), mobilizing the brachial artery. Once the brachial artery is mobilized, the anterior elbow joint capsule may be exposed. The interval between the brachialis and the biceps describes the anterolateral approach to the elbow more commonly used for exposure of the proximal aspect of the posterior interosseous nerve. The dissection interval between the brachioradialis and the pronator teres describes the proximal extent of the anterior approach to the radius.

REFERENCES: Tubiana R, McCullough CJ, Masquelet AC: *An Atlas of Surgical Exposures of the Upper Extremity*. Philadelphia, PA, JB Lippincott, 1990, p 115.

Hoppenfeld S, deBoer P: *Surgical Exposures in Orthopaedics: The Anatomic Approach*, ed 2. Philadelphia, PA, Lippincott-Raven, 1992, p 119.

A-39: A 2-year-old girl has had lethargy, fever, and abdominal pain for the past 6 months. In addition to multiple lytic lesions in the long bones and calvaria shown on the skeletal survey, the radiograph of the spine shown in Figure 21A reveals a vertebral lesion. A biopsy specimen is shown in Figure 21B. The most likely diagnosis is

1. leukemia.
2. tuberculosis.
3. Langerhans cell histiocytosis.
4. metastatic neuroblastoma.
5. multifocal osteomyelitis.

PREFERRED RESPONSE: 3

DISCUSSION: Leukemia, Langerhans cell histiocytosis, and metastatic neuroblastoma typically present with constitutional symptoms, bone pain, and multiple lytic lesions in young children. The radiographic appearance of the spinal lesion is a typical vertebra plana caused by eosinophilic granuloma (Langerhans cell histiocytosis). The biopsy specimen shows histiocytes with leukocytic infiltration, predominantly eosinophils. The clinical and other radiographic findings are also consistent with disseminated histiocytosis. Spinal tuberculosis is not usually associated with multiple osseous lesions, especially in the skull. The histology is not consistent with osteomyelitis.

REFERENCES: Campanacci M: *Bone and Soft Tissue Tumours*. Vienna, Austria, Springer-Verlag, 1990.
Springfield DS: Bone and soft tissue tumors, in Morrissy RT, Weinstein SL (eds): *Lovell and Winter's Pediatric Orthopaedics*, ed 4. Philadelphia, PA, Lippincott-Raven, 1996, vol 1, pp 423-467.

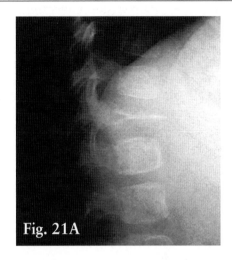

Fig. 21A

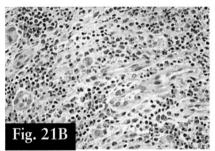

Fig. 21B

A-40: Progressive paralysis is most likely to be seen in association with what type of congenital vertebral abnormality?

1. Anterior failure of formation
2. Anterior failure of segmentation
3. Posterior failure of formation
4. Posterior failure of segmentation
5. Lateral failure of segmentation

(continued on next page)

(A-40 continued)

PREFERRED RESPONSE: 1

DISCUSSION: Anterior failure of formation results in a progressive kyphosis that may lead to cord compression and progressive neurologic deficit. Anterior failure of segmentation can also produce progressive kyphosis but usually is not severe enough to cause cord compression. Posterior failure of formation is seen in conditions such as myelomeningocele in which the neurologic deficit is generally stable. Lateral abnormalities and posterior failure of segmentation are rarely associated with progressive neurologic deficit.

REFERENCES: McMaster MJ, Singh H: Natural history of congenital kyphosis and kyphoscoliosis: A study of one hundred and twelve patients. *J Bone Joint Surg Am* 1999;81:1367-1383.
Dubousset J: Congenital kyphosis and lordosis, in Weinstein SL (ed): *The Pediatric Spine: Principles and Practice*, ed 1. New York, NY, Raven Press, 1994, pp 245-258.

A-41: Figure 22 shows the radiograph of a girl who has had a 3-month history of activity-related foot pain. She has had two previous ankle sprains on this side. Examination reveals that subtalar motion is limited and there is mild heel valgus. Which of the following studies will best confirm your diagnosis?

1. Comparison radiograph of the contralateral foot
2. Calcaneal radiograph
3. Electromyography (EMG) and a nerve conduction velocity study
4. CT scan
5. Rheumatoid factor

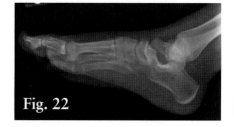

Fig. 22

PREFERRED RESPONSE: 4

DISCUSSION: The radiograph shows sclerosis in the midportion of the subtalar joint with no signs of degenerative joint disease present in any other joint. The diagnosis, based on the history and physical examination, is a tarsal coalition. Limited subtalar motion is the characteristic finding. A calcaneal view or an angled axial view parallel to the subtalar joint may show a talocalcaneal coalition. In younger children with fibrous or cartilaginous bars, radiographs may not reveal the problem. CT (or MRI) will best confirm that a coalition is present. EMG can rule out a neurologic problem causing foot deformity, but in a unilateral problem with limited subtalar motion and history of ankle sprains, a coalition is much more likely. A rheumatoid factor may be positive in isolated subtalar arthritis, but it is often negative even if arthritis is present and the history and physical examination are much more suggestive of a coalition.

REFERENCES: Westberry DE, Davids JR, Oros W: Surgical management of symptomatic talocalcaneal coalitions by resection of the sustentaculum tali. *J Pediatr Orthop* 2003;23:493-497.
Mosier KM, Asher M: Tarsal coalitions and peroneal spastic flat foot. *J Bone Joint Surg Am* 1984;66:976-984.

A-42: Figure 23 shows a newborn who has severe multiple symmetric joint contractures, including adduction/internal rotation of the shoulders, extended elbows, flexion-ulnar deviation of the wrists, thumbs in the palm of the hands, dislocated hips, knee flexion deformity, and clubfeet. The most likely diagnosis is

1. amyoplasia multiplex congenital.
2. Friedreich ataxia.
3. distal arthrogryposis.
4. spinal muscle atrophy.
5. thoracic-level myelomeningocele.

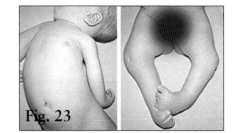
Fig. 23

PREFERRED RESPONSE: 1

DISCUSSION: There are more than 150 different types of contracture syndromes included under the category of arthrogryposis, the most common of which some authors term amyoplasia multiplex congenital. Distal arthrogryposis is a much less severe form, affecting primarily the hands and feet. Spinal muscle atrophy is generally associated with hypotonia without contracture. Friedreich ataxia has a later onset and is usually not associated with significant contractures. While myelomeningocele can exhibit similar lower extremity deformities, the upper extremities rarely have fixed contractures.

REFERENCES: Kasser JR (ed): *Orthopaedic Knowledge Update 5*. Rosemont, IL, American Academy of Orthopaedic Surgeons, 1996, pp 195-202.
Sarwark JF, MacEwen GD, Scott CI Jr: Amyoplasia (A common form of arthrogryposis). *J Bone Joint Surg Am* 1990;72:465-469.

A-43: Figure 24A shows the clinical photograph of a 2-year-old boy who has a deformity of the left leg. Examination reveals eight cutaneous markings similar to those shown in Figure 24B. Radiographs are shown in Figure 24C. Management should consist of

1. fragmentation, realignment, and intramedullary nailing of the tibia.
2. resection of the dysplastic region of the tibia and insertion of a vascularized fibula.
3. supplemental vitamin D and phosphate.
4. a clamshell orthosis.
5. observation for spontaneous remodeling.

PREFERRED RESPONSE: 4

DISCUSSION: The diagnosis of neurofibromatosis may be based on the presence of at least six café-au-lait spots larger than 5 mm in diameter and the osseous lesion shown in Figure 24C. Neurofibromatosis occurs in 50% of patients who have an anterolateral bowing deformity of the tibia, and this bowing may be the first clinical manifestation of this disorder. The patient has anterolateral bowing of the tibia and fibula that warrants concern for a possible fracture and pseudarthrosis; therefore, the limb should be protected in a total contact orthosis to prevent fracture. In contradistinction to posteromedial bowing of the tibia and fibula, spontaneous remodeling of an anterolateral bowing deformity is not expected. Intramedullary nailing or the use of a vascularized fibula is reserved for the treatment of a congenital pseudarthrosis of the tibia.

REFERENCES: Crawford AH Jr, Bagamery N: Osseous manifestations of neurofibromatosis in childhood. *J Pediatr Orthop* 1986;6:72-88.
Schoenecker PL, Rich MM: The lower extremity, in Morrissy RT, Weinstein SL (eds): *Lovell and Winter's Pediatric Orthopaedics*, ed 5. Philadelphia, PA, Lippincott Williams and Wilkins, 2001, vol 2, pp 1059-1104.

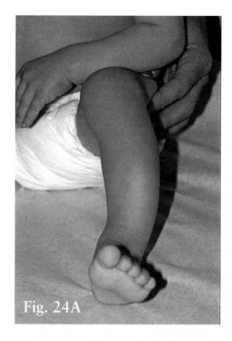

Fig. 24A

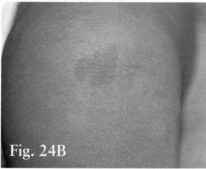

Fig. 24B

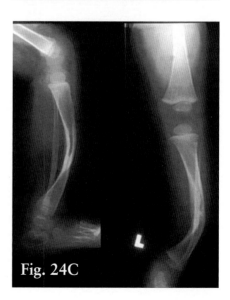

Fig. 24C

Answers: Pediatric Orthopaedics

A-44: A 10-year-old girl has had a painful 40° left thoracic scoliosis for the past 16 months. A bone scan shows a localized area of uptake in the T10 vertebra, and a CT scan of this area is shown in Figure 25. Treatment for the lesion should include

1. observation.
2. surgical excision.
3. a thoracolumbosacral orthosis.
4. posterior spinal fusion and instrumentation of T5-L3.
5. administration of nonsteroidal anti-inflammatory medication for a prolonged period.

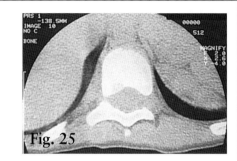

Fig. 25

PREFERRED RESPONSE: 2

DISCUSSION: Painful left thoracic scoliosis is not considered idiopathic until proven otherwise; neurologic or other causes are the typical etiology. When pain is present, either central nervous system or bony tumors are frequently the cause. The CT scan shows an osteoid osteoma. Surgical excision of the lesion offers immediate pain relief, and, if performed early, return of full mobility of the spine is likely. Although osteoid osteomas of the long bones can be treated with prolonged use of nonsteroidal anti-inflammatory medication, this treatment is not recommended for scoliosis of this magnitude, since the longer the scoliosis is present in a growing child, the more likely it will become structural and progressive. Use of orthotics alone or spinal fusion is not indicated when an underlying cause can be found.

REFERENCES: Ransford AO, Pozo JL, Hutton PA, Kirwan EO: The behaviour pattern of the scoliosis associated with osteoid osteoma or osteoblastoma of the spine. *J Bone Joint Surg Br* 1984;66:16-20.
Pettine KA, Klassen RA: Osteoid-osteoma and osteoblastoma of the spine. *J Bone Joint Surg Am* 1986;68:354-361.
Kneisl JS, Simon MA: Medical management compared with operative treatment for osteoid-osteoma. *J Bone Joint Surg Am* 1992;74:179-185.

A-45: A 6-year-old boy with spastic diplegic cerebral palsy has a crouched gait. Examination reveals hip flexion contractures of 15° and popliteal angles of 70°. Equinus contractures measure 10° with the knees extended. Which of the following surgical procedures, if performed alone, will worsen the crouching?

1. Iliopsoas release from the lesser trochanter
2. Iliopsoas release at the pelvic brim
3. Hamstring lengthening
4. Heel cord lengthening
5. Split posterior tibial tendon transfer

PREFERRED RESPONSE: 4

(continued on next page)

Answers: Pediatric Orthopaedics

(A-46 continued)

DISCUSSION: Children with spastic diplegic cerebral palsy often have contractures of multiple joints. Because the gait abnormalities can be complex, isolated surgery is rarely indicated. To avoid compensatory deformities at other joints, it is preferable to correct all deformities in a single operation. Isolated heel cord lengthening in the presence of tight hamstrings and hip flexors will lead to progressive flexion at the hips and knees, thus worsening a crouched gait. Split posterior tibial tendon transfer is used for patients with hindfoot varus, which is not present in this patient.

REFERENCES: Gage JR: Distal hamstring lengthening/release and rectus femoris transfer, in Sussman MD (ed): *The Diplegic Child*. Rosemont, IL, American Academy of Orthopaedic Surgeons, 1992, pp 324-326.

Bleck EE: Orthopaedic management of cerebral palsy, in *Saunders Monographs in Clinical Orthopaedics*. Philadelphia, PA, WB Saunders, vol 2, 1979.

A-46: Figure 26 shows the pedigree of a family with an unusual type of muscular dystrophy. This pedigree is most consistent with what type of inheritance pattern?

1. Autosomal dominant
2. Autosomal recessive
3. X-linked dominant
4. X-linked recessive
5. Mitochondrial inheritance

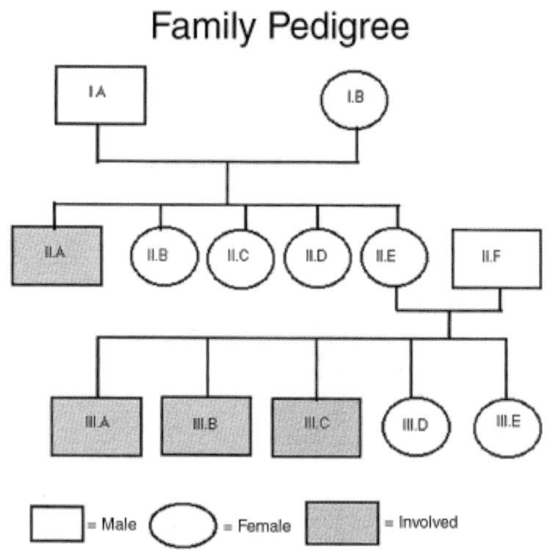

PREFERRED RESPONSE: 4

Family Pedigree

Fig. 26

DISCUSSION: The pedigree documents involvement of male offspring only, and it also shows transmission through an uninvolved female carrier. This inheritance pattern is most consistent with an X-linked recessive inheritance. It would be inconsistent with a dominant inheritance pattern unless there was incomplete penetrance. Autosomal-recessive inheritance would be possible only if the family member labeled II.F was also a carrier of the same gene; however, this is unlikely. Mitochondrial inheritance is possible, but as with autosomal patterns, mitochondrial inheritance normally affects both male and female offspring. It is transmitted only through the maternal line.

REFERENCE: Gelehrter TD, Collins FS: *Principles of Medical Genetics*. Baltimore, MD, Williams & Wilkins, 1990, pp 27-45.

A-47: A 13-year-old boy sustains a closed injury to his knee after a fall. A radiograph is shown in Figure 34. Treatment should consist of which of the following?

1. Long leg cast in extension
2. Long leg cast in 45° of flexion
3. Percutaneous pinning with smooth wires and a cylinder cast
4. Anterior cruciate ligament reconstruction and early motion
5. Open reduction and internal fixation with lag screws and a cylinder cast

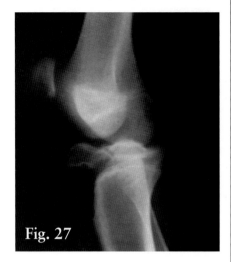

Fig. 27

PREFERRED RESPONSE: 5

DISCUSSION: The patient sustained a type III fracture of the tibial tubercle. This injury has been associated with Osgood-Schlatter disease. Treatment should consist of open reduction and internal fixation with lag screws, followed by casting for 6 weeks. Complications include meniscal tears, compartment syndrome, and leg length discrepancy.

REFERENCE: Wiss DA, Schilz JL, Zionts L: Type III fractures of the tibial tubercle in adolescents. *J Orthop Trauma* 1991;5:475-479.

A-48: An obese 4-year-old boy has infantile Blount disease. Radiographs reveal a metaphyseal-diaphyseal angle of 18° and a depression of the medial proximal tibial physis. Management should consist of

1. observation.
2. varus prevention orthoses.
3. physeal bar resection.
4. proximal tibial osteotomy that produces a neutral mechanical axis.
5. proximal tibial osteotomy that produces 10° of valgus.

PREFERRED RESPONSE: 5

DISCUSSION: The deformity is too severe for observation, and, at age 4 years, the child is too old for orthotic treatment. To prevent recurrence, surgery should be performed before irreversible changes occur in the medial physis. A proximal tibial osteotomy should overcorrect the mechanical axis to 10° of valgus. Bar resection has not been shown to be as effective in this severe deformity, especially without a concomitant osteotomy.

REFERENCES: Raney EM, Topoleski TA, Yaghoubian R, Guidera KJ, Marshall JG: Orthotic treatment of infantile tibia vara. *J Pediatr Orthop* 1998;18:670-674.
Loder RT, Johnston CE: Infantile tibia vara. *J Pediatr Orthop* 1987;7:639-646.

A-49: In girls with idiopathic scoliosis, peak height velocity (PHV) typically occurs at what point?

1. Before Risser 1 and menarche
2. After Risser 1 and menarche
3. Between Risser 1 and menarche
4. After menarche but before Risser 1
5. At Risser 2

PREFERRED RESPONSE: 1

DISCUSSION: PHV generally occurs while girls are still Risser 0; menarche typically occurs before Risser 1, which has a wide variation in its timing. The curve magnitude at the PHV is the best prognostic indicator available. Most untreated patients with curves greater than 30° at PHV require surgery, while patients with smaller curves at that stage typically do not require surgery.

REFERENCES: Little DG, Song KM, Katz D, Herring JA: Relationship of peak height velocity to other maturity indicators in idiopathic scoliosis in girls. *J Bone Joint Surg Am* 2000;82:685-693.
Anderson M, Hwang SC, Green WT: Growth of the normal trunk in boys and girls during the second decade of life; related to age, maturity, and ossification of the iliac epiphyses. *J Bone Joint Surg Am* 1965;47:1554-1564.

A-50: Which of the following pathogens are most commonly associated with neonatal septic arthritis and osteomyelitis?

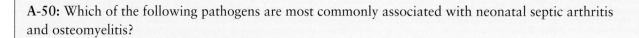

1. *Staphylococcus aureus* and *Escherichia coli*
2. *Staphylococcus aureus* and group A streptococci
3. *Staphylococcus aureus* and group B streptococci
4. *Haemophilus influenzae* and *Escherichia coli*
5. *Haemophilus influenzae* and group A streptococci

PREFERRED RESPONSE: 3

DISCUSSION: *Staphylococcus aureus* and group B streptococci have each been reported to be the most common pathogens in neonatal septic arthritis and osteomyelitis. *Haemophilus influenzae* is not seen in the neonatal period because of protective antibodies from the mother. *Escherichia coli* is an unusual pathogen, and, although seen in the neonatal period, it is still distinctly less common than *Staphylococcus aureus* or group B streptococci. Group A streptococci is an extremely uncommon pathogen in this age group.

REFERENCES: Memon IA, Jacobs NM, Yeh TF, Lilien LD: Group B streptococcal osteomyelitis and septic arthritis: Its occurrence in infants less than 2 months old. *Am J Dis Child* 1979;133:921-923.
Knudsen CJ, Hoffman EB: Neonatal osteomyelitis. *J Bone Joint Surg Br* 1990;72:846-851.

Answers: Pediatric Orthopaedics

A-51: Figure 28 shows the radiograph of a 10-year-old girl who reports chronic shoulder pain after her gymnastics classes. Examination reveals pain on internal and external rotation but no instability. What is the most likely diagnosis?

1. Acromial fracture
2. Humeral stress fracture
3. Acromioclavicular joint separation
4. Fracture of the surgical neck of the scapula
5. Triceps avulsion fracture

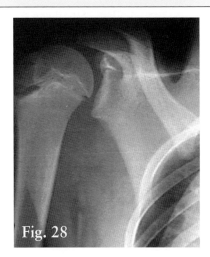

Fig. 28

PREFERRED RESPONSE: 2

DISCUSSION: The patient has a very wide humeral growth plate, indicating the presence of a proximal humeral stress fracture, an uncommon diagnosis in gymnasts. Gymnasts are prone to stress fractures of the scaphoid, distal radius, elbow, and clavicle. Proximal humeral stress fractures are more commonly seen in those participating in racket or throwing sports. Stress fractures can lead to growth arrest or inhibition, particularly in the distal radius. The radiograph shows normal findings for the acromion, acromioclavicular joint, scapula, and triceps origin.

REFERENCES: Fallon KE, Fricker PA: Stress fracture of the clavicle in a young female gymnast. *Br J Sports Med* 2001;35:448-449.
Sinha AK, Kaeding CC, Wadley GM: Upper extremity stress fractures in athletes: Clinical features of 44 cases. *Clin J Sports Med* 1999;9:199-202.
Caine D, Howe W, Ross W, Bergman G: Does repetitive physical loading inhibit radial growth in female gymnasts? *Clin J Sports Med* 1997;7:302-308.
Chan D, Aldridge MJ, Maffulli N, Davies AM: Chronic stress injuries of the elbow in young gymnasts. *Br J Radiol* 1991;64:1113-1118.

A-52: When counseling a patient with hypophosphatemic rickets, which of the following scenarios will always result in a child with the same disorder?

1. Female patient who has a female child
2. Female patient who has a male child
3. Male patient who has a female child
4. Male patient who has a male child
5. Disorder not inherited

PREFERRED RESPONSE: 3

DISCUSSION: Hypophosphatemic rickets is an inherited disorder that is transmitted by a unique sex-linked dominant gene. Therefore, if a male patient has a female offspring, his affected X chromosome will be transmitted and all of his female children will have hypophosphatemic rickets. All male offspring of a male patient will be unaffected. All offspring of a female patient have a 50% chance of having the disorder. Understanding the inheritance of hypophosphatemic rickets facilitates early diagnosis and early treatment. Medical treatment with phosphorus and some types of vitamin D (most authors recommend calcitriol) improves, but does not fully correct, the mineralization defect in hypophosphatemic rickets. However, if medical treatment is begun before the child begins walking, the growth plate is then adequately protected and a bowleg deformity will most likely be prevented.

REFERENCES: Evans GA, Arulanantham K, Gage JR: Primary hypophosphatemic rickets: Effect of oral phosphate and vitamin D on growth and surgical treatment. *J Bone Joint Surg Am* 1980;62:1130-1138. Greene WB, Kahler SG: Hypophosphatemic rickets: Still misdiagnosed and inadequately treated. *South Med J* 1985;78:1179-1184.

A-53: A 3-year-old patient with L3 myelomeningocele has bilateral dislocated hips. Management should consist of

1. observation.
2. bilateral open reduction.
3. bilateral open reduction and psoas transfers.
4. bilateral open reduction and external oblique transfers.
5. bilateral valgus osteotomies.

PREFERRED RESPONSE: 1

DISCUSSION: In patients with myelomeningocele, the presence of bilateral hip dislocation does not affect ambulation, bracing requirements, sitting ability, degree of scoliosis, or level of comfort. There is little evidence to support active treatment of bilateral hip dislocations in patients with myelomeningocele proximal to L4.

REFERENCES: Fraser RK, Hoffman EB, Sparks LT, et al: The unstable hip and mid-lumbar myelomeningocele. *J Bone Joint Surg Br* 1992;74:143-146.
Richards BS (ed): *Orthopaedic Knowledge Update: Pediatrics.* Rosemont, IL, American Academy of Orthopaedic Surgeons, 1996, pp 65-76.

A-54: During soft-tissue release for an idiopathic clubfoot, it is noted that the peroneus longus tendon has been transected in the midfoot. Failure to repair this structure may lead to

1. cavus.
2. claw toes.
3. a dorsal bunion.
4. hindfoot valgus.
5. forefoot pronation.

PREFERRED RESPONSE: 3

DISCUSSION: While a dorsal bunion was commonly seen as a sequelae of poliomyelitis, direct injury to the peroneus longus is also one of the causes. Normally, the peroneus longus opposes the tibialis anterior dorsal pull on the first ray. As the flexor hallucis longus attempts to oppose the tibialis anterior, the metatarsophalangeal joint is pulled into flexion and a dorsal bunion results. Other combinations of muscle imbalance can produce a dorsal bunion. In long-standing deformity, correction typically involves release of the plantar capsule and flexors with dorsal reefing and a possible metatarsal osteotomy. The tibialis anterior is often transferred as well. Loss of function of the peroneus longus tendon would not result in cavus, claw toes, forefoot pronation, or hindfoot valgus.

REFERENCES: Johnston CE II, Roach JW: Dorsal bunion following clubfoot surgery. *Orthopedics* 1985;8:1036-1040.
Park DB, Goldenberg EM: Dorsal bunions: A review. *J Foot Surg* 1989;28:217-219.

Answers: Pediatric Orthopaedics

A-55: A newborn with bilateral talipes equinovarus undergoes serial manipulation and casting. What is the primary goal of manipulation?

1. Rotation of the foot laterally around the fixed talus
2. Simultaneous abduction of the metatarsals and dorsiflexion of the talus
3. Lateral translation of the calcaneus
4. Anterolateral translation of the navicular
5. Dorsiflexion of the calcaneus with forefoot eversion

PREFERRED RESPONSE: 1

DISCUSSION: Manipulative treatment and casting of talipes equinovarus has become popular because of disappointing surgical results and enthusiasm for the Ponseti method of manipulation. In this technique, the primary goal is to rotate the foot laterally around a talus that is held fixed by the manipulating surgeon's hands. While the navicular may be rotated anterolaterally with this technique, the primary focus is on the calcaneus. The calcaneus is rotated laterally and superiorly, not translated. Some dorsiflexion of the calcaneus can be obtained by manipulation, but the primary focus is on the rotational relationship of the talus and calcaneus, not the degree of calcaneal dorsiflexion.

REFERENCES: Ponseti IV: Common errors in the treatment of congenital clubfoot. *Int Orthop* 1997;21:137-141.
Ponseti IV, Smoley EU: Congenital club foot: The results of treatment. *J Bone Joint Surg Am* 1963;45:261-344.

A-56: In patients with neurofibromatosis, what is the most important sign of impending rapid progression of a spinal deformity?

1. Apical curve rotation
2. Anterior vertebral body erosions
3. Cervical spine involvement
4. Penciling of three or more ribs
5. Curve magnitude of greater than 50°

PREFERRED RESPONSE: 4

DISCUSSION: Neurofibromatosis can progress very rapidly. Rib penciling is the only singular prognostic factor. Significant progression has been observed in 87% of the curves with three or more penciled ribs. The other factors are often present but do not have a high correlation with rapid, severe progression.

REFERENCES: Crawford AH, Schorry EK: Neurofibromatosis in children: The role of the orthopaedist. *J Am Acad Orthop Surg* 1999;7:217-230.
Durrani AA, Crawford AH, Chouhdry SN, Saifuddin A, Morley TR: Modulation of spinal deformities in patients with neurofibromatosis type 1. *Spine* 2000;25:69-75.

Orthopaedic Oncology and Systemic Disease

Section Editor

Kristy Weber, MD

Q-1: A 16-year-old boy has had thigh pain for the past several months. He denies any history of trauma. Examination reveals a large, deeply fixed, soft-tissue mass in the thigh. Laboratory results show an elevated erythrocyte sedimentation rate (ESR) and leukocytosis. A plain radiograph and MRI scan are shown in Figures 1A and 1B. Biopsy specimens are shown in Figures 1C and 1D. What is the most likely diagnosis?

1. Ewing sarcoma
2. Osteomyelitis
3. Osteosarcoma
4. Chondrosarcoma
5. Giant cell tumor of bone

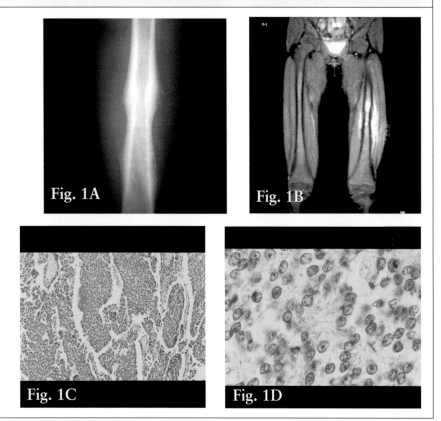

Fig. 1A   Fig. 1B

Fig. 1C   Fig. 1D

Qz: The lesion seen in Figure 2 is most likely the result of metastases from what solid organ?

1. Breast
2. Lung
3. Thyroid
4. Prostate
5. Liver

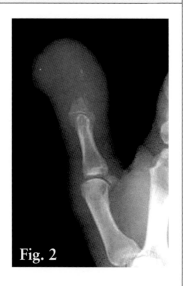

Fig. 2

Q-3: A 10-year-old child has leg discomfort with activity. A radiograph, bone scan, and biopsy specimen are shown in Figures 3A through 3C. What is the most likely diagnosis?

1. Parosteal osteosarcoma
2. Unicameral bone cyst
3. Aneurysmal bone cyst
4. Eosinophilic granuloma
5. Fibrous dysplasia

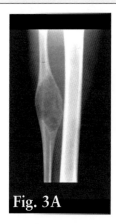
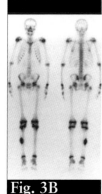
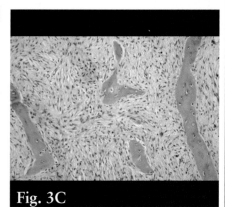

Fig. 3A   Fig. 3B   Fig. 3C

Q-4: The use of multiagent adjuvant chemotherapy is associated with a clear survival benefit in which of the following diseases?

1. Renal carcinoma
2. Osteosarcoma
3. Dedifferentiated chondrosarcoma
4. Adult soft-tissue sarcoma
5. Melanoma

Q-5: A 10-year-old boy with a history of retinoblastoma now reports right knee pain. AP and lateral radiographs are shown in Figures 4A and 4B. What is the most likely diagnosis?

1. Ewing sarcoma
2. Primitive neuroectodermal tumor
3. Osteosarcoma
4. Osteonecrosis
5. Osteomyelitis

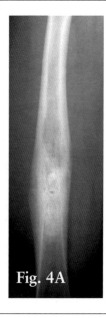
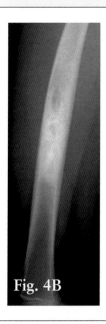

Fig. 4A   Fig. 4B

Q-6: Which of the following factors is associated with the worst prognosis in soft-tissue sarcomas?

1. Size greater than 15 cm
2. Extra-compartmental involvement
3. Number of mitotic figures per high-power field (grade)
4. Large size in a proximal location
5. Presence of metastases

Q-7: An athletic 55-year-old man reports a painless mass in the anterior aspect of the thigh that appeared 3 weeks ago and has not changed in size. The patient denies any history of trauma. Examination reveals a firm, well-defined nontender mass in the anterior thigh and no inguinal adenopathy or cutaneous changes. Plain radiographs are unremarkable. T1- and T2-weighted MRI scans are shown in Figures 5A and 5B. What is the most likely diagnosis?

1. Hematoma
2. Lipoma
3. Soft-tissue sarcoma
4. Pyomyositis
5. Hemangioma

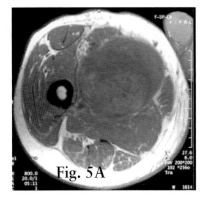
Fig. 5A

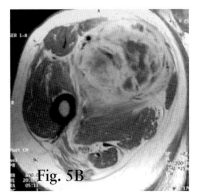
Fig. 5B

Q-8: A 77-year-old man has had increasing right knee pain for the past 3 months. A radiograph and coronal T1-weighted MRI scan are shown in Figures 6A and 6B. A biopsy specimen is shown in Figure 6C. What is the most likely diagnosis?

1. Metastatic prostate cancer
2. Enchondroma
3. Osteomyelitis
4. Dedifferentiated chondrosarcoma
5. Lymphoma

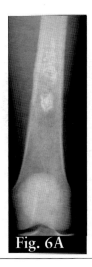
Fig. 6A

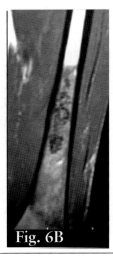
Fig. 6B

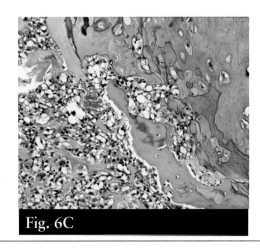
Fig. 6C

Q-9: A 47-year-old woman has an asymptomatic pelvic mass that was discovered on routine gynecologic examination. A radiograph, CT scan, MRI scan, and biopsy specimen are shown in Figures 7A through 7D. Metastatic work-up is negative. Treatment should consist of

1. observation.
2. primary wide resection.
3. intralesional curettage.
4. radiation therapy.
5. preoperative chemotherapy.

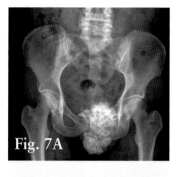

Fig. 7A

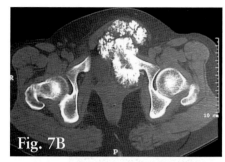

Fig. 7B

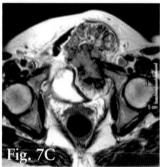

Fig. 7C

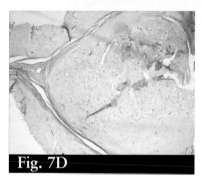

Fig. 7D

Q-10: A 20-year-old patient has foot pain. A radiograph and T1-weighted MRI scan are shown in Figures 8A and 8B. A biopsy specimen is shown in Figure 8C. Treatment should consist of

1. extended curettage and cementation.
2. amputation of the first ray.
3. wide resection and chemotherapy.
4. extended curettage, radiation therapy, and chemotherapy.
5. Syme amputation.

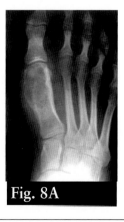

Fig. 8A

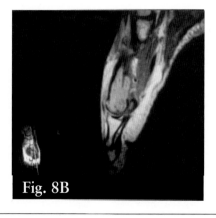

Fig. 8B

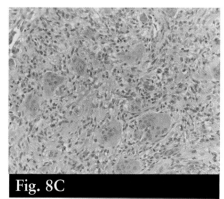

Fig. 8C

Q-11: A 69-year-old man has a painful slow-growing lesion of the distal phalanx of his thumb. History reveals that he has had chronic osteomyelitis of the thumb for the past 12 years. The radiograph and biopsy specimens are seen in Figures 9A through 9C. Treatment should consist of

1. intralesional curettage.
2. wrist disarticulation.
3. amputation.
4. chemotherapy.
5. radiation therapy.

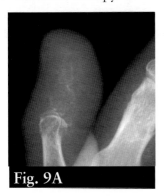

Fig. 9A

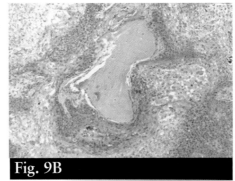

Fig. 9B

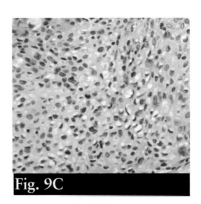

Fig. 9C

Q-12: What is the most common presentation of a benign bone tumor in childhood?

1. Pain
2. Deformity
3. Pathologic fracture
4. Presence of a mass
5. Incidental finding

Q-13: Soft-tissue sarcomas most commonly metastasize to the

1. liver.
2. lung.
3. bone.
4. regional nodes.
5. distant nodes.

Q-14: A 43-year-old woman has had pain in the left hip for the past 2 months. A radiograph, CT scan, MRI scan, and biopsy specimens are shown in Figures 10A through 10E. What is the most likely diagnosis?

1. Osteosarcoma
2. Osteochondroma
3. Chondrosarcoma
4. Chordoma
5. Enchondroma

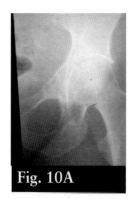

Fig. 10A

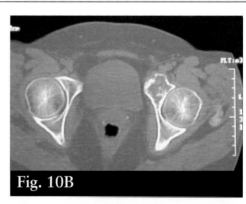

Fig. 10B

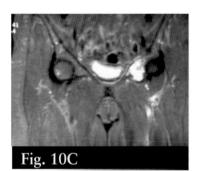

Fig. 10C

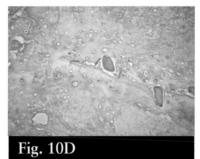

Fig. 10D

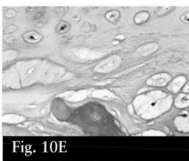

Fig. 10E

Q-15: Following preoperative chemotherapy, the percent of tumor necrosis has been shown to be of prognostic value for which of the following tumors?

1. Rhabdomyosarcoma
2. Chondrosarcoma
3. Metastatic adenocarcinoma
4. Osteosarcoma
5. Giant cell tumor of bone

Q-16: What is the most common clinical presentation of a patient with a malignant bone tumor?

1. Incidental finding
2. Pain
3. Pathologic fracture
4. Deformity
5. Presence of a mass

Q-17: What is the current 5-year survival rate for patients with classic nonmetastatic, high-grade osteo-sarcoma of the extremity?

1. 10%
2. 20%
3. 40%
4. 70%
5. 90%

Q-18: What malignant disease most commonly develops in conjunction with chronic osteomyelitis?

1. Fibrosarcoma
2. Basal cell carcinoma
3. Lymphoma
4. Osteosarcoma
5. Squamous cell carcinoma

Q-19: A 10-year-old girl reports activity-related bilateral arm pain. Examination reveals no soft-tissue masses in either arm, and she has full painless range of motion in both shoulders and elbows. The radiograph and bone scan are shown in Figures 11A and 11B, and biopsy specimens are shown in Figures 11C and 11D. What is the most likely diagnosis?

1. Enchondroma
2. Fibrous dysplasia
3. Osteogenic sarcoma
4. Aneurysmal bone cyst
5. Periosteal chondroma

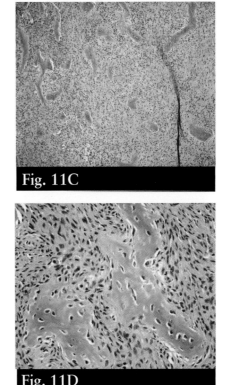

Fig. 11C

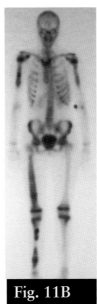

Fig. 11B

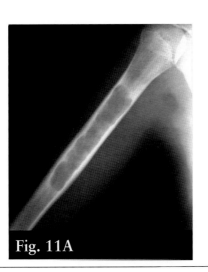

Fig. 11A

Fig. 11D

Q-20: Chemotherapy is routinely included in the treatment of which of the following soft-tissue sarcomas?

1. Angiosarcoma
2. Malignant fibrous histiocytoma
3. Liposarcoma
4. Rhabdomyosarcoma
5. Clear cell sarcoma

Q-21: An 83-year-old man has a painful mass of the great toe. Radiographs and a biopsy specimen are seen in Figures 12A and 12B. What is the most likely diagnosis?

1. Gout
2. Pseudogout
3. Infection
4. Epidermal inclusion cyst
5. Charcot joint

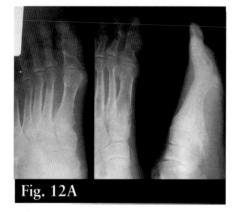
Fig. 12A

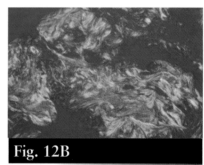
Fig. 12B

Q-22: Eosinophilic granuloma frequently occurs as a solitary lesion in the tubular long bones. After biopsy, what is the best course of action?

1. Neoadjuvant chemotherapy
2. En bloc resection
3. Observation
4. Amputation
5. Chemotherapy followed by radiation therapy

Q-23: A 10-year-old child reports acute leg pain after wrestling with his brother. AP and lateral radiographs are shown in Figures 13A and 13B. What is the best course of action?

1. Biopsy, curettage, and plating
2. Wide segmental resection
3. Hip disarticulation
4. Closed reduction and a long leg cast
5. Tibial traction and MRI

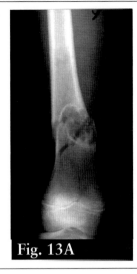

Fig. 13A

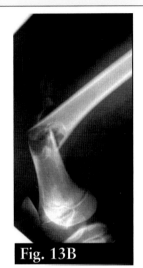

Fig. 13B

Q-24: A 15-year-old boy has had pain in the right shoulder for the past 3 months. He denies any history of trauma and has no constitutional symptoms. Examination reveals a large firm mass in the proximal arm. A radiograph and MRI scan are shown in Figures 14A and 14B. Biopsy specimens are shown in Figures 14C and 14D. Management should consist of

1. observation.
2. steroid injection.
3. curettage and bone grafting.
4. wide resection with neoadjuvant chemotherapy.
5. débridement, irrigation, and intravenous antibiotics.

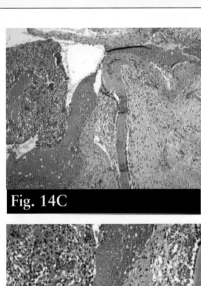

Fig. 14C

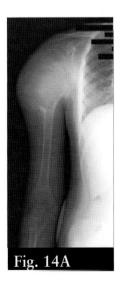

Fig. 14A

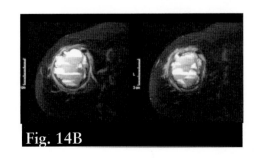

Fig. 14B

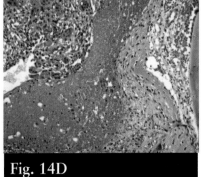

Fig. 14D

Q-25: Which of the following tumors is most likely to present with a pathologic fracture in a child?

1. Unicameral bone cyst
2. Fibrous cortical defect
3. Osteosarcoma
4. Ewing sarcoma
5. Giant cell tumor

Q-26: A previously healthy 14-year-old boy now reports fatigue, and has a bilateral Trendelenburg gait, right hip pain, and bilateral knee and foot pain. Biopsy of a right sacral mass reveals intermediate grade osteosarcoma. There are no metastases. Laboratory studies reveal a serum calcium level of 7.7 mg/dL (normal 8.5 to 10.5), a phosphate level of 2.0 mg/dL (normal 2.7 to 4.5), a 1,25-dihydroxyvitamin D level of less than 10 pg/mL (normal 18 to 62), a parathyroid hormone level of 19 pg/mL (normal 10 to 60), and an alkaline phosphatase level of 428 U/L (normal 15 to 351). What is the most likely cause of the patient's symptoms?

1. Oncogenic rickets
2. Calcium sequestration by the tumor
3. Elevated alkaline phosphatase level
4. Tumor cachexia
5. L5 neuropathy

Q-27: A 12-year-old girl has painless bowing of the tibia. Radiographs and a biopsy specimen are shown in Figures 15A through 15C. What is the most likely diagnosis?

1. Osteofibrous dysplasia
2. Adamantinoma
3. Osteosarcoma
4. Ewing sarcoma
5. Fibrous dysplasia

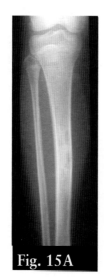
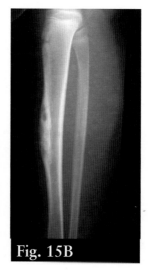
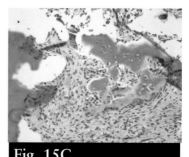

Fig. 15A   Fig. 15B   Fig. 15C

Q-28: A 16-year-old girl has had pain in the left groin for the past 4 months. She notes that the pain is worse at night; however, she denies any history of trauma and has no constitutional symptoms. There is no history of steroid or alcohol use. Examination reveals pain in the left groin with rotation of the hip. There is no associated soft-tissue mass. A radiograph and MRI scan are shown in Figures 16A and 16B, and biopsy specimens are shown in Figures 16C and 16D. What is the most likely diagnosis?

1. Clear cell chondrosarcoma
2. Chondroblastoma
3. Giant cell tumor
4. Aneurysmal bone cyst
5. Osteonecrosis of the femoral head

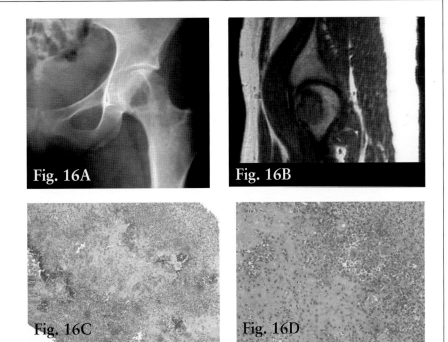

Fig. 16A   Fig. 16B

Fig. 16C   Fig. 16D

Q-29: A 52-year-old man has had back pain radiating to the left leg for the past 5 weeks. A radiograph, MRI scans, and biopsy specimens are shown in Figures 17A through 17F. What is the most likely diagnosis?

1. Metastatic renal cell carcinoma
2. Metastatic adenocarcinoma
3. Chordoma
4. Osteoblastoma
5. Chondrosarcoma

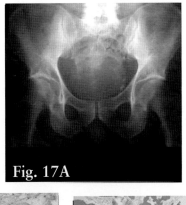

Fig. 17A

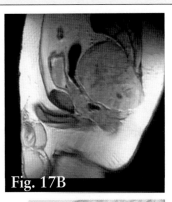

Fig. 17B

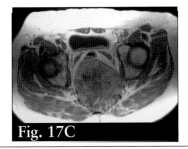

Fig. 17C

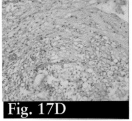

Fig. 17D

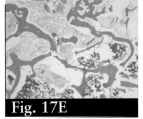

Fig. 17E

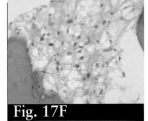

Fig. 17F

Q-30: An 18-year-old boy has had pain in the right knee for the past 6 months. Examination reveals some fullness behind the knee but no significant palpable soft-tissue mass. There is no effusion, and he has full knee range of motion. The remainder of the examination is unremarkable. A radiograph and MRI scans are shown in Figures 18A through 18C, and biopsy specimens are shown in Figures 18D and 18E. What is the most likely diagnosis?

1. Parosteal osteosarcoma
2. Classic osteogenic sarcoma
3. Ewing sarcoma
4. Osteochondroma
5. Chondrosarcoma

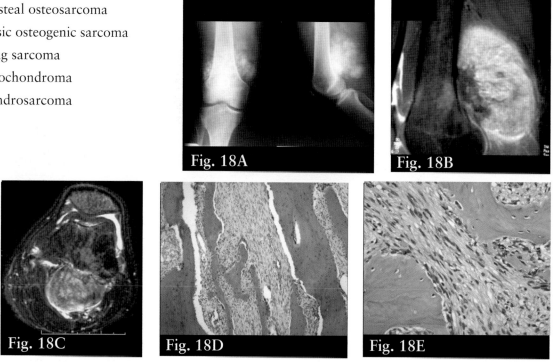

Fig. 18A
Fig. 18B
Fig. 18C
Fig. 18D
Fig. 18E

Q-31: A 47-year-old woman has had a 1-month history of left hip and medial thigh pain that is exacerbated by sitting. Laboratory studies show a total protein level of 8.2 g/dL (normal 6.0 to 8.0) and an immunoglobulin G (IGG) level of 2,130 mg/dL (normal 562 to 1,835). A radiograph, CT scan, and biopsy specimen are shown in Figures 19A through 19C. What is the most likely diagnosis?

1. Osteomyelitis
2. Lymphoma
3. Myeloma
4. Ewing sarcoma
5. Osteosarcoma

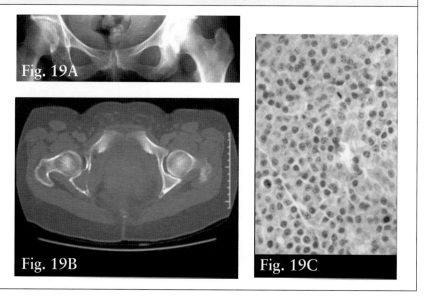

Fig. 19A
Fig. 19B
Fig. 19C

Q-32: A 19-year-old girl has had pain and swelling in the right ankle for the past 4 months. She denies any history of trauma. Examination reveals a small soft-tissue mass over the anterior aspect of the ankle and slight pain with range of motion of the ankle joint. The examination is otherwise unremarkable. A radiograph and MRI scan are shown in Figures 20A and 20B, and biopsy specimens are shown in Figures 20C and 20D. What is the most likely diagnosis?

1. Osteogenic sarcoma
2. Ewing sarcoma
3. Giant cell tumor of bone
4. Aneurysmal bone cyst
5. Metastatic adenocarcinoma

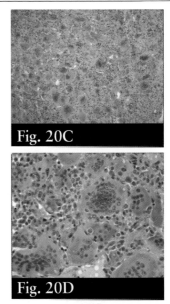

Fig. 20C

Fig. 20D

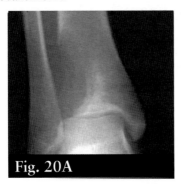

Fig. 20A

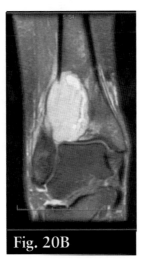

Fig. 20B

Q-33: A 13-year-old patient has foot drop and lateral knee pain. AP and lateral radiographs and an MRI scan are shown in Figures 21A through 21C. A biopsy specimen is shown in Figure 21D. What is the preferred method of treatment?

1. Wide resection alone
2. Chemotherapy and radiation therapy
3. Chemotherapy and wide resection
4. Above-knee amputation
5. Through-knee amputation

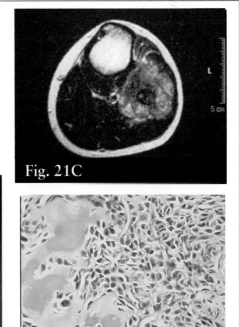

Fig. 21C

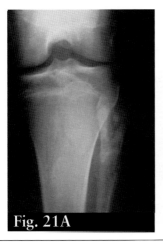

Fig. 21A

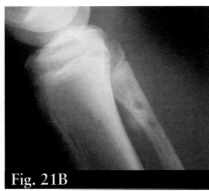

Fig. 21B

Fig. 21D

Q-34: A 23-year-old woman has had vague left knee pain for the past 6 months. A radiograph and CT scan are shown in Figures 22A and 22B. What is the most likely diagnosis?

1. Myositis ossificans
2. Osteochondroma
3. Parosteal osteosarcoma
4. Dedifferentiated chondrosarcoma
5. Tumoral calcinosis

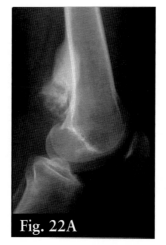
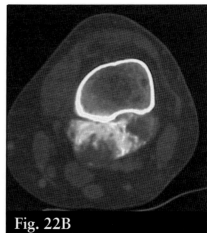

Fig. 22A

Fig. 22B

Q-35: Figures 23A through 23C show the radiograph, CT scan, and biopsy specimen of a 44-year-old man who underwent chemotherapy and radiation therapy for lymphoma of the distal femur 20 years ago. His current problem is most likely related to

1. steroid-induced osteonecrosis.
2. radiation therapy with secondary malignancy.
3. recurrence of the lymphoma.
4. radiation osteitis.
5. a primary lung tumor.

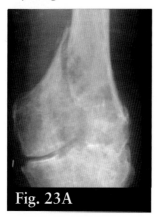
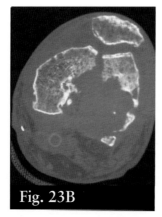
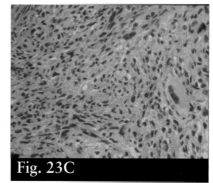

Fig. 23A

Fig. 23B

Fig. 23C

A-1: A 16-year-old boy has had thigh pain for the past several months. He denies any history of trauma. Examination reveals a large, deeply fixed, soft-tissue mass in the thigh. Laboratory results show an elevated erythrocyte sedimentation rate (ESR) and leukocytosis. A plain radiograph and MRI scan are shown in Figures 1A and 1B. Biopsy specimens are shown in Figures 1C and 1D. What is the most likely diagnosis?

1. Ewing sarcoma
2. Osteomyelitis
3. Osteosarcoma
4. Chondrosarcoma
5. Giant cell tumor of bone

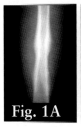 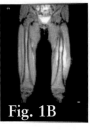 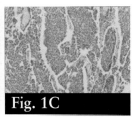 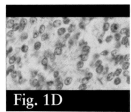

Fig. 1A　　Fig. 1B　　Fig. 1C　　Fig. 1D

PREFERRED RESPONSE: 1

DISCUSSION: Ewing sarcoma typically can occur in the diaphysis of the long bones (50% to 55%). It is often accompanied by a large soft-tissue mass. Abnormal findings are common, including a low-grade fever, an elevated ESR, and leukocytosis. The histology is consistent with a small round blue cell tumor. The unique pathology and other findings exclude osteosarcoma. Giant cell tumor and chondrosarcoma have a different histologic appearance and typically are more metaphyseal in location. Chondrosarcoma typically is found in older age groups, has a different histologic pattern, and rarely occurs in the midshaft of the femur.

REFERENCE: Simon MA, Springfield DS, et al: *Ewing's Sarcoma: Surgery for Bone and Soft Tissue Tumors.* Philadelphia, PA, Lippincott Raven, 1998, pp 287-297.

A-2: The lesion seen in Figure 2 is most likely the result of metastases from what solid organ?

1. Breast
2. Lung
3. Thyroid
4. Prostate
5. Liver

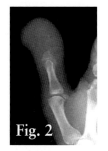

Fig. 2

PREFERRED RESPONSE: 2

DISCUSSION: The primary carcinoma most likely to metastasize distal to the elbow and knees is lung carcinoma. Renal cell carcinoma can also metastasize to distal sites. Most metastatic bone disease occurs in the vertebral bodies, pelvis, and proximal long bones.

REFERENCES: Simon MA, Bartucci EJ: The search for the primary tumor in patients with skeletal metastases of unknown origin. *Cancer* 1986;58:1088-1095.
Leeson MC, Makley JT, Carter JR: Metastatic skeletal disease distal to the elbow and knee. *Clin Orthop Relat Res* 1986;206:94-99.

A-3: A 10-year-old child has leg discomfort with activity. A radiograph, bone scan, and biopsy specimen are shown in Figures 3A through 3C. What is the most likely diagnosis?

1. Parosteal osteosarcoma
2. Unicameral bone cyst
3. Aneurysmal bone cyst
4. Eosinophilic granuloma
5. Fibrous dysplasia

Surface lesion

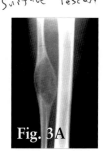
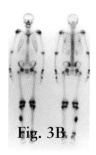
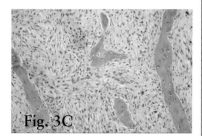

Fig. 3A   Fig. 3B   Fig. 3C

PREFERRED RESPONSE: 5

DISCUSSION: The ground glass appearance on the radiograph, the hot bone scan, and histologic findings of bony spicules without osteoblastic rimming in a background of bland fibrous tissue all suggest fibrous dysplasia. Stress-related pain is common with activity because of the dysplastic bone. Parosteal osteosarcomas are surface lesions. Simple cysts, aneurysmal bone cysts, and eosinophilic granuloma are all possible radiographically; however, the histology is most consistent with fibrous dysplasia.

REFERENCES: Harris WH, Dudley HR Jr, Barry RS: The natural history of fibrous dysplasia: An orthopaedic, pathological and roentgenographic study. *J Bone Joint Surg Am* 1962;44:207.
Campanacci M: *Bone and Soft Tissue Tumors.* Vienna, Austria, Springer-Verlag, 1990.

A-4: The use of multiagent adjuvant chemotherapy is associated with a clear survival benefit in which of the following diseases?

1. Renal carcinoma
2. Osteosarcoma
3. Dedifferentiated chondrosarcoma
4. Adult soft-tissue sarcoma
5. Melanoma

PREFERRED RESPONSE: 2

DISCUSSION: The use of multiagent chemotherapy has been shown to be associated with a survival benefit in patients with osteosarcoma. The use of chemotherapy in adults with soft-tissue sarcoma remains somewhat controversial. It has not been associated with improved survival rates in patients with renal carcinoma, dedifferentiated chondrosarcoma, or melanoma.

REFERENCES: Menendez LR (ed): *Orthopaedic Knowledge Update: Musculoskeletal Tumors.* Rosemont, IL, American Academy of Orthopaedic Surgeons, 2002, p 53.
Link M, Goorin A, Miser A, et al: The effect of adjuvant chemotherapy and relapse free survival in patients with osteosarcoma of the extremity. *N Engl J Med* 1986;314:1600-1606.

A-5: A 10-year-old boy with a history of retinoblastoma now reports right knee pain. AP and lateral radiographs are shown in Figures 4A and 4B. What is the most likely diagnosis?

1. Ewing sarcoma
2. Primitive neuroectodermal tumor
3. Osteosarcoma
4. Osteonecrosis
5. Osteomyelitis

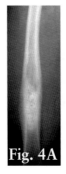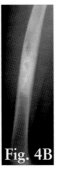

Fig. 4A   Fig. 4B

PREFERRED RESPONSE: 3

DISCUSSION: The radiographs show a bone-producing lesion in the femoral diaphysis. The radiographic appearance of small round cell tumors is more permeative with an elevated periosteum and no matrix production. The appearance of this lesion is most consistent with osteosarcoma. Patients who carry the Rb gene are predisposed to osteosarcoma. However, Ewing sarcoma, primitive neuroectodermal tumor, and osteomyelitis can all occur in this location.

REFERENCES: Unni KK: *Dahlin's Bone Tumors: General Aspects and Data on 11,087 Cases*, ed 5. Philadelphia, PA, Lippincott-Raven, 1996, pp 143-160.
Chauveinc L, Mosseri V, Quintana E, Desjardins L, Schlienger P, Doz F, Dutrillaux B: Osteosarcoma following retinoblastoma: Age at onset and latency period. *Ophthalmic Genet* 2001;22:77-88.

A-6: Which of the following factors is associated with the worst prognosis in soft-tissue sarcomas?

1. Size greater than 15 cm
2. Extra-compartmental involvement
3. Number of mitotic figures per high-power field (grade)
4. Large size in a proximal location
5. Presence of metastases

PREFERRED RESPONSE: 5

DISCUSSION: Although factors such as a high-grade tumor and large size are associated with decreased survival, the presence of metastases carries the worst prognosis. Good results are very rare when metastases are present. Soft-tissue sarcomas, as a whole, respond poorly to chemotherapy, leading to a poor prognosis when metastases are present.

REFERENCES: Collin C, Goobold J, Hadju SI, Brennan MF: Localized extremity soft tissue sarcoma: An analysis of factors affecting survival. *J Clin Oncol* 1987;5:601-612.
Eilber FC, Rosen G, Nelson SE, et al: High-grade extremity soft tissue sarcomas: Factors predictive of local recurrence and its effect on morbidity and mortality. *Ann Surg* 2003;237:218-226.

A-7: An athletic 55-year-old man reports a painless mass in the anterior aspect of the thigh that appeared 3 weeks ago and has not changed in size. The patient denies any history of trauma. Examination reveals a firm, well-defined nontender mass in the anterior thigh and no inguinal adenopathy or cutaneous changes. Plain radiographs are unremarkable. T1- and T2-weighted MRI scans are shown in Figures 5A and 5B. What is the most likely diagnosis?

1. Hematoma
2. Lipoma
3. Soft-tissue sarcoma
4. Pyomyositis
5. Hemangioma

PREFERRED RESPONSE: 3

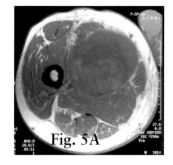

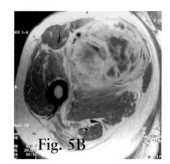

Fig. 5A   Fig. 5B

DISCUSSION: The presence of a painless soft-tissue mass that is greater than 5 cm and deep to the fascia should be considered a soft-tissue sarcoma until proven otherwise. The diagnosis of a hematoma should be made with great caution because the absence of a history of trauma, pain, or presence of ecchymosis makes it unlikely. A diagnosis of pyomyositis is unlikely because of the absence of warmth, erythema, or adenopathy. The MRI scans are not consistent with lipoma or hemangioma. The MRI signal characteristics of a lipoma should be the same as subcutaneous fat on all sequences. Soft-tissue hemangiomas are not well defined and have an infiltrative appearance on MRI scans, as does pyomyositis.

REFERENCES: Sim FH, Frassica FJ, Frassica DA: Soft-tissue tumors: Diagnosis, evaluation and management. *J Am Acad Orthop Surg* 1994;2:202-211.
Kransdorf MJ, Jelinek JS, Moser RP Jr, et al: Soft-tissue masses: Diagnosis using MR imaging. *Am J Roentgenol* 1989;153:541-547.

A-8: A 77-year-old man has had increasing right knee pain for the past 3 months. A radiograph and coronal T1-weighted MRI scan are shown in Figures 6A and 6B. A biopsy specimen is shown in Figure 6C. What is the most likely diagnosis?

1. Metastatic prostate cancer
2. Enchondroma
3. Osteomyelitis
4. Dedifferentiated chondrosarcoma
5. Lymphoma

PREFERRED RESPONSE: 4

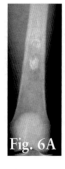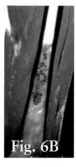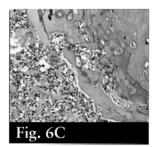

Fig. 6A   Fig. 6B   Fig. 6C

(continued on next page)

(A-8: *continued*)

DISCUSSION: The radiograph shows a calcified lesion in the medullary canal of the distal femoral diaphysis. The MRI scan shows extensive marrow change distal to the lesion, which is not consistent with an enchondroma. The histology shows a biphasic pattern with low-grade cartilage just apposed to high-grade spindle cell sarcoma. The overall appearance is consistent with dedifferentiated chondrosarcoma. The radiographic appearance is not consistent with enchondroma, and the histologic appearance is not consistent with the other choices.

REFERENCES: Mitchell AD, Ayoub K, Mangham DC, et al: Experience in the treatment of dedifferentiated chondrosarcoma. *J Bone Joint Surg Br* 2000;82:55-61.
Frassica FJ, Unni KK, Beabout JW, Sim FH: Dedifferentiated chondrosarcoma: A report of the clinicopathological features and treatment of seventy-eight cases. *J Bone Joint Surg Am* 1986;68:1197-1205.

A-9: A 47-year-old woman has an asymptomatic pelvic mass that was discovered on routine gynecologic examination. A radiograph, CT scan, MRI scan, and biopsy specimen are shown in Figures 7A through 7D. Metastatic work-up is negative. Treatment should consist of

1. observation.
2. primary wide resection.
3. intralesional curettage.
4. radiation therapy.
5. preoperative chemotherapy.

PREFERRED RESPONSE: 2

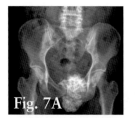

Fig. 7A

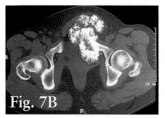

Fig. 7B

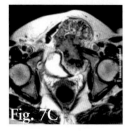

Fig. 7C

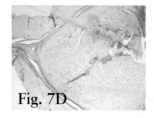

Fig. 7D

DISCUSSION: The imaging studies show a chondrosarcoma; therefore, surgical treatment is indicated. There is no role for intralesional treatment of an exophytic lesion, particularly in the pelvis. Even obtaining a biopsy specimen risks intrapelvic contamination, although many surgeons would still perform a biopsy prior to a resection to confirm the diagnosis. Chondrosarcoma is considered resistant to both radiation therapy and chemotherapy; therefore, radiation therapy generally is not used except for unresectable lesions. Chemotherapy would be used only for metastatic disease or in patients with high-grade chondrosarcoma. The grade would not be known until after resection, and in this patient, the histology slide showed a grade I neoplasm. Chemotherapy would not be used preoperatively because a cartilage tumor is unlikely to shrink, and in this patient, the lesion is resectable.

REFERENCES: Springfield DS, Gebhardt MS, Mcguire MH: Chondrosarcoma: A review. *J Bone Joint Surg Am* 1996;78:141-149.
Marco RA, Gitelis S, Brebach GT, Healey JH: Cartilage tumors: Evaluation and treatment. *J Am Acad Orthop Surg* 2000;8:292-304.

A-10: A 20-year-old patient has foot pain. A radiograph and T1-weighted MRI scan are shown in Figures 8A and 8B. A biopsy specimen is shown in Figure 8C. Treatment should consist of

1. extended curettage and cementation.
2. amputation of the first ray.
3. wide resection and chemotherapy.
4. extended curettage, radiation therapy, and chemotherapy.
5. Syme amputation.

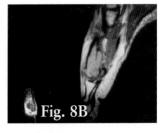
Fig. 8A   Fig. 8B

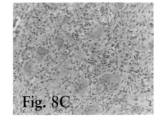
Fig. 8C

PREFERRED RESPONSE: 1

DISCUSSION: Giant cell tumors occur near articular surfaces in young adults. The histology shows abundant giant cells with nuclei resembling the surrounding cells. Although the MRI scan shows soft-tissue involvement, curettage is still the preferred treatment. Chemotherapy is not necessary for benign lesions, and amputation is too aggressive. Cementation, phenol, and cryosurgery (liquid nitrogen) are all acceptable local adjuvants to curettage. Packing the cavity with bone graft rather than cement is also acceptable.

REFERENCES: Dahlin DC, Unni KK: *Bone Tumors: General Aspects and Data on 8,542 Cases.* Springfield, IL, Charles C. Thomas, 1986.
Gitelis S, Mallin BA, Piasecki P, Turner F: Intralesional excision compared with en bloc resection for giant cell tumor of bone. *J Bone Joint Surg Am* 1993;75:1648-1655.

A-11: A 69-year-old man has a painful slow-growing lesion of the distal phalanx of his thumb. History reveals that he has had chronic osteomyelitis of the thumb for the past 12 years. The radiograph and biopsy specimens are seen in Figures 9A through 9C. Treatment should consist of

1. intralesional curettage.
2. wrist disarticulation.
3. amputation.
4. chemotherapy.
5. radiation therapy.

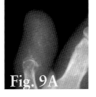 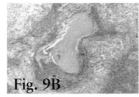 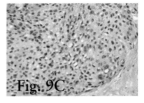
Fig. 9A   Fig. 9B   Fig. 9C

PREFERRED RESPONSE: 3

DISCUSSION: The diagnosis is squamous cell carcinoma. The radiograph shows a destructive lesion, and the histologic slides demonstrate squamous cells invading bone. The preferred treatment for squamous cell carcinoma is wide resection; however, in this location a wide margin can be achieved only with amputation. Overall survival in patients with squamous cell carcinoma secondary to chronic osteomyelitis is not significantly worse than that expected for age-matched controls.

(continued on next page)

(A-11: *continued*)

REFERENCES: Dell PC: Hand, in Simon MA, Springfield D (eds): *Surgery for Bone and Soft Tissue Tumors*. Philadelphia, PA, Lippincott-Raven, 1998, pp 405-420.
McGrory JE, Pritchard DJ, Unni KK, Ilstrup D, Rowland CM: Malignant lesion arising in chronic osteomyelitis. *Clin Orthop Relat Res* 1998;362:181-189.

A-12: What is the most common presentation of a benign bone tumor in childhood?

1. Pain
2. Deformity
3. Pathologic fracture
4. Presence of a mass
5. Incidental finding

PREFERRED RESPONSE: 5

DISCUSSION: The most common benign bone tumors in childhood are discovered incidentally and include single bone cysts, fibrous cortical defects, nonossifying fibroma, and osteochondroma. Benign bone tumors can be classified as latent, active, or aggressive. Aggressive bone tumors usually present with pain, whereas active lesions present with pain or pathologic fracture. Only aggressive benign bone tumors are associated with a soft-tissue mass, and they are far less common than indolent bone tumors, especially in children.

REFERENCES: Aboulafia AJ, Kennon RE, Jelinek JS: Benign bone tumors of childhood. *J Am Acad Orthop Surg* 1999;7:377-388.
Biermann JS: Common benign lesions of bone in children and adolescents. *J Pediatr Orthop* 2002;22:268-273.

A-13: Soft-tissue sarcomas most commonly metastasize to the

1. liver.
2. lung.
3. bone.
4. regional nodes.
5. distant nodes.

PREFERRED RESPONSE: 2

(continued on next page)

(A-13: *continued*)

DISCUSSION: The most common location for soft-tissue tumors to metastasize is the lungs. Depending on the grade of the sarcoma, metastases develop in as many as 50% of patients with soft-tissue sarcomas. Tumor grade is considered the most significant prognostic factor in predicting risk of metastases, with high-grade lesions at greatest risk. Staging CT of the chest should be performed once the diagnosis of a soft-tissue sarcoma is suspected or confirmed. Regular surveillance of patients treated for soft-tissue sarcomas includes follow-up CT scans at regular intervals. Intra-abdominal metastases are uncommon but may occur, particularly in patients with myxoid liposarcoma. Regional metastases are relatively uncommon and occur in approximately 5% of all patients with soft-tissue sarcoma. The incidence of regional nodal metastases is higher for synovial sarcoma and epithelioid sarcomas than other soft-tissue sarcomas.

REFERENCES: Sim FH, Frassica FJ, Frassica DA: Soft-tissue tumors: Diagnosis, evaluation, and management. *J Am Acad Orthop Surg* 1994;2:202-211.
Enzinger FM, Weiss SW, Goldblum F: *Soft Tissue Tumors*, ed 4. Washington, DC, Mosby/AFIP, 2001.

A-14: A 43-year-old woman has had pain in the left hip for the past 2 months. A radiograph, CT scan, MRI scan, and biopsy specimens are shown in Figures 10A through 10E. What is the most likely diagnosis?

1. Osteosarcoma
2. Osteochondroma
3. Chondrosarcoma
4. Chordoma
5. Enchondroma

PREFERRED RESPONSE: 3

DISCUSSION: The imaging studies are consistent with a chondrosarcoma. The radiograph shows a radiolucent lesion in the pelvis, and there are stippled calcifications on the CT scan. The histology shows a low-grade cellular hyaline cartilage neoplasm with stellate, occasionally binucleated chondrocytes. Enchondroma has a more benign histologic appearance.

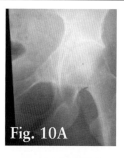
Fig. 10A

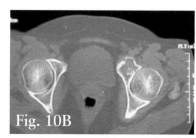
Fig. 10B

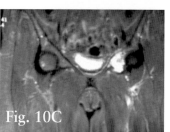
Fig. 10C

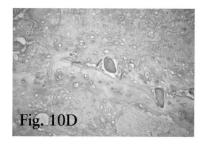
Fig. 10D

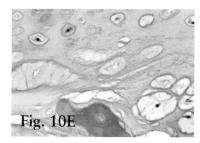
Fig. 10E

REFERENCE: Mirra JM, Gold R, Downs J, Eckardt JJ: A new histologic approach to the differentiation of enchondroma and chondrosarcoma of the bones: A clinicopathologic analysis of 51 cases. *Clin Orthop Relat Res* 1985;201:214-237.

A-15: Following preoperative chemotherapy, the percent of tumor necrosis has been shown to be of prognostic value for which of the following tumors?

1. Rhabdomyosarcoma
2. Chondrosarcoma
3. Metastatic adenocarcinoma
4. Osteosarcoma
5. Giant cell tumor of bone

PREFERRED RESPONSE: 4

Chemotherapy

DISCUSSION: The grading of response to chemotherapy for osteosarcoma was introduced by Huvos and associates. Patients with tumors that show more than 90% necrosis after neoadjuvant chemotherapy are considered to have had a good response and have better survival rates than those with less than 90% necrosis. However, it should be noted that survival rates for patients with a poor response are still better than in patients who do not receive neoadjuvant chemotherapy. More recently, similar results have been reported in patients with Ewing sarcoma. Chemotherapy is not typically used for giant cell tumor of bone.

REFERENCES: Meyers PA, Heller G, Healey J, Huvos A, Lane J, Marcove R, et al: Chemotherapy for nonmetastatic osteogenic sarcoma: The Memorial Sloan- Kettering experience. *J Clin Oncol* 1992;10:5-15.
Wunder JS, Paulian G, Huvos AG, Heller G, Meyers PA, Healey JH: The histological response to chemotherapy as a predictor of the oncological outcome of operative treatment of Ewing sarcoma. *J Bone Joint Surg Am* 1998;80:1020-1033.

A-16: What is the most common clinical presentation of a patient with a malignant bone tumor?

1. Incidental finding
2. Pain
3. Pathologic fracture
4. Deformity
5. Presence of a mass

PREFERRED RESPONSE: 2

DISCUSSION: The most common clinical presentation of a patient with a malignant bone tumor is pain. Malignant bone tumors rarely are diagnosed as an incidental finding or pathologic fracture. In patients who have a pathologic fracture on initial presentation, a history of increasing pain prior to the fracture is typical. While 90% of malignant bone tumors are associated with a soft-tissue mass, in many patients the soft-tissue component of the tumor is not clinically apparent.

(continued on next page)

(A-16: *continued*)

REFERENCES: Buckwalter JA: Musculoskeletal neoplasms and disorders that resemble neoplasms, in Weinstein SL, Buckwalter JA (eds): *Turek's Orthopaedics: Principles and Their Application*, ed 5. Philadelphia, PA, JB Lippincott, 1994, pp 290-295.
Mehlman CT, Crawford AH, McMath JA: Pediatric vertebral and spinal cord tumors: A retrospective study of musculoskeletal aspects of presentation, treatment, and complications. *Orthopedics* 1999;22:49-55.

A-17: What is the current 5-year survival rate for patients with classic nonmetastatic, high-grade osteosarcoma of the extremity?

1. 10%
2. 20%
3. 40%
4. 70%
5. 90%

PREFERRED RESPONSE: 4

DISCUSSION: Multidisciplinary treatment combining systemic chemotherapy and adequate surgical resection has resulted in a 5-year survival rate of 70% in patients with nonmetastatic osteosarcoma of the extremity. The advent of effective chemotherapy has increased the overall survival rate from 20% to 70% in current studies.

REFERENCES: Arndt CA, Crist WM: Common musculoskeletal tumors of childhood and adolescence. *N Engl J Med* 1999;341:342-352.
Glasser DB, Lane JM, Huvos AG, Marcove RC, Rosen G: Survival, prognosis, and therapeutic response in osteogenic sarcoma: The Memorial Hospital experience. *Cancer* 1992;69:698-708.

A-18: What malignant disease most commonly develops in conjunction with chronic osteomyelitis?

1. Fibrosarcoma
2. Basal cell carcinoma
3. Lymphoma
4. Osteosarcoma
5. Squamous cell carcinoma

PREFERRED RESPONSE: 5

(*continued on next page*)

(A-18: *continued*)

REFERENCES: Dell PC: Hand, in Simon MA, Springfield D (eds): *Surgery for Bone and Soft Tissue Tumors.* Philadelphia, PA, Lippincott-Raven, 1998, pp 405-420.
McGrory JE, Pritchard DJ, Unni KK, Ilstrup D, Rowland CM: Malignant lesion arising in chronic osteomyelitis. *Clin Orthop Relat Res* 1998;362:181-189.

A-19: A 10-year-old girl reports activity-related bilateral arm pain. Examination reveals no soft-tissue masses in either arm, and she has full painless range of motion in both shoulders and elbows. The radiograph and bone scan are shown in Figures 11A and 11B, and biopsy specimens are shown in Figures 11C and 11D. What is the most likely diagnosis?

1. Enchondroma
2. Fibrous dysplasia
3. Osteogenic sarcoma
4. Aneurysmal bone cyst
5. Periosteal chondroma

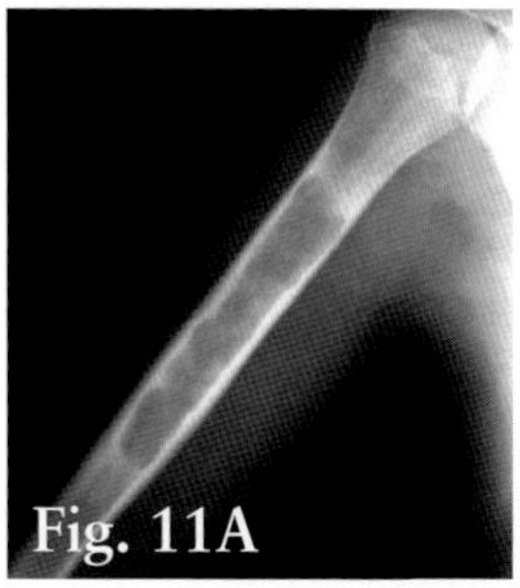

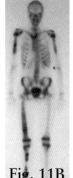
Fig. 11A

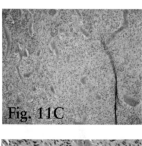
Fig. 11C

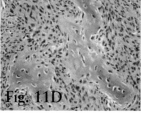
Fig. 11D

Fig. 11B

PREFERRED RESPONSE: 2

DISCUSSION: Based on these findings, the most likely diagnosis is fibrous dysplasia. Twenty percent of patients with fibrous dysplasia have multifocal disease. The lesions show a typical ground glass appearance. Fibrous dysplasia frequently involves the diaphysis of the long bones. There is no associated soft-tissue mass and no periosteal reactions to these lesions, suggesting a benign lesion. The histology shows proliferating fibroblasts in a dense collagen matrix. Trabeculae are arranged in an irregular or "Chinese letter" appearance. Osteogenic sarcoma and Ewing sarcoma have a much different radiographic appearance of malignant osteoid and small round blue cells. Periosteal chondroma does occur in the proximal humerus but is not typically multifocal. It appears as a surface lesion with saucerization of the underlying bone and a bony buttress adjacent to the lesion. Some patients with multifocal lesions have associated endocrine abnormalities (McCune-Albright syndrome).

REFERENCES: Wold LA, et al: *Atlas of Orthopaedic Pathology.* Philadelphia, PA, WB Saunders, 1990, pp 118-119.
Simon M, et al: *Surgery for Bone and Soft Tissue Tumors.* Philadelphia, PA, Lippincott Raven, 1998, p 197.

Answers: Orthopaedic Oncology and Systemic Disease

A-20: Chemotherapy is routinely included in the treatment of which of the following soft-tissue sarcomas?

1. Angiosarcoma
2. Malignant fibrous histiocytoma
3. Liposarcoma
4. Rhabdomyosarcoma
5. Clear cell sarcoma

radiation c̄ wide resection

PREFERRED RESPONSE: 4

DISCUSSION: Most soft-tissue sarcomas are treated with a combination of radiation therapy and wide resection. Rhabdomyosarcomas are an exception, where chemotherapy is included in all treatment plans. Chemotherapy for other soft-tissue sarcomas is controversial.

REFERENCES: Enzinger FM, Weiss SW: Rhabdomyosarcoma, in *Soft Tissue Tumors*, ed 3. St Louis, MO, CV Mosby, 1995, p 539.
Hays DM: Rhabdomyosarcoma. *Clin Orthop Relat Res* 1993;289:36-49.

A-21: An 83-year-old man has a painful mass of the great toe. Radiographs and a biopsy specimen are seen in Figures 12A and 12B. What is the most likely diagnosis?

1. Gout — *negative Birefringent*
2. Pseudogout
3. Infection
4. Epidermal inclusion cyst
5. Charcot joint

PREFERRED RESPONSE: 1

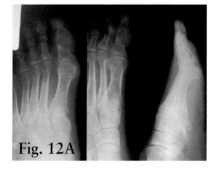
Fig. 12A

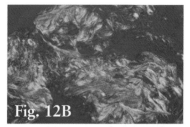
Fig. 12B

DISCUSSION: Gouty arthritis, pseudogout, and infection can all present with inflammatory arthritis and periarticular erosions. Strongly negative birefringent crystals are seen in gout. The histologic image shows elongated "needle-like" crystals of gout. Epidermal inclusion cysts are rarely painful and usually have a history of localized penetrating trauma.

REFERENCES: Hamilton W, Breedman KB, Haupt HM, Lackman R: Knee pain in a 40-year-old man. *Clin Orthop Relat Res* 2001;383:282-285,290-292.
Mizel M, Miller R, Scioli M (eds): *Orthopaedic Knowledge Update: Foot and Ankle 2*. Rosemont, IL, American Academy of Orthopaedic Surgeons, 1998, pp 301-302.

A-22: Eosinophilic granuloma frequently occurs as a solitary lesion in the tubular long bones. After biopsy, what is the best course of action?

1. Neoadjuvant chemotherapy
2. En bloc resection
3. Observation
4. Amputation
5. Chemotherapy followed by radiation therapy

PREFERRED RESPONSE: 3

DISCUSSION: Most lesions of eosinophilic granuloma are simply observed, but larger aggressive lesions may require curettage and bone grafting. Frequently, biopsy is required to rule out a malignant diagnosis. The differential diagnosis of eosinophilic granuloma is osteomyelitis, Ewing sarcoma of bone, or osteogenic sarcoma. The biopsy alone can be followed by spontaneous resolution. In some patients, low-dose radiation therapy is used. Chemotherapy or amputation is not indicated for these benign lesions.

REFERENCE: Simon M, Springfield D, et al: *Common Benign Bone Tumors: Surgery for Bone and Soft Tissue Tumors.* Philadelphia, PA, Lippincott Raven, 1998, p 200.

A-23: A 10-year-old child reports acute leg pain after wrestling with his brother. AP and lateral radiographs are shown in Figures 13A and 13B. What is the best course of action?

1. Biopsy, curettage, and plating
2. Wide segmental resection
3. Hip disarticulation
4. Closed reduction and a long leg cast
5. Tibial traction and MRI

PREFERRED RESPONSE: 4

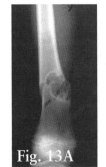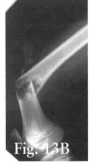
Fig. 13A   Fig. 13B

DISCUSSION: The radiographs show an eccentric metaphyseal lesion with a well-defined reactive rim of bone that is consistent with a nonossifying fibroma. Pathologic fractures through benign lesions should be treated as appropriate for the fracture, allowing the fracture to heal. Biopsy is not needed when the radiographic diagnosis is benign. MRI, in the presence of a fracture, is not particularly helpful because of the hematoma. If radiographic findings reveal that the lesion appears aggressive, a biopsy should be performed, obtaining tissue away from the fracture site.

REFERENCES: Marks KE, Bauer TW: Fibrous tumors of bone. *Orthop Clin North Am* 1989;20:377. Ponseti IV, Friedman B: Evaluation of metaphyseal fibrous defects. *J Bone Joint Surg Am* 1949;31:582.

Answers: Orthopaedic Oncology and Systemic Disease

A-24: A 15-year-old boy has had pain in the right shoulder for the past 3 months. He denies any history of trauma and has no constitutional symptoms. Examination reveals a large firm mass in the proximal arm. A radiograph and MRI scan are shown in Figures 14A and 14B. Biopsy specimens are shown in Figures 14C and 14D. Management should consist of

1. observation.
2. steroid injection.
3. curettage and bone grafting.
4. wide resection with neoadjuvant chemotherapy.
5. débridement, irrigation, and intravenous antibiotics.

PREFERRED RESPONSE: 3

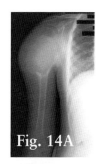
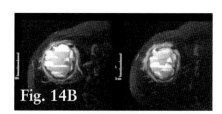

Fig. 14A   Fig. 14B

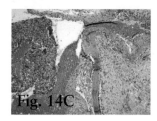
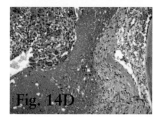

Fig. 14C   Fig. 14D

DISCUSSION: The patient has an aneurysmal bone cyst. The fluid-fluid levels seen on the MRI scan are typical for aneurysmal bone cyst, and the histology is consistent with a cystic lining. Vascular lakes, multinucleated giant cells, reactive bone, fibrovascular tissue, and an absence of atypical cells or numerous mitoses are seen histologically. Aneurysmal bone cysts will typically continue to grow and cause further bone destruction; therefore, observation is not recommended. Steroid injections are not effective. A thorough curettage of the cyst lining and bone grafting are required. Wide resection and chemotherapy are reserved for more aggressive tumors. There is no evidence of infection radiographically or histologically. Telangiectatic osteosarcoma should also be considered in the differential diagnosis; therefore, biopsy is an important part of the work-up.

REFERENCES: Wold LA, et al: *Atlas of Orthopaedic Pathology.* Philadelphia, PA, WB Saunders, 1990, pp 232-233.
Simon M, et al: *Surgery for Bone and Soft Tissue Tumors.* Philadelphia, PA, Lippincott Raven, 1998, pp 194-196.

A-25: Which of the following tumors is most likely to present with a pathologic fracture in a child?

1. Unicameral bone cyst
2. Fibrous cortical defect
3. Osteosarcoma
4. Ewing sarcoma
5. Giant cell tumor

PREFERRED RESPONSE: 1

(continued on next page)

(A-25: *continued*)

DISCUSSION: In nearly 50% of patients with a unicameral bone cyst, the lesion remains asymptomatic until a fracture occurs, usually as the result of relatively minor trauma. If the lesion expands, the bone is weakened and may cause pain. Fibrous cortical defects are usually an incidental finding and typically asymptomatic. Malignant bone tumors such as osteosarcoma and Ewing sarcoma most commonly cause pain, and pathologic fracture occurs in less than 10% of patients. Giant cell tumors are uncommon in children and usually are painful.

REFERENCES: Wilkins RM: Unicameral bone cysts. *J Am Acad Orthop Surg* 2000;8:217-224.
Dormans JP, Pill SG: Fractures through bone cysts: Unicameral bone cysts, aneurysmal bone cysts, fibrous cortical defects, and nonossifying fibromas. *Instr Course Lect* 2002;51:457-467.
Hecht AC, Gebhardt MC: Diagnosis and treatment of unicameral and aneurysmal bone cysts in children. *Curr Opin Pediatr* 1998;10:87-94.

A-26: A previously healthy 14-year-old boy now reports fatigue, and has a bilateral Trendelenburg gait, right hip pain, and bilateral knee and foot pain. Biopsy of a right sacral mass reveals intermediate grade osteosarcoma. There are no metastases. Laboratory studies reveal a serum calcium level of 7.7 mg/dL (normal 8.5 to 10.5), a phosphate level of 2.0 mg/dL (normal 2.7 to 4.5), a 1,25-dihydroxyvitamin D level of less than 10 pg/mL (normal 18 to 62), a parathyroid hormone level of 19 pg/mL (normal 10 to 60), and an alkaline phosphatase level of 428 U/L (normal 15 to 351). What is the most likely cause of the patient's symptoms?

1. Oncogenic rickets
2. Calcium sequestration by the tumor
3. Elevated alkaline phosphatase level
4. Tumor cachexia
5. L5 neuropathy

PREFERRED RESPONSE: 1

DISCUSSION: The laboratory findings are typical for rickets. Oncogenic rickets is a paraneoplastic syndrome that results from a substance secreted by the tumor that interferes with renal tubule reabsorption of phosphate. This substance previously had been called phosphatonin but recently has been identified as fibroblast growth factor 23. Nutritional rickets is rare in developed countries. Delayed onset familial hypophosphatemic rickets is possible, but the likelihood of having two rare diseases is unlikely. Osteosarcoma does not sequester calcium. Alkaline phosphatase levels can be elevated in osteosarcoma, but this does not cause muscle weakness. Tumor cachexia would occur only with advanced metastatic disease. A unilateral sacral mass would not cause a bilateral L5 neuropathy or the abnormal laboratory findings.

REFERENCES: Case records of the Massachusetts General Hospital. Weekly clinicopathological exercises. Case 29-2001. A 14-year-old with abnormal bones and a sacral mass. *N Engl J Med* 2001;345:903-908.
Jonsson KB, Zahradnik R, Larsson T, White KE, Sugimoto T, Imanishi Y, et al: Fibroblast growth factor 23 in oncogenic osteomalacia and X-linked hypophosphatemia. *N Engl J Med* 2003;348:1656-1663.

Answers: Orthopaedic Oncology and Systemic Disease

A-27: A 12-year-old girl has painless bowing of the tibia. Radiographs and a biopsy specimen are shown in Figures 15A through 15C. What is the most likely diagnosis?

1. Osteofibrous dysplasia
2. Adamantinoma — *Soap Bubble appearance*
3. Osteosarcoma
4. Ewing sarcoma
5. Fibrous dysplasia

PREFERRED RESPONSE: 1

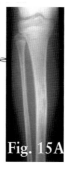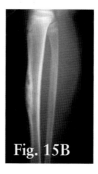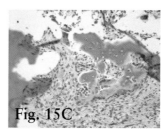

Fig. 15A   Fig. 15B   Fig. 15C

DISCUSSION: The patient has osteofibrous dysplasia. The radiographic differential diagnosis includes osteofibrous dysplasia, fibrous dysplasia, and adamantinoma. Histology shows a fibro-osseous lesion with prominent osteoblastic rimming but a lack of epithelial nests. Adamantinoma is a low-grade malignancy that typically is located in the anterior tibial cortex and has a soap bubble appearance. Histologically, it is similar to osteofibrous dysplasia but includes epithelial nests of cells. Treatment requires resection. Fibrous dysplasia usually does not require biopsy; however, in this patient the radiographs do not distinguish it from adamantinoma. The radiographic findings are not typical of Ewing sarcoma or osteosarcoma. Repeat biopsy should be considered if clinical or radiographic features change.

REFERENCE: Mirra J: *Bone Tumors: Clinical, Radiologic, and Pathologic Correlations.* Philadelphia, PA, Lea & Febiger, 1989, vol 2, ch 18.

A-28: A 16-year-old girl has had pain in the left groin for the past 4 months. She notes that the pain is worse at night; however, she denies any history of trauma and has no constitutional symptoms. There is no history of steroid or alcohol use. Examination reveals pain in the left groin with rotation of the hip. There is no associated soft-tissue mass. A radiograph and MRI scan are shown in Figures 16A and 16B, and biopsy specimens are shown in Figures 16C and 16D. What is the most likely diagnosis?

1. Clear cell chondrosarcoma
2. Chondroblastoma — *epiphyseal location*
3. Giant cell tumor
4. Aneurysmal bone cyst
5. Osteonecrosis of the femoral head

PREFERRED RESPONSE: 2

DISCUSSION: Based on the epiphyseal location and sharp, well-defined borders, the radiograph suggests chondroblastoma. Histologically, multinucleated giant cells are scattered among mononuclear cells. The nuclei are homogeneous and contain a characteristic longitudinal groove.

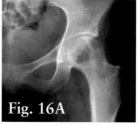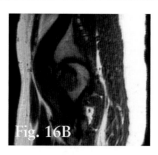

Fig. 16A   Fig. 16B

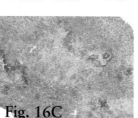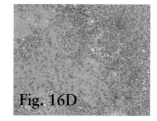

Fig. 16C   Fig. 16D

(continued on next page)

(A-28: *continued*)

Although not seen here, "chicken-wire calcification" with a bland giant cell-rich matrix is also typical for chondroblastoma. Clear cell chondrosarcoma occurs in epiphyseal locations but has a more aggressive histologic pattern and occurs in an older age group. Giant cell tumors occur in the epiphysis but have a more uniform giant cell population histologically. Aneurysmal bone cyst often results in bone remodeling and has a different pathologic appearance. Osteonecrosis has a typical histologic pattern of empty lacunae and necrotic bone.

REFERENCES: Springfield DS, Capanna R, Gherlinzoni F, et al: Chondroblastoma: A review of seventy cases. *J Bone Joint Surg Am* 1985;67:748-755.
Simon M, Springfield D, et al: *Chrondroblastoma: Surgery for Bone and Soft Tissue Tumors*. Philadelphia, PA, Lippincott Raven, 1998, p 190.
Wold LA, et al: *Atlas of Orthopaedic Pathology*. Philadelphia, PA, WB Saunders, 1990, pp 62-67.

⊛ Chondroblastoma
 ~ epiphyseal location
 ~ chicken wire calcifications
 ~ Giant cell rich matrix

A-29: A 52-year-old man has had back pain radiating to the left leg for the past 5 weeks. A radiograph, MRI scans, and biopsy specimens are shown in Figures 17A through 17F. What is the most likely diagnosis?

1. Metastatic renal cell carcinoma
2. Metastatic adenocarcinoma
3. Chordoma
4. Osteoblastoma
5. Chondrosarcoma

PREFERRED RESPONSE: 3

DISCUSSION: The histology shows cells with bubbly, abundant clear cytoplasm typical of physaliphorous cells; therefore, the most likely diagnosis is chordoma. These tumors arise from notocord rests in the upper and lower spine.

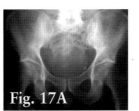
Fig. 17A

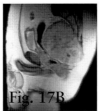
Fig. 17B

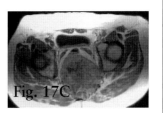
Fig. 17C

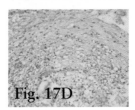
Fig. 17D

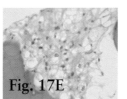
Fig. 17E

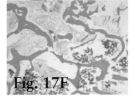
Fig. 17F

REFERENCE: Mirra J: *Bone Tumors: Clinical, Radiologic, and Pathologic Correlations*. Philadelphia, PA, Lea and Febiger, 1989, vol 1, ch 8.

Answers: Orthopaedic Oncology and Systemic Disease

A-30: An 18-year-old boy has had pain in the right knee for the past 6 months. Examination reveals some fullness behind the knee but no significant palpable soft-tissue mass. There is no effusion, and he has full knee range of motion. The remainder of the examination is unremarkable. A radiograph and MRI scans are shown in Figures 18A through 18C, and biopsy specimens are shown in Figures 18D and 18E. What is the most likely diagnosis?

1. Parosteal osteosarcoma
2. Classic osteogenic sarcoma
3. Ewing sarcoma
4. Osteochondroma
5. Chondrosarcoma

PREFERRED RESPONSE: 1

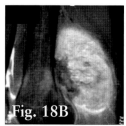

Fig. 18A

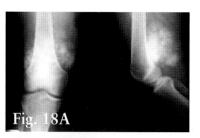

Fig. 18B

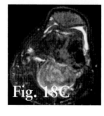

Fig. 18C

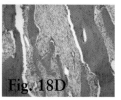

Fig. 18D

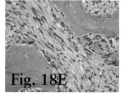

Fig. 18E

DISCUSSION: The patient has parosteal osteosarcoma. The posterior aspect of the distal femur is the typical location for this variant of osteogenic sarcoma. The imaging studies indicate a surface lesion with no involvement of the adjacent intramedullary canal. The histologic appearance is that of a low-grade fibroblastic osteosarcoma, consisting of relatively mature bone and a bland fibroblastic stroma lacking cytologic atypia and mitotic activity. A cartilaginous component is also frequently seen. Classic osteosarcoma typically has a more aggressive radiologic and histologic appearance. Sessile osteochondromas, while common behind the knee, have a presence of hematopoietic marrow and fat. The cartilage found in the associated cartilaginous cap is oriented. Chondrosarcomas are more typical in an older age group and have a histologic pattern consisting of malignant chondroid.

REFERENCES: Wold LA, et al: *Atlas of Orthopaedic Pathology.* Philadelphia, PA, WB Saunders, 1990, pp 20-21.
Unni KK, Dahlin DC, Beabout JW, Ivins JC: Parosteal osteogenic sarcoma. *Cancer* 1976;37:2466-2475.

A-31: A 47-year-old woman has had a 1-month history of left hip and medial thigh pain that is exacerbated by sitting. Laboratory studies show a total protein level of 8.2 g/dL (normal 6.0 to 8.0) and an immunoglobulin G (IGG) level of 2,130 mg/dL (normal 562 to 1,835). A radiograph, CT scan, and biopsy specimen are shown in Figures 19A through 19C. What is the most likely diagnosis?

1. Osteomyelitis
2. Lymphoma
3. Myeloma
4. Ewing sarcoma
5. Osteosarcoma

PREFERRED RESPONSE: 3

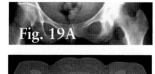

Fig. 19A

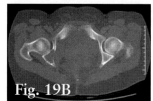

Fig. 19B

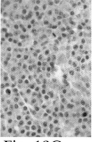

Fig. 19C

(continued on next page)

(A-31: *continued*)

DISCUSSION: The laboratory studies and histology are both consistent with myeloma. Infection should show white blood cells other than plasma cells on histology. Lymphoma would show lymphocytes, not plasma cells. The lack of bone formation on the imaging studies and the lack of osteoid on histology rule out osteosarcoma. The cells have too much cytoplasm and nuclear chromatin to be Ewing sarcoma cells.

REFERENCE: Mirra J: *Bone Tumors: Clinical, Radiologic, and Pathologic Correlations.* Philadelphia, PA, Lea & Febiger, 1989, vol 2, ch 16.

A-32: A 19-year-old girl has had pain and swelling in the right ankle for the past 4 months. She denies any history of trauma. Examination reveals a small soft-tissue mass over the anterior aspect of the ankle and slight pain with range of motion of the ankle joint. The examination is otherwise unremarkable. A radiograph and MRI scan are shown in Figures 20A and 20B, and biopsy specimens are shown in Figures 20C and 20D. What is the most likely diagnosis?

1. Osteogenic sarcoma
2. Ewing sarcoma
3. Giant cell tumor of bone
4. Aneurysmal bone cyst
5. Metastatic adenocarcinoma

PREFERRED RESPONSE: 3

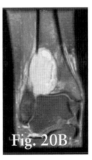
Fig. 20A

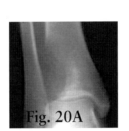
Fig. 20B

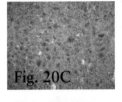
Fig. 20C

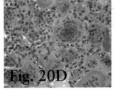
Fig. 20D

DISCUSSION: Giant cell tumors typically occur in a juxta-articular location involving the epiphysis and metaphysis of long bones, usually eccentric in the bone. The radiographs show a destructive process within the distal tibia and an associated soft-tissue mass. The histology shows multinucleated giant cells in a bland matrix with a few scattered mitoses. Osteosarcoma can have a similar destructive appearance but a very different histologic pattern with osteoid production. Ewing sarcoma also can have a diffuse destructive process in the bone. The histologic pattern of Ewing sarcoma is diffuse round blue cells. Aneurysmal bone cysts typically are seen as a fluid-filled lesion on imaging studies and have only a scant amount of giant cells histologically. Metastatic adenocarcinoma does not demonstrate the pattern shown in the patient's histology specimen.

REFERENCES: Wold LA, et al: *Atlas of Orthopaedic Pathology.* Philadelphia, PA, WB Saunders, 1990, pp 198-199.
Simon M, et al: *Surgery for Bone and Soft Tissue Tumors.* Philadelphia, PA, Lippincott Raven, 1998, pp 200-202.

Answers: Orthopaedic Oncology and Systemic Disease

A-33: A 13-year-old patient has foot drop and lateral knee pain. AP and lateral radiographs and an MRI scan are shown in Figures 21A through 21C. A biopsy specimen is shown in Figure 21D. What is the preferred method of treatment?

1. Wide resection alone
2. Chemotherapy and radiation therapy
3. Chemotherapy and wide resection
4. Above-knee amputation
5. Through-knee amputation

PREFERRED RESPONSE: 3

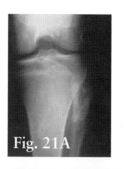
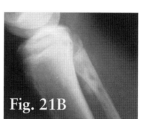

Fig. 21A

Fig. 21B

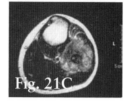
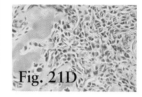

Fig. 21C

Fig. 21D

DISCUSSION: The "sunburst" radiographic appearance suggests an osteosarcoma, and the histologic findings confirm the diagnosis with malignant cells surrounded by pink osteoid. MRI scans are not particularly helpful in the diagnosis of osteosarcoma but are mandatory for surgical planning. Osteosarcomas are high-grade sarcomas that are best treated with chemotherapy and wide resection. Even though the peroneal nerve is involved, limb salvage is indicated. Survival after limb salvage is equivalent to amputation, with better function.

REFERENCES: Goorin AM, Abelson HT, Frei E: Osteosarcoma: Fifteen years later. *N Engl J Med* 1985;313:1637.
Link MP, Goorin AM, Miser AW, et al: The effect of adjuvant chemotherapy on relapse-free survival in patients with osteosarcoma of the extremity. *N Engl J Med* 1986;314:1600.
Davis AM, Bell RS, Goodwin PJ: Prognostic factors in osteosarcoma: A critical review. *J Clin Oncol* 1994;12:423.

A-34: A 23-year-old woman has had vague left knee pain for the past 6 months. A radiograph and CT scan are shown in Figures 22A and 22B. What is the most likely diagnosis?

1. Myositis ossificans
2. Osteochondroma
3. Parosteal osteosarcoma
4. Dedifferentiated chondrosarcoma
5. Tumoral calcinosis

PREFERRED RESPONSE: 3

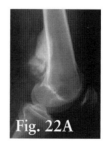
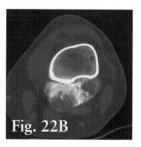

Fig. 22A

Fig. 22B

(continued on next page)

(A-34: *continued*)

DISCUSSION: The radiographic appearance of the lesion emanating from the posterior cortex of the left distal femur is consistent with a surface bone-producing lesion; therefore, the most likely diagnosis is a parosteal osteosarcoma. In an osteochondroma, the cortex and medullary cavity of the lesion are in continuity with that of the native bone. A dedifferentiated chondrosarcoma has histologic components of a high-grade sarcoma plus a benign or low-grade malignant cartilage tumor. Tumoral calcinosis is characterized by amorphous calcium in the soft tissues and does not emanate from the bone itself. While often confused with parosteal osteosarcoma, myositis ossificans is usually more mature at the periphery of the lesion rather than the center. In addition, myositis ossificans does not involve the underlying cortex but remains separate from the bone.

REFERENCES: Unni KK: *Dahlin's Bone Tumors: General Aspects and Data on 11,087 Cases*, ed 5. Philadelphia, PA, Lippincott-Raven, 1996, pp 185-196.
Okada K, Frassica FJ, Sim FH, Beabout JW, Bond JR, Unni KK: Parosteal osteosarcoma. A clinicopathological study. *J Bone Joint Surg Am* 1994;76:366-378.

A-35: Figures 23A through 23C show the radiograph, CT scan, and biopsy specimen of a 44-year-old man who underwent chemotherapy and radiation therapy for lymphoma of the distal femur 20 years ago. His current problem is most likely related to

1. steroid-induced osteonecrosis.
2. radiation therapy with secondary malignancy.
3. recurrence of the lymphoma.
4. radiation osteitis.
5. a primary lung tumor.

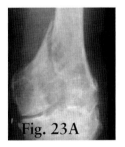
Fig. 23A

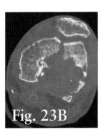
Fig. 23B

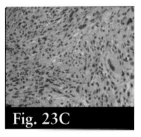
Fig. 23C

PREFERRED RESPONSE: 2

DISCUSSION: The patient has changes consistent with radiation therapy to the femur, including osteopenia and an aggressive appearing neoplasm. The tumor is most likely a radiation-induced sarcoma. This is more likely than recurrent lymphoma at this late date. It is not related to steroid use or a primary lung tumor.

REFERENCES: Mirra J (ed): *Bone Tumors: Clinical, Radiologic and Pathologic Correlations*. Philadelphia, PA, Lea and Febiger, 1989, p 353.
Huvos A, Woodard H, Cahan W, et al: Postradiation osteogenic sarcoma of bone and soft tissue. A clinical pathologic study of 66 Patients. *Cancer* 1985;55:1244.

Sports Medicine

Section Editor

Kurt P. Spindler, MD

Q-1: Which fibers of the anterior cruciate ligament are tight in flexion?

1. Anteromedial
2. Anterolateral
3. Posteromedial
4. Posterolateral
5. Middle

Q-2: After making a tackle, a football player is found prone and unconscious without spontaneous respirations. Initial management should consist of

1. log roll to a supine position, helmet removal, and initiation of assisted breathing.
2. log roll to a supine position, head and neck stabilization, face mask removal, and CPR.
3. log roll onto a spine board, head and neck stabilization, face mask removal, and CPR.
4. head and neck stabilization, log roll to a supine position, helmet removal, and initiation of assisted breathing.
5. head and neck stabilization, log roll to a supine position, face mask removal, and initiation of assisted breathing.

Q-3: Following harvesting of patellar tendon autograft, paresthesia most commonly occurs in which of the following locations?

1. Medial to the incision
2. Lateral to the incision
3. First web space of the foot
4. Medial foot
5. Dorsal foot

Q-4: Patients with hip disease may report knee pain, which is primarily caused by irritation of which of the following branches of the obturator nerve?

1. Cutaneous continuation of the branch to the gracilis muscle
2. Continuation of the branch to the adductor magnus
3. Accessory obturator nerve branch
4. Branch within the sartorius muscle
5. Branch within the linea aspera

Q-5: A posterior approach to the knee with an incision of the superficial fascia medial to the small saphenous vein avoids injury to what structure that lies just lateral and adjacent to the small saphenous vein?

1. Popliteal vein
2. Popliteal artery
3. Tibial nerve
4. Common peroneal nerve
5. Medial sural cutaneous nerve

Q-6: Which of the following tendons are typically harvested when performing anterior cruciate ligament reconstruction with double loop hamstring autograft?

1. Semitendinosus and semimembranosus
2. Sartorius and semitendinosus
3. Gracilis and semimembranosus
4. Gracilis and semitendinosus
5. Biceps and semimembranosus

Q-7: What tendon has an intra-articular (intrasynovial) location in the knee joint?

1. Patellar
2. Popliteal
3. Semitendinosus
4. Semimembranosus
5. Biceps femoris

Q-8: What is the most anatomic location for placement of the femoral tunnel in anterior cruciate ligament reconstruction?

1. As far superior in the notch as possible
2. As far posterior as possible on the lateral femoral condyle
3. As far posterior as possible on the medial femoral condyle
4. Directly across from the posterior cruciate femoral insertion
5. At resident's ridge

Q-9: What neurovascular structure is most at risk when performing an inside-out repair of the posterior horn of the medial meniscus?

1. Popliteal artery
2. Peroneal nerve
3. Saphenous nerve
4. Tibial nerve
5. Sciatic nerve

Q-10: Within the menisci, most of the large collagen fiber bundles are oriented in what configuration?

1. Radially
2. Circumferentially
3. Vertically
4. Obliquely
5. Randomly

Q-11: A 12-year-old boy reports knee discomfort after prolonged strenuous activities. He denies knee swelling or catching and has no pain with activities of daily living. A radiograph is shown in Figure 1. Prognosis for the pathology shown is most influenced by

1. weight.
2. gender.
3. the knee compartment involved.
4. open or closed growth plates.
5. limb alignment.

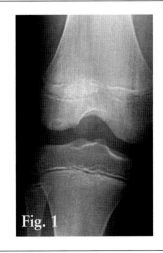

Fig. 1

Q-12: A patient with no history of patellar instability sustains a traumatic lateral patellar dislocation. What structure most likely has been torn?

1. Vastus medialis obliquus
2. Medial patellofemoral ligament
3. Medial patellotibial ligament
4. Medial retinaculum
5. Quadriceps tendon

Q-13: A 17-year-old high school long distance runner is seeking advice before running a marathon for the first time. What advice should be given regarding his fluid, carbohydrate, and electrolyte intake around the time of the race?

1. Restrict fluid intake 2 hours before the start of the race to avoid abdominal cramping.
2. Drink low osmolality (less than 10%) solutions before, during, and after the race.
3. Drink fruit juice, such as orange juice, instead of water to replenish essential carbohydrates.
4. Drink high osmolality (greater than 10%) solutions before and during the race and low osmolality solutions after the race.
5. Avoid the use of glucose polymers because they slow down gastric emptying and may lead to abdominal cramping.

A-1: Which fibers of the anterior cruciate ligament are tight in flexion?

1. Anteromedial
2. Anterolateral
3. Posteromedial
4. Posterolateral
5. Middle

PREFERRED RESPONSE: 1

DISCUSSION: There are two bundles of the anterior cruciate ligament, the anteromedial and posterolateral. The anteromedial bundle is tight in flexion; in extension, all fibers are tensioned.

REFERENCE: Sapega AA, Moyer RA, Schneck C, et al: Testing for isometry during reconstruction of the anterior cruciate ligament: Anatomical and biomechanical considerations. *J Bone Joint Surg Am* 1990;72:259-267.

A-2: After making a tackle, a football player is found prone and unconscious without spontaneous respirations. Initial management should consist of

1. log roll to a supine position, helmet removal, and initiation of assisted breathing.
2. log roll to a supine position, head and neck stabilization, face mask removal, and CPR.
3. log roll onto a spine board, head and neck stabilization, face mask removal, and CPR.
4. head and neck stabilization, log roll to a supine position, helmet removal, and initiation of assisted breathing.
5. head and neck stabilization, log roll to a supine position, face mask removal, and initiation of assisted breathing.

PREFERRED RESPONSE: 5

DISCUSSION: The on-field evaluation and management of a seriously injured athlete requires that health care teams have a game plan in place and proper equipment that is readily available. The initial step, which consists of stabilizing the head and neck by manually holding them in a neutral position, is then followed by assessment of breathing, pulses, and level of consciousness. If the athlete is breathing, management should consist of mouth guard removal and airway maintenance. If the athlete is not breathing, the face mask should be removed, with the chin strap left in place. The airway must be established, followed by initiation of assisted breathing. CPR is instituted only when breathing and circulation are compromised. In the unconscious athlete or if a cervical spine injury is suspected, the helmet must not be removed until the athlete has been transported to an appropriate facility and the cervical spine has been completely evaluated.

REFERENCES: McSwain NE, Garnelli, RL: Helmet removal from injured patients. *Bull of Am Coll Surg* 1997;82:42-44.
Vegso JJ: Field evaluation and management of head and neck injuries. *Post Grad Adv Sport Med* 1987;10:2-10.

A-3: Following harvesting of patellar tendon autograft, paresthesia most commonly occurs in which of the following locations?

1. Medial to the incision
2. Lateral to the incision
3. First web space of the foot
4. Medial foot
5. Dorsal foot

PREFERRED RESPONSE: 2

DISCUSSION: The infrapatellar branch of the saphenous nerve often crosses over the anterior aspect of the knee and innervates the skin lateral to the anterior midline of the knee. An anterior midline incision often results in incision of the terminal branches, resulting in lateral numbness. The superficial peroneal, deep peroneal, and saphenous nerves that provide sensation to the foot are not at risk.

REFERENCE: Hoppenfeld S, deBoer P (ed): *Surgical Exposures in Orthopaedics: The Anatomic Approach.* Philadelphia, PA, JB Lippincott, 1984, pp 407-410.

A-4: Patients with hip disease may report knee pain, which is primarily caused by irritation of which of the following branches of the obturator nerve?

1. Cutaneous continuation of the branch to the gracilis muscle
2. Continuation of the branch to the adductor magnus
3. Accessory obturator nerve branch
4. Branch within the sartorius muscle
5. Branch within the linea aspera

PREFERRED RESPONSE: 2

DISCUSSION: The branch of the obturator nerve to the knee is the continuation of the motor branch to the adductor magnus.

REFERENCE: Basmajian JV: *Grant's Method of Anatomy,* ed 8. Baltimore, Williams & Wilkins, 1971, p 357.

A-5: A posterior approach to the knee with an incision of the superficial fascia medial to the small saphenous vein avoids injury to what structure that lies just lateral and adjacent to the small saphenous vein?

1. Popliteal vein
2. Popliteal artery
3. Tibial nerve
4. Common peroneal nerve
5. Medial sural cutaneous nerve

PREFERRED RESPONSE: 5

DISCUSSION: The posterior approach to the knee has recently become popular for a variety of indications, such as repair of avulsions to the posterior cruciate ligament, repair of neurovascular structures, open reduction and internal fixation of posteromedial tibial plateau fragments, and excision of popliteal cysts. The small saphenous vein is the landmark for the incision of the superficial popliteal fascia, and the medial sural cutaneous nerve lies just lateral to the small saphenous vein. The popliteal artery and vein and the tibial nerve lie deep to the fascia. The common peroneal nerve is located much further lateral.

REFERENCE: Hoppenfeld S, deBoer P: *Surgical Exposures in Orthopaedics: The Anatomic Approach.* Philadelphia, PA, JB Lippincott, 1984, pp 427-436.

A-6: Which of the following tendons are typically harvested when performing anterior cruciate ligament reconstruction with double loop hamstring autograft?

1. Semitendinosus and semimembranosus
2. Sartorius and semitendinosus
3. Gracilis and semimembranosus
4. Gracilis and semitendinosus
5. Biceps and semimembranosus

PREFERRED RESPONSE: 4

DISCUSSION: Because of the availability of long tendons and the minimal donor morbidity associated with the gracilis and semitendinosus tendons, they are currently considered the structures of choice for hamstring tendon autograft anterior cruciate ligament reconstruction by most authors. The gracilis and semitendinosus are beneath and behind the sartorius (not a hamstring) at the tibial insertion of the pes anserinus. They have long tendons and relatively small muscle bellies typical of vestigial muscles (in contrast to the biceps and semimembranosus). With approximately 20 cm of tendon typically available, this allows the double loop technique to provide a graft of sufficient strength.

REFERENCES: Aglietti P, Buzzi R, Zaccheratti G, et al: Patellar tendon versus doubled semitendinosus and gracilis tendon for anterior cruciate ligament reconstruction. *Am J Sports Med* 1994;22:211-218. Last RJ: *Anatomy: Regional and Applied*, ed 6. New York, NY, Churchill Livingstone, 1975, p 116.

Answers: Sports Medicine

A-7: What tendon has an intra-articular (intrasynovial) location in the knee joint?

1. Patellar
2. Popliteal
3. Semitendinosus
4. Semimembranosus
5. Biceps femoris

PREFERRED RESPONSE: 2

DISCUSSION: The popliteal tendon arises from the posterior aspect of the tibia and courses through the knee joint through the popliteus hiatus of the lateral meniscus before attaching on the lateral femur anterior to the lateral collateral ligament. It is the only tendon in the knee joint that can be viewed directly on arthroscopy.

REFERENCES: Kimura M, Shirakura K, Hasegawa A, Kobayashi Y, Udagawa E: Anatomy and pathophysiology of the popliteal tendon area in the lateral meniscus: 1. Arthroscopic and anatomical investigation. *Arthroscopy* 1992;8:419-423.
Arnoczky SP, Skyhar MJ, Wickiewicz TL: Basic science of the knee, in McGinty JB (ed): *Operative Arthroscopy.* New York, NY, Raven Press, 1991, pp 155-182.

A-8: What is the most anatomic location for placement of the femoral tunnel in anterior cruciate ligament reconstruction?

1. As far superior in the notch as possible
2. As far posterior as possible on the lateral femoral condyle
3. As far posterior as possible on the medial femoral condyle
4. Directly across from the posterior cruciate femoral insertion
5. At resident's ridge

PREFERRED RESPONSE: 2

DISCUSSION: It is critical for graft isometry and knee stability that the femoral tunnel be placed as far posterior as possible on the lateral femoral condyle. Superiorly, the graft should be at the one o'clock position on the left knee. Resident's ridge is a false posterior shelf that often seems like the extreme posterior cortex. Abnormal tunnel placement results in a variety of complications, including an unstable knee, early graft failure, and joint stiffness.

REFERENCES: Johnson RJ, Beynnon BD, Nichols CE, Renstrom PA: The treatment of injuries of the anterior cruciate ligament. *J Bone Joint Surg Am* 1992;74:140-151.
Beaty JH (ed): *Orthopaedic Knowledge Update 6.* Rosemont, IL, American Academy of Orthopaedic Surgeons, 1999, pp 533-557.

A-9: What neurovascular structure is most at risk when performing an inside-out repair of the posterior horn of the medial meniscus?

1. Popliteal artery
2. Peroneal nerve
3. Saphenous nerve
4. Tibial nerve
5. Sciatic nerve

[handwritten note: Nerves at risk with meniscal Repairs]

PREFERRED RESPONSE: 3

DISCUSSION: The saphenous nerve is located on the posterior medial aspect of the knee and must be protected when performing an inside-out repair of the medial meniscus. The peroneal nerve is most at risk with lateral meniscal repairs. The other structures usually are not at risk with meniscal repair.

REFERENCES: Cannon WD Jr, Morgan CD: Meniscal repair: Arthroscopic repair techniques. *Instr Course Lect* 1994;43:77-96.
Scott GA, Jolly BL, Henning CE: Combined posterior incision and arthroscopic intra-articular repair of the meniscus: An examination of factors affecting healing. *J Bone Joint Surg Am* 1986;68:847-861.

A-10: Within the menisci, most of the large collagen fiber bundles are oriented in what configuration?

1. Radially
2. Circumferentially
3. Vertically
4. Obliquely
5. Randomly

PREFERRED RESPONSE: 2

DISCUSSION: The majority of large collagen fibers within the menisci are oriented circumferentially. It is these fibers that develop the hoop stress with compressive loading of the menisci. Most meniscal tears are longitudinal and occur between these circumferential fibers.

REFERENCES: Mow VC, et al: Structure and function relations of the menisci of the knee, in Mow VC, Arnoczky SP, Jackson DW (eds): *Knee Meniscus: Basic and Clinical Foundations.* New York, NY, Raven Press, 1992, pp 37-57.
De Haven KE, Arnoczky SP: Mensicus repair: Basic science, indications for repair, and open repair. *Instr Course Lect* 1994;43:65-76.

A-11: A 12-year-old boy reports knee discomfort after prolonged strenuous activities. He denies knee swelling or catching and has no pain with activities of daily living. A radiograph is shown in Figure 1. Prognosis for the pathology shown is most influenced by

1. weight.
2. gender.
3. the knee compartment involved.
4. open or closed growth plates.
5. limb alignment.

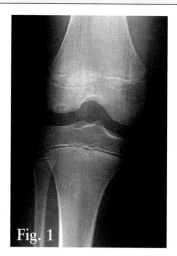

Fig. 1

PREFERRED RESPONSE: 4

DISCUSSION: While many factors play a role in the outcome of osteochondritis dissecans, ample evidence has shown that the prognosis is most influenced by the growth status of the plates. If the growth plates are open, the chance of a successful outcome is significantly greater than if they are closed.

REFERENCES: Federico DJ, Lynch JK, Jokl P: Osteochondritis dissecans of the knee: A historical review of etiology and treatment. *Arthroscopy* 1990;6:190-197.
Linden B: Osteochondritis dissecans of the femoral condyles: A long-term follow-up study. *J Bone Joint Surg Am* 1977;59:769-776.

A-12: A patient with no history of patellar instability sustains a traumatic lateral patellar dislocation. What structure most likely has been torn?

1. Vastus medialis obliquus
2. Medial patellofemoral ligament
3. Medial patellotibial ligament
4. Medial retinaculum
5. Quadriceps tendon

PREFERRED RESPONSE: 2

DISCUSSION: Any of the above structures may be involved in a lateral patellar dislocation. However, biomechanic studies have found that the medial patellofemoral ligament is the major soft-tissue static restraint of lateral patellar displacement, providing at least 50% of this function.

REFERENCES: Desio SM, Burks RT, Bachus KN: Soft tissue restraints to lateral patellar translation in the human knee. *Am J Sports Med* 1998;26:59-65.
Conlan T, Garth WP Jr, Lemons JE: Evaluation of the medial soft-tissue restraints of the extensor mechanism of the knee. *J Bone Joint Surg Am* 1993;75:682-693.
Warren LF, Marshall JL: The supporting structures and layers on the medial compartment of the knee: An anatomical analysis. *J Bone Joint Surg Am* 1979;61:56-62.

A-13: A 17-year-old high school long distance runner is seeking advice before running a marathon for the first time. What advice should be given regarding his fluid, carbohydrate, and electrolyte intake around the time of the race?

1. Restrict fluid intake 2 hours before the start of the race to avoid abdominal cramping.

2. Drink low osmolality (less than 10%) solutions before, during, and after the race.

3. Drink fruit juice, such as orange juice, instead of water to replenish essential carbohydrates.

4. Drink high osmolality (greater than 10%) solutions before and during the race and low osmolality solutions after the race.

5. Avoid the use of glucose polymers because they slow down gastric emptying and may lead to abdominal cramping.

PREFERRED RESPONSE: 2

DISCUSSION: The goal of fluid replenishment should be to replace the sweat that has been lost. Sweat is mostly water, with a small concentration of salts and other electrolytes. Absorption is enhanced by solutions of low osmolality. Scientific research has also shown that adding carbohydrates to the drink improves athletic performance. Carbohydrates such as glucose and maltodextrins (glucose polymers) stimulate fluid absorption by the intestines. Fructose slows intestinal absorption of fluids. Drinks that are high in fructose, such as orange juice, can lead to gastrointestinal distress and osmotic diarrhea.

REFERENCES: Kirkendall D: Fluids and electrolytes, in *The U.S. Soccer Sports Medicine Book.* Baltimore, MD, Williams and Wilkins, 1996.
Gisolfi CV, Duchman SM: Guidelines for optimal replacement beverages for different athletic events. *Med Sci Sports Exerc* 1992;24:679-687.

Trauma

Section Editor

Kenneth J. Koval, MD

Q-1: Figures 1A and 1B show the radiographs of a 51-year-old woman who injured her left leg after falling off a stepladder. Surgical reconstruction was performed with a compression screw and side plate; the postoperative radiograph is shown in Figure 1C. Following gradual progression of weight bearing, she reports that she slipped again and placed full weight on the extremity. She now notes a new onset of increased pain in her left thigh and hip region. Follow-up radiographs are shown in Figures 1D and 1E. Reconstruction should consist of

1. conversion to a longer side plate with the same compression screw and tube angle.

2. in situ bone grafting.

3. hardware removal and reconstruction with an intramedullary device that provides fixation into the femoral head and neck.

4. hardware removal and retrograde femoral nailing.

5. revision reconstruction with cerclage wiring.

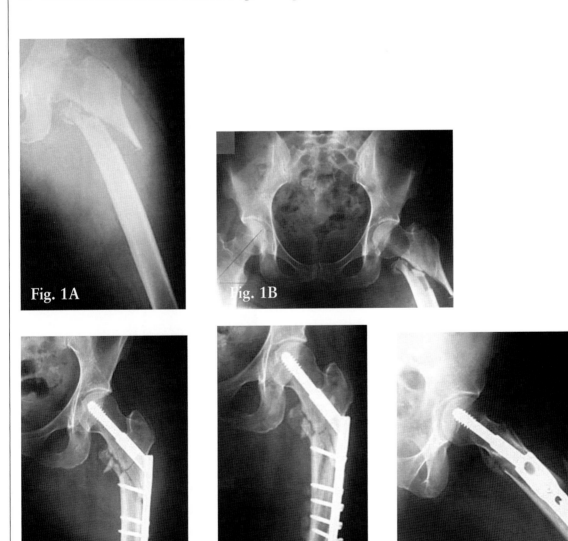

Fig. 1A

Fig. 1B

Fig. 1C

Fig. 1D

Fig. 1E

Q-2: Seven hours ago, a 32-year-old man who was not wearing a seat belt was injured when his car struck a power pole. He needed to be extricated from the vehicle. Examination reveals absent pulses in the left foot, the thigh is swollen and tender, and a closed fracture is noted. Radiographs are shown in Figures 2A and 2B. Doppler examination reveals no significant flow distal to the fracture site. Treatment should include which of the following?

1. Immediate angiography

2. Insertion of a distal femoral traction pin in the emergency department and angiography

3. Surgical exploration of the femoral and popliteal artery through a medial approach

4. Manipulative reduction in the emergency department and angiography

5. Urgent reduction of the fracture, followed by an on-table angiogram or arterial exploration

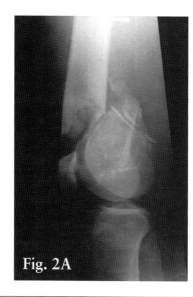
Fig. 2A

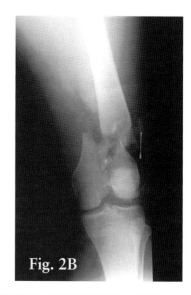
Fig. 2B

Q-3: A 36-year-old man sustains the injury seen in Figure 3A and 3B. Examination reveals a 3-cm wound overlying the site of the ulnar fracture. The neurovascular status of the limb is normal. In addition to tetanus prophylaxis, IV antibiotics, and urgent débridement, treatment should include which of the following?

1. Splint immobilization without an attempt at fracture reduction

2. Closed reduction and splint immobilization

3. Open reduction and internal fixation of both bones of the forearm

4. External fixation of the ulna with splint supplementation

5. External fixation of the ulna, and open reduction and plate fixation of the radius

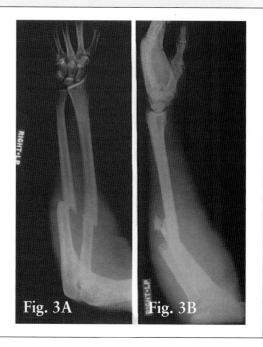
Fig. 3A   Fig. 3B

Q-4: What artery is the primary blood supply to the humeral head?

1. Thoracoacromial
2. Posterior humeral circumflex
3. Anterior humeral circumflex
4. Suprascapular
5. Suprahumeral

Q-5: What nerve lies in the subcutaneous tissue immediately lateral to the cephalic vein at the elbow?

1. Radial
2. Ulnar
3. Median
4. Lateral antebrachial cutaneous
5. Medial antebrachial cutaneous

Q-6: A 25-year-old man has a midshaft femoral fracture with 25% comminution and is undergoing closed intramedullary nailing. Proximal locking is performed uneventfully; however, during distal locking screw insertion, only one of the screws is noted to have bone purchase. Which of the following procedures is the best solution to this problem?

1. Leave only one distal screw; this will provide adequate fixation.
2. Exchange the nail for one either longer or shorter, and relock at a new level.
3. Insert methylmethacrylate cement into the hole and redrill when the cement hardens.
4. Insert a screw through the hole either anterior or posterior to the intramedullary nail locking hole.
5. Insert a small-diameter threaded pin at a different angle through the locking hole.

Q-7: Which of the following organisms is most commonly isolated in acute necrotizing fasciitis?

1. Group A streptococcus
2. Group D streptococcus
3. *Pseudomonas aeruginosa*
4. *Staphylococcus aureus*
5. *Clostridium difficile*

Q-8: A 23-year-old man sustains the injury shown in Figures 4A and 4B. In association with this injury, which of the following nerves is most commonly injured?

1. Axillary
2. Median
3. Musculocutaneous
4. Radial
5. Ulnar

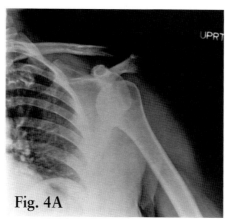

Fig. 4A

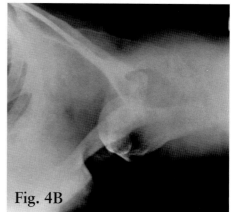

Fig. 4B

Q-9: A 23-year-old man has an isolated open tibial fracture without distal neurologic or vascular compromise following a motorcycle accident. After undergoing skeletal stabilization and several debridements, a clean 6 x 6-cm wound remains over the anteromedial surface of the distal third of the tibia. The tibia is exposed throughout the length of the wound and the periosteum has been stripped. What is the best option for wound management at this time?

1. Split-thickness skin graft
2. Free muscle transfer
3. Soleus muscle flap
4. Medial gastrocnemius muscle flap
5. Cross-leg gastrocnemius flap

Q-10: What is the main disadvantage of using antibiotic-impregnated polymethylmethacrylate beads to treat infected or contaminated wounds?

1. Local toxicity
2. Systemic toxicity
3. Inadequate antibiotic elution
4. Foreign body reaction
5. Allergic reaction

Q-11: Which of the following preoperative findings correlates best with results after operative fixation of the calcaneus?

1. Displacement of the sustentaculum tali
2. Displacement of the lateral wall
3. Number of major fragments of the posterior facet
4. Diminution of Bohler's angle
5. Amount of heel varus

Q-12: A 30-year-old man underwent an intramedullary nailing for a closed midthird tibial fracture 2 months ago. He has had pain and erythema in the area of the fracture for the past 3 days, and radiographs show a midthird tibia fracture with an interlocking nail in place. Which of the following tests would be most appropriate to obtain a diagnosis?

1. Erythrocyte sedimentation rate
2. MRI scan
3. CT scan
4. Aspiration of the fracture site
5. Indium-labeled white blood cell scan

Q-13: A patient with a type IIIB open tibia fracture is treated with intravenous gentamicin and ceftazidime for an infection. The patient experiences frequent, loose, and watery stools, and a stool assay for *Clostridium difficile* toxin is positive. Which of the following antibiotics should be administered?

1. Tobramycin
2. Ampicillin
3. Metronidazole
4. Cefazolin
5. Clindamycin

Q-14: A 21-year-old man sustained a displaced pelvic fracture after falling 40 feet from a scaffold. Examination reveals the presence of blood in the urethral meatus. Which of the following measures is most likely to complicate urologic management?

1. Intravenous pyelography
2. Placement of a Foley catheter
3. Placement of suprapubic catheter
4. Rectal examination
5. Retrograde cystogram

Q-15: Which of the following is the most appropriate treatment for an acute comminuted radial head fracture, in association with an Essex-Lopresti injury (radioulnar dissociation)?

1. Radial head preservation
2. Radial head excision
3. Sauvé-Kapandji procedure
4. Darrach procedure
5. Radioulnar synostosis

Q-16: Which of the following nerves is most likely to be injured during percutaneous pinning of pediatric supracondylar humeral fractures?

1. Ulnar
2. Median
3. Radial
4. Lateral antebrachial
5. Medial antebrachial

Q-17: A 23-year-old man is experiencing impotence and penile numbness following intramedullary nailing for a femoral shaft fracture. Which of the following conditions is a likely cause of these symptoms?

1. Unrecognized urologic trauma
2. Injury to S2-S3
3. Injury to the penis from the traction post
4. Pudendal nerve palsy
5. Posttraumatic stress

Q-18: A 37-year-old man sustains an isolated injury to his right arm as the result of being struck by a car. Examination reveals that the radial and ulnar pulses are normal, and the neurologic examination reveals that he is unable to extend the wrist, fingers, or thumb. A radiograph of the right humerus is shown in Figure 4. Management should consist of

1. plate osteosynthesis via an anterolateral approach.
2. external fixation.
3. closed reduction and application of a splint.
4. exploration of the radial nerve and a locked intramedullary nail.
5. electrodiagnostic studies of the radial nerve.

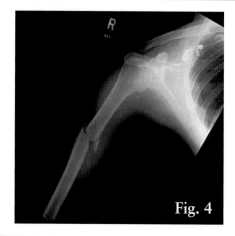

Fig. 4

Q-19: During four-compartment fasciotomy for compartment syndrome of the leg, what nerves are decompressed in the anterior and lateral compartments, respectively?

1. Posterior tibial and superficial peroneal
2. Superficial peroneal and sural
3. Deep peroneal and sural
4. Deep peroneal and saphenous
5. Deep peroneal and superficial peroneal

Q-20: An iliosacral screw that exits just anterior to the S1 body is most likely to injure which of the following structures?

1. L4 nerve root
2. L5 nerve root
3. S1 nerve root
4. S2 nerve root
5. External iliac artery

Q-21: Which of the following is considered the most common complication following intramedullary nailing of a closed tibial fracture?

1. Infection
2. Nonunion
3. Malunion
4. Knee pain
5. Compartment syndrome

Q-22: A patient has a swollen, tender hindfoot with focal tenderness beneath the heel after falling 12 feet. Radiographs and a CT scan are negative. An MRI scan would most likely reveal which of the following conditions?

1. Occult subcortical fracture of the calcaneus
2. Acute osteonecrosis
3. Compression of the tibial nerve (tarsal tunnel syndrome)
4. Rupture of the posterior tibial tendon
5. Rupture of the plantar fascia

Q-23: Which of the following treatment principles for tarsometatarsal joint (Lisfranc) injuries has resulted in improved clinical outcomes?

1. Early treatment of compartment syndrome
2. Early treatment of dorsal nerve injury
3. Closed reduction and percutaneous pin fixation
4. Open joint reduction and internal fixation
5. Rigid transarticular fixation

Q-24: Which of the following is considered the most common cause of a poor functional prognosis after an unstable posterior pelvic ring injury?

1. Residual displacement causing a leg-length discrepancy of less than 1.0 cm
2. Persistent neurologic deficit
3. Malreduced sacroiliac joint
4. Genitourinary dysfunction
5. Fracture nonunion

Q-25: The acute mortality rate after multiple trauma is most frequently related to involvement of which of the following systems?

1. Pulmonary
2. Cardiac
3. Central nervous system
4. Multiple open long-bone fractures (musculoskeletal)
5. Genitourinary

Q-26: Which of the following is considered the most reliable early clinical finding for hemorrhagic shock?

1. Decreased systolic blood pressure
2. Decreased diastolic blood pressure
3. Decreased hemoglobin level
4. Low urine output
5. Tachycardia

Q-27: After undergoing a closed unreamed tibial nailing, a patient is diagnosed with an isolated anterior leg compartment syndrome. However, no treatment is initiated because the patient is thought to have a nerve palsy. Which of the following findings should be present at 2 weeks when the cast is removed?

1. Drop foot and numbness in the first web space of the foot
2. Calcaneal deformity of the ankle
3. Rigid equinus deformity
4. Plantar foot numbness
5. Supple claw toes

Q-28: Which of the following nerve roots is at risk during anterior placement of the iliosacral screw in the treatment of sacroiliac disruptions?

1. L3
2. L4
3. L5
4. S1
5. S2

Q-29: Which of the following CT scans will best help evaluate a calcaneal fracture?

1. 3-D reconstructions
2. Sagittal reconstructions
3. Axial and semicoronal planes
4. Sections parallel to the posterior facet of the calcaneus
5. Sections perpendicular to the anterior facet of the calcaneus

Q-30: A patient with an acromioclavicular dislocation has a very prominent distal clavicle. Examination reveals that the deformity increases rather than reduces with an isometric shoulder shrug. Which of the following structures is most likely intact?

1. Trapezoid ligament
2. Conoid ligament
3. Acromioclavicular ligament
4. Deltoid muscle origin
5. Trapezius muscle insertion

Q-31: Posterior sternoclavicular dislocations are most commonly associated with which of the following complications?

1. Chronic instability
2. Brachial plexus palsy
3. Pneumothorax
4. Esophageal compression
5. Tracheal compression

Q-32: During an anterior approach to the shoulder, excessive traction on the conjoined tendon is most likely to result in loss of

1. elbow flexion.
2. shoulder flexion.
3. shoulder internal rotation.
4. shoulder abduction.
5. forearm pronation.

Q-33: Which of the following nerves is most commonly injured when obtaining a bone graft from the posterior ilium?

1. Lateral femoral cutaneous
2. Superior gluteal
3. Cluneal
4. L5 nerve root
5. S1 nerve root

Q-34: Which of the following ligaments is most commonly involved in posterolateral rotatory instability of the elbow?

1. Annular
2. Lateral ulnar collateral
3. Anterior band of the medial collateral
4. Radial part of the lateral collateral
5. Posterior capsular

Q-35: A 28-year-old man sustains the closed injury shown in Figures 6A through 6C after falling 8 feet while rock climbing. Management should consist of

1. open reduction and internal fixation via an anteromedial arthrotomy.

2. talectomy.

3. primary tibiotalocalcaneal arthrodesis.

4. open reduction and internal fixation via a medial malleolar osteotomy and limited anterior lateral arthrotomy.

5. closed reduction and a non-weight-bearing cast.

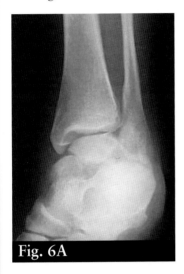

Fig. 6A

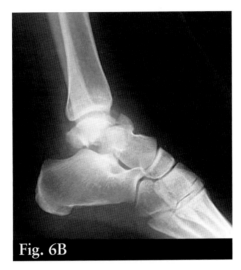

Fig. 6B

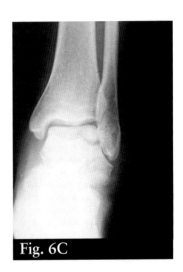

Fig. 6C

Q-36: A 20-year-old man sustains the injury shown in Figures 7A and 7B in a motorcycle accident. In addition to a prompt closed reduction, his outcome might be optimized by

1. a subtalar arthrodesis.

2. screw fixation of the talar neck.

3. repair of the medial subtalar capsule.

4. temporary transarticular pin fixation.

5. evaluation for and excision or fixation of osteochondral fractures.

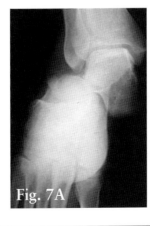

Fig. 7A

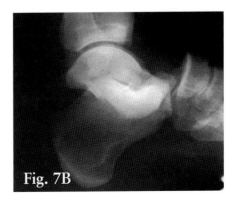

Fig. 7B

Q-37: Which of the following types of displaced posterior pelvic disruptions must undergo anatomic reduction and internal fixation to ensure the best clinical outcome?

1. Sacral fracture through the foramen
2. Sacral fracture through the ala
3. Sacroiliac joint dislocation
4. Reverse fracture-dislocation of the sacroiliac joint through the ilium
5. Iliac wing fracture

Q-38: A 28-year-old woman who is training for the New York Marathon reports pain in the postero-medial aspect of her right ankle. Examination reveals tenderness just posterior to the medial malleolus. Radiographs are normal. An MRI scan is shown in Figure 8. What is the most likely diagnosis?

1. Posterior tibial tendinitis
2. Osteoid osteoma
3. Posterior ankle impingement
4. Tibial stress fracture
5. Flexor hallucis longus tendinitis

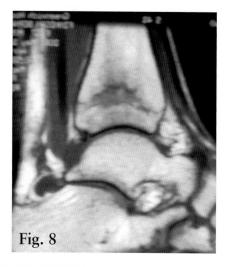

Fig. 8

Q-39: A 10-year-old boy has a painful, swollen knee after falling off his bicycle. Examination reveals that the knee is held in 45° of flexion, and any attempt to actively or passively extend the knee produces pain and muscle spasms. A lateral radiograph is shown in Figure 9. What is the most likely diagnosis?

1. Patellar sleeve fracture
2. Avulsion of the tibial tubercle
3. Avulsion of the anterior tibial spine
4. Osteochondral fracture of the femoral condyle
5. Osteochondral fracture of the patella

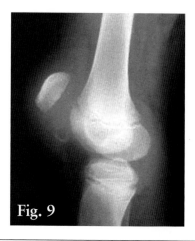

Fig. 9

Q-40: Which of the following factors is considered most important when assessing an ankle fracture for surgical treatment?

1. Level of the fibular fracture
2. Displacement of the fibular fracture
3. Size of the posterior malleolus
4. Position of the talus in the mortise
5. Rupture of the deltoid ligament

Q-41: A 35-year-old woman who underwent open reduction and internal fixation of a calcaneal fracture 14 months ago reports pain that has failed to respond to nonsurgical management. Examination reveals limited painful subtalar motion but no hindfoot deformity. A lateral radiograph is shown in Figure 10. Surgical reconstruction is best accomplished with

1. calcaneal osteotomy.
2. subtalar joint arthrodesis.
3. triple arthrodesis.
4. pantalar arthrodesis.
5. distraction bone-block arthrodesis.

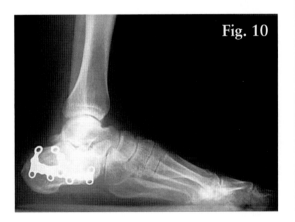

Fig. 10

Q-42: After stabilizing a bimalleolar ankle fracture with a plate and lag screws for the fibula and two interfragmental compression screws for the medial malleolus, a syndesmosis screw is indicated in which of the following situations?

1. In all suprasyndesmotic fibular fractures
2. In all transsyndesmotic fibular fractures
3. When there is increased medial clear space with external rotation stress
4. If the deltoid ligament is ruptured
5. If the posterior malleolus is fractured

Q-43: The primary stabilizer to valgus stress in the elbow is the

1. radiocapitellar joint.
2. anterior oblique band of the medial collateral ligament.
3. transverse band of the medial collateral ligament.
4. posterior oblique band of the medial collateral ligament.
5. ulnar trochlear articulation.

Q-44: A 32-year-old man sustains an iliac wing fracture and a contralateral femur fracture. Twelve hours later he has shortness of breath with tachypnea, hypoxia, and confusion. A chest radiograph is normal. What is the most likely diagnosis?

1. Fat emboli syndrome
2. Adult respiratory distress syndrome
3. Pulmonary embolus
4. Tension pneumothorax
5. Sepsis

Q-45: The nerve that traverses the triangular interval (bounded by the teres major superiorly, the long head of the triceps medially, and the humeral shaft laterally) supplies which of the following muscles?

1. Brachioradialis
2. Flexor pollicis longus
3. Deltoid
4. Teres major
5. Pronator teres

Q-46: A 24-year-old woman has a spleen laceration and hypotension. Radiographs reveal a pulmonary contusion and a displaced mid-diaphyseal fracture of the femur. The trauma surgeon clears the patient for stabilization of the femoral fracture. What technique will offer the least potential for initial complications?

1. External fixation
2. Plate fixation
3. Unreamed unlocked intramedullary nailing
4. Reamed statically locked intramedullary nailing
5. Reamed unlocked nailing

Q-47: The use of nasotracheal intubation for airway management is contraindicated in the acute multiply injured patient when the patient has

1. suspected cervical spine trauma.
2. head injuries and spontaneous respirations.
3. respiratory arrest.
4. a need for prolonged ventilatory support.
5. a hemopneumothorax.

Q-48: A 26-year-old man is brought to the emergency department unresponsive and intubated after being found lying on the side of the road. He has a Glasgow Coma Scale score of 6. A chest tube has been inserted on the right side of the chest for a pneumothorax. An abdominal CT scan reveals a small liver laceration and minimal intraperitoneal hematoma. A pneumatic antishock garment (PASG) is on but not inflated. He has bilateral tibia fractures. A pelvic CT scan shows an anterior minimally displaced left sacral ala fracture and left superior and inferior rami fractures. He has received 2 L of saline solution and 4 units of blood but remains hemodynamically unstable. What is the next most appropriate step in management?

1. Inflation of the abdominal portion of the PASG
2. Application of a pelvic clamp
3. Application of a pelvic external fixator
4. Rapid infusion of 4 more units of blood
5. Angiography and embolization

Q-49: Figure 11 shows the radiograph of a 23-year-old man who has severe right shoulder pain after his motorcyle hit a bridge guardrail. He is neurologically intact. Nonsurgical management will most likely result in

1. nonunion of the clavicle or glenoid.
2. thoracic outlet syndrome.
3. less than 50% range of motion compared with the contralateral shoulder.
4. less than 50% strength compared with the contralateral houlder.
5. high patient satisfaction and good shoulder function.

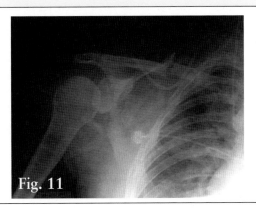

Fig. 11

Q-50: A left-handed 23-year-old man who fell 5 feet from a ladder onto his left elbow sustained the closed injury shown in Figure 12. Management should consist of

1. percutaneous pin fixation.
2. a percutaneous 6.5-mm screw.
3. long arm casting in flexion.
4. open reduction and internal fixation with a tension band plate.
5. closed reduction and long arm casting in extension.

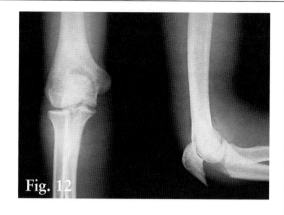

Fig. 12

Q-51: Which of the following is a long-term complication of ankle arthrodesis for posttraumatic arthritis?

1. Progressive limb-length discrepancy
2. Contralateral ankle arthritis
3. Ipsilateral hindfoot and midfoot arthritis
4. Ipsilateral knee arthritis
5. Talar osteonecrosis

Q-52: In displaced calcaneal fractures, what fragment is the only one that remains in its anatomic position?

1. Posterior tubercle
2. Posterior articular facet
3. Anterior process
4. Sustentaculum tali
5. Lateral wall

Q-53: What is the most common clinically significant preventable complication secondary to the treatment of a displaced talar neck fracture?

1. Osteonecrosis
2. Nonunion
3. Malunion
4. Infection
5. Osteoarthritis of the ankle joint

Q-54: Figure 13 shows the radiograph of an 8-year-old boy who has a swollen forearm after falling out of a tree. Examination reveals that all three nerves are functionally intact, and there is no evidence of circulatory embarrassment. Management should consist of

1. open reduction of both the radius and ulna with plate and screw fixation.

2. closed reduction and a long arm cast, with the elbow in 90° of flexion and the forearm in neutral rotation.

3. closed reduction and a long arm cast, with the elbow in 120° of flexion and the forearm in full supination.

4. closed reduction and a long arm cast, with the elbow extended and the forearm pronated.

5. closed reduction and intramedullary pin fixation of both the radius and ulna.

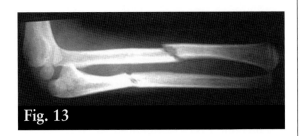

Fig. 13

Q-55: An 18-year-old man has a simple oblique fracture of the humeral shaft that requires surgical stabilization to maintain reduction and facilitate mobilization. Which of the following methods will provide the best outcome?

1. Unreamed intramedullary nail
2. Reamed statically locked intramedullary nail
3. External fixation
4. Plate fixation and interfragmentary compression
5. Bridge plate stabilization

Q-56: Injury to which of the following structures has been reported following iliac crest bone graft harvest?

1. Superior gluteal artery from an anterior crest harvest
2. Superior cluneal nerve from an anterior crest harvest
3. Inferior gluteal artery from a posterior crest harvest
4. Ilioinguinal nerve from a posterior crest harvest
5. Lateral femoral cutaneous nerve from an anterior crest harvest

Q-57: A 17-year-old patient sustains a supracondylar/intercondylar humerus fracture and examination reveals a complete motor and sensory ulnar nerve palsy. At surgery for internal fixation, the nerve is found to be contused but in continuity. In the early postoperative period, examination reveals a mild flexion deformity of the ulnar two digits "clawing." At 10 weeks after surgery, the patient's mother reports that the clawing deformity is progressively worsening. What is the next most appropriate step in management?

1. Surgical exploration of the ulnar nerve

2. Hardware removal

3. Emergent office evaluation

4. Reassurance of the mother and patient

5. Tendon transfers to restore intrinsic function

Q-58: A 23-year-old man is seen in your office after crashing his bicycle in a regional semipro race 2 days ago. Immediately after the crash, he was taken to the emergency department where he was diagnosed with a right clavicle fracture and placed in a sling. He is right hand dominant. Examination reveals no shortness of breath and he is neurovascularly intact. He has an obvious deformity of the clavicle, but the skin is intact and there is no evidence of an open fracture. A radiograph is shown in Figure 14. What should he be told about his treatment options?

1. Surgical and nonsurgical treatment programs have similar rates of nonunion.

2. Surgical treatment does not reduce the time to radiographic union.

3. Patients who are age 18 to 25 years have an increased risk of nonunion.

4. Fracture displacement is not a risk factor in developing a nonunion.

5. The most common complication of surgical treatment is related to the hardware.

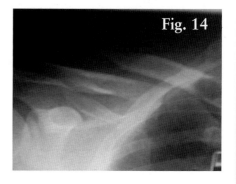

Fig. 14

Q-59: A 13-year-old hockey player reports a 1-week history of left medial clavicle pain and dysphagia. A chest radiograph obtained at the emergency department on the day of injury was negative. Examination reveals swelling and tenderness along the medial edge of the left clavicle. The upper extremity neurologic examination is normal. What is the next most appropriate test to best define the patient's injury?

1. CT of the sternoclavicular joint

2. Barium swallowing study

3. Electromyography of the upper extremity

4. MRI of the glenohumeral joint

5. Bone scan

A-1: Figures 1A and 1B show the radiographs of a 51-year-old woman who injured her left leg after falling off a stepladder. Surgical reconstruction was performed with a compression screw and side plate; the postoperative radiograph is shown in Figure 1C. Following gradual progression of weight bearing, she reports that she slipped again and placed full weight on the extremity. She now notes a new onset of increased pain in her left thigh and hip region. Follow-up radiographs are shown in Figures 1D and 1E. Reconstruction should consist of

1. conversion to a longer side plate with the same compression screw and tube angle.

2. in situ bone grafting.

3. hardware removal and reconstruction with an intramedullary device that provides fixation into the femoral head and neck.

4. hardware removal and retrograde femoral nailing.

5. revision reconstruction with cerclage wiring.

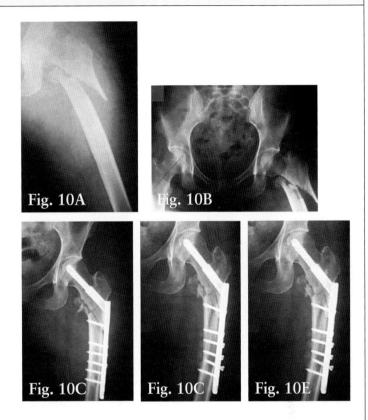

Fig. 10A   Fig. 10B

Fig. 10C   Fig. 10C   Fig. 10E

PREFERRED RESPONSE: 3

DISCUSSION: The initial fracture was an unstable reverse oblique intertrochanteric fracture with subtrochanteric extension. Initial fixation with a high-angled screw and side plate construct may not provide stability as well as a 95° fixed-angle device or a intramedullary hip screw device. The follow-up radiographs show loss of fixation and further propagation of the fracture distally. Reconstruction would best be accomplished with hardware removal and conversion to a long intramedullary nail with femoral head fixation or a 95° angled plate and screw device. Conversion to a longer plate does not improve the biomechanical situation at the primary fracture site. In situ bone grafting would not provide any additional stability and would not correct the deformity. The proximal femoral fracture is not amenable to retrograde nailing. Cerclage wiring will not sufficiently enhance stability and is not indicated.

REFERENCES: Bridle SH, Patel AD, Bircher M, Calvert PT: Fixation of intertrochanteric fractures of the femur: A randomized prospective comparison of a gamma nail and dynamic hip screw. *J Bone Joint Surg Br* 1991;73:330-334.

DeLee JC: Fractures and dislocations of the hip, in Rockwood CA Jr, Green DP, Bucholz RW, Heckman JD (eds): *Rockwood and Green's Fractures in Adults*, ed 4. Philadelphia, PA, Lippincott-Raven, 1996, pp 1659-1825.

Haidukewych GJ, Israel TA, Berry DJ: Reverse obliquity fractures of the intertrochanteric region of the femur. *J Bone Joint Surg Am* 2001;83:643-650.

Sanders RW, Regazzoni P: Treatment of subtrochanteric femur fractures using the dynamic condylar screw. *J Orthop Trauma* 1989;3:206-213.

A-2: Seven hours ago, a 32-year-old man who was not wearing a seat belt was injured when his car struck a power pole. He needed to be extricated from the vehicle. Examination reveals absent pulses in the left foot, the thigh is swollen and tender, and a closed fracture is noted. Radiographs are shown in Figures 2A and 2B. Doppler examination reveals no significant flow distal to the fracture site. Treatment should include which of the following?

1. Immediate angiography
2. Insertion of a distal femoral traction pin in the emergency department and angiography
3. Surgical exploration of the femoral and popliteal artery through a medial approach
4. Manipulative reduction in the emergency department and angiography
5. Urgent reduction of the fracture, followed by an on-table angiogram or arterial exploration

PREFERRED RESPONSE: 5

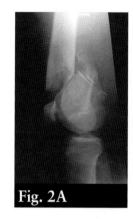 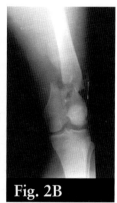

Fig. 2A   Fig. 2B

DISCUSSION: This patient has a probable vascular injury based on absent pulses and a Doppler examination. Since 7 hours have elapsed since the injury, immediate restoration of blood flow is imperative. Angiography with the fracture in a displaced position will be misleading. The patient should undergo urgent reduction of the fracture and an on-table angiogram or arterial exploration, followed by fracture and vascular repair.

REFERENCES: Johnson KD: Femur: Trauma, in Frymoyer JW (ed): *Orthopaedic Knowledge Update 4: Home Study Syllabus.* Rosemont, IL, American Academy of Orthopaedic Surgeons, 1993, pp 559-567. Johnson KD: Femoral shaft fractures, in Browner BD, Jupiter JB, Levine AM, et al (eds): *Skeletal Trauma.* Philadelphia, PA, WB Saunders, 1992, vol 2, pp 1575-1576.

A-3: A 36-year-old man sustains the injury seen in Figure 3A and 3B. Examination reveals a 3-cm wound overlying the site of the ulnar fracture. The neurovascular status of the limb is normal. In addition to tetanus prophylaxis, IV antibiotics, and urgent débridement, treatment should include which of the following?

1. Splint immobilization without an attempt at fracture reduction
2. Closed reduction and splint immobilization
3. Open reduction and internal fixation of both bones of the forearm
4. External fixation of the ulna with splint supplementation
5. External fixation of the ulna, and open reduction and plate fixation of the radius

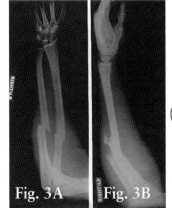

Fig. 3A   Fig. 3B

PREFERRED RESPONSE: 3

DISCUSSION: The patient has a type II open fracture of the forearm, and assuming treatment takes place less than 24 hours after the injury, open reduction and plate fixation is the preferred method for stabilization of types I, II, and IIIA open forearm fractures.

REFERENCES: Moed BR, Kellam JF, Foster RJ, et al: Immediate internal fixation of open fractures of the diaphysis of the forearm. *J Bone Joint Surg Am* 1986;68:1008-1017.
Duncan R, Geissler W, Freeland AE, et al: Immediate internal fixation of open fractures of the diaphysis of the forearm. *J Orthop Trauma* 1992;6:25-31.

A-4: What artery is the primary blood supply to the humeral head?

1. Thoracoacromial
2. Posterior humeral circumflex
3. Anterior humeral circumflex
4. Suprascapular
5. Suprahumeral

PREFERRED RESPONSE: 3

DISCUSSION: The primary blood supply to the humeral head is the arcuate artery, which is a continuation of the ascending branch of the anterior humeral circumflex artery. All five vessels mentioned and the subscapular artery supply blood to the rotator cuff.

REFERENCES: Bigliani LU: Fractures of the proximal humerus, in Rockwood CA Jr, Matsen FA III: *The Shoulder.* Philadelphia, PA, WB Saunders, 1990, vol 1, pp 280-281.
Rothman RH, Parke WW: The vascular anatomy of the rotator cuff. *Clin Orthop Relat Res* 1965;41:176-186.

A-5: What nerve lies in the subcutaneous tissue immediately lateral to the cephalic vein at the elbow?

1. Radial
2. Ulnar
3. Median
4. Lateral antebrachial cutaneous
5. Medial antebrachial cutaneous

PREFERRED RESPONSE: 4

DISCUSSION: The lateral antebrachial cutaneous nerve is a continuation of the musculocutaneous nerve after it has supplied three muscles in the arm. As it emerges laterally from between the biceps and brachialis at the elbow, the nerve is now purely sensory and passes lateral to the cephalic vein.

REFERENCE: Netter FH: *Atlas of Human Anatomy*. Summit, NJ, Ciba-Geigy Corp, 1989, plate 423.

A-6: A 25-year-old man has a midshaft femoral fracture with 25% comminution and is undergoing closed intramedullary nailing. Proximal locking is performed uneventfully; however, during distal locking screw insertion, only one of the screws is noted to have bone purchase. Which of the following procedures is the best solution to this problem?

1. Leave only one distal screw; this will provide adequate fixation.
2. Exchange the nail for one either longer or shorter, and relock at a new level.
3. Insert methylmethacrylate cement into the hole and redrill when the cement hardens.
4. Insert a screw through the hole either anterior or posterior to the intramedullary nail locking hole.
5. Insert a small-diameter threaded pin at a different angle through the locking hole.

PREFERRED RESPONSE: 1

DISCUSSION: For the majority of femoral diaphyseal fractures above the distal third, one distal locking screw is sufficient. Fractures located in the distal third will often require the addition of a second locking screw.

REFERENCES: Hajek PD, Bicknell HR Jr, Bronson WE, et al: The use of one compared with two distal screws in the treatment of femoral shaft fractures with interlocking intramedullary nailing: A clinical and biomechanical analysis. *J Bone Joint Surg Am* 1993;75:519-525.
Grover J, Wiss DA: A prospective study of fractures of the femoral shaft treated with a static, intramedullary, interlocking nail comparing one versus two distal screws. *Orthop Clin North Am* 1995;26:139-146.

A-7: Which of the following organisms is most commonly isolated in acute necrotizing fasciitis?

1. Group A streptococcus
2. Group D streptococcus
3. *Pseudomonas aeruginosa*
4. *Staphylococcus aureus*
5. *Clostridium difficile*

PREFERRED RESPONSE: 1

DISCUSSION: Many cases of acute necrotizing fasciitis involve a synergy of several organisms. The most commonly isolated organism, singly or in combination, is a group A streptococcus.

REFERENCES: Wang KC, Shih CH: Necrotizing fasciitis of the extremities. *J Trauma* 1992;32:179-182. Meleney FL: Hemolytic streptococcus gangrene. *Arch Surg* 1924;9:317-364.

A-8: A 23-year-old man sustains the injury shown in Figures 4A and 4B. In association with this injury, which of the following nerves is most commonly injured?

1. Axillary
2. Median
3. Musculocutaneous
4. Radial
5. Ulnar

PREFERRED RESPONSE: 1

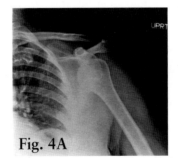 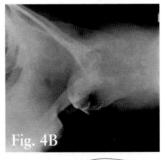

Fig. 4A   Fig. 4B

DISCUSSION: An anterior dislocation of the shoulder is shown in Figures 4A and 4B. The axillary nerve is the most commonly involved nerve, having an incidence ranging from 5% to 33% for first-time anterior glenohumeral dislocations. The likelihood of injury to the axillary nerve increases with age and the duration of the dislocation. It is usually a traction neurapraxia but the prognosis for recovery is good.

REFERENCES: Blom S, Dahlback LO: Nerve injuries in dislocations of the shoulder joint and fractures of the neck of the humerus: A clinical and electromyographical study. *Acta Chir Scand* 1970;136:461-466. Rockwood CA Jr, Thomas SC, Matsen FA III: Subluxation and dislocations about the glenohumeral joint, in Rockwood CA Jr, Green DP, Bucholz RW (eds): *Rockwood & Green's Fractures in Adults*, ed 3. Philadelphia, PA, JB Lippincott, 1991, pp 1021-1179.

Answers: Trauma

A-9: A 23-year-old man has an isolated open tibial fracture without distal neurologic or vascular compromise following a motorcycle accident. After undergoing skeletal stabilization and several débridements, a clean 6 x 6-cm wound remains over the anteromedial surface of the distal third of the tibia. The tibia is exposed throughout the length of the wound and the periosteum has been stripped. What is the best option for wound management at this time?

1. Split-thickness skin graft
2. Free muscle transfer
3. Soleus muscle flap
4. Medial gastrocnemius muscle flap
5. Cross-leg gastrocnemius flap

PREFERRED RESPONSE: 2

DISCUSSION: Exposed bone cannot be adequately covered by a skin graft alone. The medial gastrocnemius muscle is preferred for coverage of exposed bone in the proximal third of the tibia, and the soleus muscle flap is preferred for coverage of exposed bone in the middle third of the tibia. Neither of these pedicle grafts, however, can adequately reach the distal third of the tibia. Cross-leg gastrocnemius flaps have been previously used with some success in the treatment of contralateral leg soft-tissue defects; however, this technique is awkward and uncomfortable for the patient and requires prolonged hospitalization. In the United States, free muscle transfer is more frequently used.

REFERENCES: Trafton PG: Tibial shaft fractures, in Browner BD, Jupiter JB, Levine AM, et al (eds): *Skeletal Trauma*. Philadelphia, PA, WB Saunders, 1992, vol 2, pp 1800-1803.
Wood MB, Cooney WP, Irons GB: Lower extremity salvage and reconstruction by free-tissue transfer: Analysis of results. *Clin Orthop Relat Res* 1985;201:151-161.

A-10: What is the main disadvantage of using antibiotic-impregnated polymethylmethacrylate beads to treat infected or contaminated wounds?

1. Local toxicity
2. Systemic toxicity
3. Inadequate antibiotic elution
4. Foreign body reaction
5. Allergic reaction

PREFERRED RESPONSE: 4

DISCUSSION: The main disadvantage is that the polymethylmethacrylate beads act as a foreign body. Antibiotic elution, low toxicity, and minimal allergic reactions are considered advantages.

REFERENCE: Patzakis MJ, Mazur K, Wilkins J, et al: Septopal beads and autogenous bone grafting for bone defects in patients with chronic osteomyelitis. *Clin Orthop Relat Res* 1993;295:112-118.

A-11: Which of the following preoperative findings correlates best with results after operative fixation of the calcaneus?

1. Displacement of the sustentaculum tali
2. Displacement of the lateral wall
3. Number of major fragments of the posterior facet
4. Diminution of Bohler's angle
5. Amount of heel varus

PREFERRED RESPONSE: 3

DISCUSSION: Satisfactory results correlate with fewer fragments of the posterior facet. Two-part fractures have a good outcome, whereas four-part fractures tend to do poorly. Varus and lateral wall displacement that occur postoperatively predict a poor result, but the presence of these findings preoperatively is common and indicate a need for surgery.

REFERENCE: Sanders R, Fortin P, DiPasquale T, Walling A: Operative treatment in 120 displaced intra-articular calcaneal fractures: Results using a prognostic computed tomography scan classification. *Clin Orthop Relat Res* 1993;290:87-95.

A-12: A 30-year-old man underwent an intramedullary nailing for a closed midthird tibial fracture 2 months ago. He has had pain and erythema in the area of the fracture for the past 3 days, and radiographs show a midthird tibia fracture with an interlocking nail in place. Which of the following tests would be most appropriate to obtain a diagnosis?

1. Erythrocyte sedimentation rate
2. MRI scan
3. CT scan
4. Aspiration of the fracture site
5. Indium-labeled white blood cell scan

PREFERRED RESPONSE: 4

DISCUSSION: Aspiration of the fracture site and testing the aspiration fluid by Gram stain, culture, and sensitivities is the best way to confirm the diagnosis. The other tests are either nondiagnostic or do not make a specific diagnosis.

REFERENCES: Patzakis MJ: Management of osteomyelitis, in *Operative Orthopaedics*, ed 2. Philadelphia, PA, JB Lippincott, 1993, p 3335.
Zych GA, Hutson JJ Jr: Diagnosis and management of infection after tibial intramedullary nailing. *Clin Orthop Relat Res* 1995;315:153-162.

Answers: Trauma

A-13: A patient with a type IIIB open tibia fracture is treated with intravenous gentamicin and ceftazidime for an infection. The patient experiences frequent, loose, and watery stools, and a stool assay for *Clostridium difficile* toxin is positive. Which of the following antibiotics should be administered?

1. Tobramycin
2. Ampicillin
3. Metronidazole
4. Cefazolin
5. Clindamycin

PREFERRED RESPONSE: 3

DISCUSSION: The antibiotics associated with *Clostridium difficile* colitis in orthopaedic patients include clindamycin, cefazolin, and aminoglycosides. The recommended treatment is either oral metronidazole or vancomycin, administered for 72 hours.

REFERENCE: Clarke HJ, Jinnah RH, Byank RP, Cox QG: Clostridium difficile infection in orthopaedic patients. *J Bone Joint Surg Am* 1990;72:1056-1059.

A-14: A 21-year-old man sustained a displaced pelvic fracture after falling 40 feet from a scaffold. Examination reveals the presence of blood in the urethral meatus. Which of the following measures is most likely to complicate urologic management?

1. Intravenous pyelography
2. Placement of a Foley catheter
3. Placement of suprapubic catheter
4. Rectal examination
5. Retrograde cystogram

PREFERRED RESPONSE: 2

DISCUSSION: The incidence of urologic injury in association with pelvic fractures is 30%, and the finding of blood in the urethral meatus suggests the presence of a urethral tear. Placement of a urethral catheter may precipitate further dissection of a preexisting urethral tear. Appropriate evaluation would include a rectal examination and retrograde cystogram prior to catheter placement. Intravenous pyelography may also be an appropriate part of the evaluation of hematuria. A suprapubic catheter may be appropriate treatment for an isolated urethral tear; however, it may complicate any required or planned pelvic internal fixation.

REFERENCE: Colapinto V: Trauma to the pelvis: Urethral injury. *Clin Orthop Relat Res* 1980;151:46-55.

Answers: Trauma

A-15: Which of the following is the most appropriate treatment for an acute comminuted radial head fracture, in association with an Essex-Lopresti injury (radioulnar dissociation)?

1. Radial head preservation
2. Radial head excision
3. Suavé-Kapandji procedure
4. Darrach procedure
5. Radioulnar synostosis

PREFERRED RESPONSE: 1

DISCUSSION: An Essex-Lopresti injury consists of a fracture of the radial head, disruption of the radioulnar interosseous membrane, and dislocation of the distal radioulnar joint. The diagnosis is frequently made late, ie, after excision of a comminuted radial head fracture, after pain develops at the distal radioulnar joint, and radiographs show progressive positive ulnar variance and/or dislocation due to proximal migration of the radial shaft. Patients who have undergone reduction and internal fixation of the radial head or replacement have done better than those who have had excision. Concurrent treatment should include reduction of the distal radioulnar joint and temporary stabilization.

REFERENCES: Trousdale RT, Amadio PC, Cooney WP, et al: Radio-ulnar dissociation: A review of twenty cases. *J Bone Joint Surg Am* 1992;74:1486-1497.
Bruckner JD, Alexander AH, Lichtman DM: Acute dislocations of the distal radioulnar joint. *Instr Course Lect* 1996;45:27-36.

A-16: Which of the following nerves is most likely to be injured during percutaneous pinning of pediatric supracondylar humeral fractures?

1. Ulnar
2. Median
3. Radial
4. Lateral antebrachial
5. Medial antebrachial

PREFERRED RESPONSE: 1

DISCUSSION: Although radial nerve injury has been reported as a result of direct pin trauma, the ulnar nerve is most susceptible to injury because of its proximity to the supracondylar humeral region in the cubital tunnel.

REFERENCE: Royce RO, Dutkowsky JP, Kasser JR, et al: Neurologic complications after K-wire fixation of supracondylar humerus fractures in children. *J Pediatr Orthop* 1991;11:191-194.

Answers: Trauma

A-17: A 23-year-old man is experiencing impotence and penile numbness following intramedullary nailing for a femoral shaft fracture. Which of the following conditions is a likely cause of these symptoms?

1. Unrecognized urologic trauma
2. Injury to S2-S3
3. Injury to the penis from the traction post
4. Pudendal nerve palsy
5. Posttraumatic stress

PREFERRED RESPONSE: 4

DISCUSSION: The pudendal nerve is vulnerable to injury during intramedullary nailing of the femur. This has been attributed to prolonged traction or improper positioning.

REFERENCE: Kao JT, Burton D, Comstock C, McClellan RT, Carragee E: Pudendal nerve palsy after femoral intramedullary nailing. *J Orthop Trauma* 1993;7:58-63.

A-18: A 37-year-old man sustains an isolated injury to his right arm as the result of being struck by a car. Examination reveals that the radial and ulnar pulses are normal, and the neurologic examination reveals that he is unable to extend the wrist, fingers, or thumb. A radiograph of the right humerus is shown in Figure 5. Management should consist of

1. plate osteosynthesis via an anterolateral approach.
2. external fixation.
3. closed reduction and application of a splint.
4. exploration of the radial nerve and a locked intramedullary nail.
5. electrodiagnostic studies of the radial nerve.

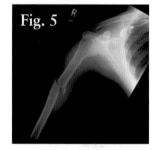
Fig. 5

PREFERRED RESPONSE: 3

DISCUSSION: The patient has a high-energy closed humeral shaft fracture with an immediate complete radial nerve palsy. Closed reduction and application of a splint yield excellent results in closed humeral shaft fractures. With observation, the prognosis of the nerve injury is favorable for return of extension. Indications for surgical treatment, such as open an fracture, vascular injury, a floating elbow, or associated intra-articular fractures, are not present. Exploration of radial nerve injuries has not been shown to improve the neurologic outcome.

REFERENCES: Levine AM (ed): *Orthopaedic Knowledge Update: Trauma.* Rosemont, IL, American Academy of Orthopaedic Surgeons, 1996, pp 25-34.
Zagorski JB, Latta LL, Zych GA, Finnieston AR: Diaphyseal fractures of the humerus: Treatment with prefabricated braces. *J Bone Joint Surg Am* 1988;70:607-610.

A-19: During four-compartment fasciotomy for compartment syndrome of the leg, what nerves are decompressed in the anterior and lateral compartments, respectively?

1. Posterior tibial and superficial peroneal
2. Superficial peroneal and sural
3. Deep peroneal and sural
4. Deep peroneal and saphenous
5. Deep peroneal and superficial peroneal

PREFERRED RESPONSE: 5

DISCUSSION: The leg has four fascial compartments. The anterior compartment contains the anterior tibial artery and deep peroneal nerve. The lateral compartment contains the superficial peroneal nerve until it exits superficially distally. The deep posterior compartment contains the posterior tibial artery and tibial nerve, as well as the peroneal artery. The superficial posterior compartment contains the sural nerve. The saphenous nerve is subcutaneous or outside the crural fascia.

REFERENCE: Last RJ: *Anatomy, Regional and Applied*, ed 6. Edinburgh, Scotland, Churchill Livingstone, 1978, pp 170-175.

A-20: An iliosacral screw that exits just anterior to the S1 body is most likely to injure which of the following structures?

1. L4 nerve root
2. L5 nerve root
3. S1 nerve root
4. S2 nerve root
5. External iliac artery

PREFERRED RESPONSE: 2

DISCUSSION: The fifth lumbar nerve root with its continuation as the lumbosacral trunk is relatively fixed to the sacral ala with fibrous connective tissue and is the structure at greatest risk along the path described. A screw that is too long and is aimed at and penetrates the sacral ala anterior to S1 or a screw aimed into the body of S1 that misses anteriorly may result in injury to the L5 nerve root. Vascular structures are also at risk, but the internal iliac vein is closer to the sacrum.

REFERENCES: Ebraheim NA, Lu J, Biyani A, Huntoon M, Yeasting RA: The relationship of lumbosacral plexus to the sacrum and the sacroiliac joint. *Am J Orthop* 1997;26:105-110.
Dietemann JL, Sick H, Wolfram-Gabel R, et al: Anatomy and computed tomography of the normal lumbosacral plexus. *Neuroradiology* 1987;29:58-68.
Kellam JF, Browner BD: Fractures of the pelvic ring, in Browner BD, Jupiter JB, Levine AM, et al (eds): *Skeletal Trauma*. Philadelphia, PA, WB Saunders, 1992, pp 849-897.

A-21: Which of the following is considered the most common complication following intramedullary nailing of a closed tibial fracture?

1. Infection
2. Nonunion
3. Malunion
4. Knee pain
5. Compartment syndrome

PREFERRED RESPONSE: 4

DISCUSSION: Knee pain has been recognized as a significant complication after tibial nailing and was first described by Court-Brown and associates. Its incidence has been reported at a rate of 40% to 56% in some studies, and it is considered a significant complication that often leads to removal of the hardware. The other complications all occur much less frequently, with infection occurring at a rate of 1% to 3%, nonunion at 2% to 5%, malunion at 2% to 5%, and compartment syndrome at a rate of 0% to 10%.

REFERENCES: Court-Brown CM, Gustilo T, Shaw AD: Knee pain after intramedullary tibial nailing: Its incidence, etiology, and outcome. *J Orthop Trauma* 1997;11:103-105.
Keating JF, Orfaly R, O'Brien PJ: Knee pain after tibial nailing. *J Orthop Trauma* 1997;11:10-13.

A-22: A patient has a swollen, tender hindfoot with focal tenderness beneath the heel after falling 12 feet. Radiographs and a CT scan are negative. An MRI scan would most likely reveal which of the following conditions?

1. Occult subcortical fracture of the calcaneus
2. Acute osteonecrosis
3. Compression of the tibial nerve (tarsal tunnel syndrome)
4. Rupture of the posterior tibial tendon
5. Rupture of the plantar fascia

PREFERRED RESPONSE: 5

DISCUSSION: Falls from a height may damage the plantar fascia near the origin on the calcaneus or in the midfascia, and an MRI scan would most likely reveal this condition. An MRI scan is unlikely to reveal a fracture not seen on a CT scan. Acute osteonecrosis (bone bruise) has not been correlated with symptoms in patients who have sustained blunt trauma to the heel. The patient's symptoms are not consistent with a tarsal tunnel syndrome, and the physical findings do not support a diagnosis of posterior tibial tendon injury.

REFERENCES: Weinstabl R, Stiskal M, Neuhold A, et al: Classifying calcaneal tendon injury according to MRI findings. *J Bone Joint Surg Br* 1991;73:683-685.
Levine AM (ed): *Orthopaedic Knowledge Update: Trauma.* Rosemont, IL, American Academy of Orthopaedic Surgeons, 1996, pp 191-209.

A-23: Which of the following treatment principles for tarsometatarsal joint (Lisfranc) injuries has resulted in improved clinical outcomes?

1. Early treatment of compartment syndrome
2. Early treatment of dorsal nerve injury
3. Closed reduction and percutaneous pin fixation
4. Open joint reduction and internal fixation
5. Rigid transarticular fixation

PREFERRED RESPONSE: 4

DISCUSSION: Restoration of joint alignment via open reduction and transarticular fixation for displaced tarsometatarsal fracture-dislocations has resulted in a clinical success rate of 70%. Fixation with screws or Kirschner wires does not appreciably change the radiographic and clinical results. There are not enough reported cases of nerve injury or untreated compartment syndrome to know if they contribute significantly to poor clinical results. There is ample evidence that early restoration of joint congruity has improved outcomes over nonanatomic treatments.

REFERENCES: Brunet JA, Wiley JJ: The late results of tarsometatarsal joint injuries. *J Bone Joint Surg Br,* 1987;69:437-440.
Arntz CT, Veith RG, Hansen ST Jr: Fractures and fracture-dislocations of the tarsometatarsal joint. *J Bone Joint Surg Am* 1988;70:173-181.

A-24: Which of the following is considered the most common cause of a poor functional prognosis after an unstable posterior pelvic ring injury?

1. Residual displacement causing a leg-length discrepancy of less than 1.0 cm
2. Persistent neurologic deficit
3. Malreduced sacroiliac joint
4. Genitourinary dysfunction
5. Fracture nonunion

PREFERRED RESPONSE: 3

DISCUSSION: It has been long recognized that the persistent malreduction of a sacroiliac (SI) dislocation leads to a high degree of debilitating pain. A study by Dujardin and associates confirms that exact reduction of pure SI lesions is critical for good functional results. Small leg-length discrepancies are generally well tolerated. Persistent neurologic deficits often are not associated with pain, and despite previous reports, have shown improvement over time. Long-term genitourinary dysfunction and fracture nonunion are uncommon.

REFERENCES: Dujardin FH, Hossenbaccus M, Duparc F, Biga N, Thomine JM: Long-term functional prognosis of posterior injuries in high-energy pelvic disruption. *J Orthop Trauma* 1998;12:145-151.
Tornetta P III, Matta JM: Outcome of operatively treated unstable posterior pelvic ring disruptions. *Clin Orthop Relat Res* 1996;329:186-193.

Answers: Trauma

A-25: The acute mortality rate after multiple trauma is most frequently related to involvement of which of the following systems?

1. Pulmonary
2. Cardiac
3. Central nervous system
4. Multiple open long-bone fractures (musculoskeletal)
5. Genitourinary

PREFERRED RESPONSE: 3

DISCUSSION: Acute mortality secondary to multiple injuries is most frequently associated with severe head injuries.

REFERENCES: Swiontkowski MF: The multiply injured patient with musculoskeletal injuries, in Rockwood CA, Green DP, Bucholz RW (eds): *Rockwood and Green's Fractures in Adults.* Philadelphia, PA, Lippincott-Raven, 1996, pp 121-157.
Copes WS, Champion HR, Sacco WJ, et al: The Injury Severity Score revisited. *J Trauma* 1988;28:69-77.

A-26: Which of the following is considered the most reliable early clinical finding for hemorrhagic shock?

1. Decreased systolic blood pressure
2. Decreased diastolic blood pressure
3. Decreased hemoglobin level
4. Low urine output
5. Tachycardia

PREFERRED RESPONSE: 5

DISCUSSION: Because there are no laboratory tests to diagnose shock, the initial treatment of hemorrhagic shock is recognizing the problem. In most patients with hemorrhagic shock, tachycardia is the earliest measurable sign. Cutaneous vasoconstriction is also an early clinical finding. A drop in systolic blood pressure is often a late finding in hemorrhagic shock. As much as 30% of circulatory blood volume can be lost prior to any change in the systolic blood pressure. In an early state of shock, diastolic blood pressure is increased because of arterial vasoconstriction, which leads to a narrow pulse pressure. A decreased hemoglobin level is an uncommon finding in an early state of hemorrhagic shock. If present, it may indicate massive hemorrhage or preexisting anemia. Blood flow to the kidneys, heart, and brain is relatively preserved in the early state of shock.

REFERENCES: Collicott PE: Initial management of the trauma patient, in Moore EE, Mattox KL, Felician DV (eds): *Trauma*, ed 2. East Norwalk, CT, Appleton & Lange, 1991, pp 114-115.
Advanced Trauma Life Support for Doctors: Student Course Manual, ed 6. Chicago, IL, American College of Surgeons, 1997, pp 89-91.

Answers: Trauma

A-27: After undergoing a closed unreamed tibial nailing, a patient is diagnosed with an isolated anterior leg compartment syndrome. However, no treatment is initiated because the patient is thought to have a nerve palsy. Which of the following findings should be present at 2 weeks when the cast is removed?

1. Drop foot and numbness in the first web space of the foot
2. Calcaneal deformity of the ankle
3. Rigid equinus deformity
4. Plantar foot numbness
5. Supple claw toes

PREFERRED RESPONSE: 1

DISCUSSION: In the acute phase, anterior leg compartment syndrome may look identical to a peroneal nerve palsy; however, with removal of the cast, the patient will most likely have a drop foot and numbness in the first web space of the foot. Calcaneal deformity of the ankle is unlikely to develop following anterior leg compartment syndrome. Deep posterior compartment syndrome most often results in a rigid equinus deformity or claw toes.

REFERENCES: Moed BR, Strom DE: Compartment syndrome after closed intramedullary nailing of the tibia: A canine model and report of two cases. *J Orthop Trauma* 1991;5:71-77.
Tischenko GJ, Goodman SB: Compartment syndrome after intramedullary nailing of the tibia. *J Bone Joint Surg Am* 1990;72:41-44.
Tornetta P III, French BG: Compartment pressures during nonreamed tibial nailing without traction. *J Orthop Trauma* 1997;11:24-27.

A-28: Which of the following nerve roots is at risk during anterior placement of the iliosacral screw in the treatment of sacroiliac disruptions?

1. L3
2. L4
3. L5
4. S1
5. S2

PREFERRED RESPONSE: 3

DISCUSSION: The L5 root exits between the L5-S1 junction and travels anterior to the sacral alar surface. A screw directed into the sacral vertebral body that is out of the bone can endanger this root.

REFERENCES: Levine AM (ed): *Orthopaedic Knowledge Update: Trauma.* Rosemont, IL, American Academy of Orthopaedic Surgeons, 1996, pp 241-248.
Matta JM, Saucedo T: Internal fixation of pelvic ring fractures. *Clin Orthop Relat Res* 1989;242:83-97.

Answers: Trauma

A-29: Which of the following CT scans will best help evaluate a calcaneal fracture?

1. 3-D reconstructions
2. Sagittal reconstructions
3. Axial and semicoronal planes
4. Sections parallel to the posterior facet of the calcaneus
5. Sections perpendicular to the anterior facet of the calcaneus

PREFERRED RESPONSE: 3

DISCUSSION: The most information is obtained with a CT scan performed in the axial and semicoronal planes. Only the surface of the bone is illustrated with 3-D reconstructions. Sagittal reconstructions are rarely of value. The semicoronal plane should be perpendicular to the posterior facet of the calcaneus, not parallel to it.

REFERENCES: Benirschke SK, Sangeorzan BJ: Extensive intra-articular fractures of the foot: Surgical management of calcaneal fractures. *Clin Orthop Relat Res* 1993;292:128-134.
Crosby LA, Fitzgibbons T: Computerized tomography scanning of acute intra-articular fractures of the calcaneus: A new classification system. *J Bone Joint Surg Am* 1990;72:852-859.
Sanders R: Trauma to the calcaneus and its tendon: Fractures of the calcaneus, in Jahss MH (ed): *Disorders of the Foot and Ankle: Medical and Surgical Management*, ed 2. Philadelphia, PA, WB Saunders, 1991, pp 2326-2354.

A-30: A patient with an acromioclavicular dislocation has a very prominent distal clavicle. Examination reveals that the deformity increases rather than reduces with an isometric shoulder shrug. Which of the following structures is most likely intact?

1. Trapezoid ligament
2. Conoid ligament
3. Acromioclavicular ligament
4. Deltoid muscle origin
5. Trapezius muscle insertion

PREFERRED RESPONSE: 5

DISCUSSION: Severely displaced acromioclavicular injuries disrupt the deltotrapezial fascia and muscular origin in addition to the ligaments (acromioclavicular and coracoclavicular or trapezoid and conoid). When the deltoid is still attached to the clavicle, an isometric shoulder shrug will tend to reduce the displacement. When the deltoid is detached but the trapezius is attached, this manuever will increase the deformity and surgery may be indicated.

REFERENCE: Weinstein DM, McCann PD, McIlveen SJ, Flatow EL, Bigliani LU: Surgical treatment of complete acromioclavicular dislocations. *Am J Sports Med* 1995;23:324-331.

A-31: Posterior sternoclavicular dislocations are most commonly associated with which of the following complications?

1. Chronic instability
2. Brachial plexus palsy
3. Pneumothorax
4. Esophageal compression
5. Tracheal compression

PREFERRED RESPONSE: 5

DISCUSSION: Posterior sternoclavicular dislocations are commonly associated with tracheal compression, which can be a life-threatening condition requiring immediate reduction. The other listed complications are less common.

REFERENCES: Brooks AL, Henning GD: Injury to the proximal clavicular epiphysis, abstracted. *J Bone Joint Surg Am* 1972;54:1347-1348.
Mooney JF III: Shoulder and arm: Pediatric aspects, in Beaty JH (ed): *Orthopaedic Knowledge Update 6*. Rosemont, IL, American Academy of Orthopaedic Surgeons, 1999, pp 255-260.

A-32: During an anterior approach to the shoulder, excessive traction on the conjoined tendon is most likely to result in loss of

1. elbow flexion.
2. shoulder flexion.
3. shoulder internal rotation.
4. shoulder abduction.
5. forearm pronation.

PREFERRED RESPONSE: 1

DISCUSSION: The musculocutaneous nerve travels through the conjoined tendon approximately 8 cm distal to the tip of the acromion. The musculocutaneous nerve innervates the biceps muscle and the brachialis muscle, both of which are responsible for elbow flexion. Shoulder flexion is facilitated by the anterior fibers of the deltoid muscle (axillary nerve) and the supraspinatus muscle (suprascapular nerve). The subscapular muscle facilitates internal rotation of the shoulder (upper and lower subscapularis nerve). Shoulder abduction is performed by the deltoid muscle (axillary nerve), and forearm pronation is facilitated by the pronator teres (median nerve).

REFERENCES: Hollinshead WH: *Anatomy for Surgeons: The Back and Limbs*, ed 3. Philadelphia, PA, Harper and Row, 1982, pp 391-393.
Hoppenfeld S, deBoer P: *Surgical Exposures in Orthopaedics: The Anatomic Approach*, ed 2. Philadelphia, PA, Lippincott-Raven, 1992, pp 2-49.

Answers: Trauma

A-33: Which of the following nerves is most commonly injured when obtaining a bone graft from the posterior ilium?

1. Lateral femoral cutaneous
2. Superior gluteal
3. Cluneal
4. L5 nerve root
5. S1 nerve root

PREFERRED RESPONSE: 3

DISCUSSION: Cutaneous sensation to the buttock is provided by the superior, middle, and inferior cluneal nerves. The superior cluneal nerves are the lateral branches of the dorsal rami of the upper three lumbar nerves and penetrate deep fascia just proximal to the iliac crest. They pass distally to the skin of the buttock and will be injured if the exposure extends more than 8 cm anterolateral to the posterior superior iliac spine. The lateral femoral cutaneous nerve can be injured in an anterior ilium bone graft. The superior gluteal nerve or even the sciatic nerve can be injured if bone is removed from the sciatic notch or dissection is not kept subperiosteal; however, the rate of injury is far less than cluneal nerve injury. The L5 and S1 nerve roots are anterior and can be injured if the inner table bone is harvested and the dissection is not kept subperiosteal or is too medial; however, the rate of injury still is far less than cluneal nerve injury.

REFERENCES: Hoppenfeld S, deBoer P: *Surgical Exposures in Orthopaedics: The Anatomic Approach.* Philadelphia, PA, JB Lippincott, 1984, pp 295-297.
Hollinshead WH: *Textbook of Anatomy,* ed 3. Hagerstown, MD, Harper and Row, 1974, p 379.
Last RJ: *Anatomy: Regional and Applied,* ed 6. London, England, Churchill Livingstone, 1978, p 23.
Ebraheim NA, Elgafy H, Xu R: Bone-graft harvesting from iliac and fibular donor sites: Techniques and complications. *J Am Acad Orthop Surg* 2001;9:210-218.

A-34: Which of the following ligaments is most commonly involved in posterolateral rotatory instability of the elbow?

1. Annular
2. Lateral ulnar collateral
3. Anterior band of the medial collateral
4. Radial part of the lateral collateral
5. Posterior capsular

PREFERRED RESPONSE: 2

(continued on next page)

Answers: Trauma

(A-34: *continued*)

DISCUSSION: Recurrent posterolateral rotatory instability of the elbow is difficult to diagnose. Such instability can be demonstrated only by the lateral pivot-shift test. The cause for this condition is laxity of the ulnar part of the lateral collateral ligament, which allows a transient rotatory subluxation of the ulnohumeral joint and a secondary dislocation of the radiohumeral joint. The annular ligament remains intact, so the radioulnar joint does not dislocate. Treatment consists of surgical reconstruction of the lax ulnar part of the lateral collateral ligament. The anterior band is the most important part of the medial collateral ligament which is lax in valgus instability of the elbow.

REFERENCES: Morrey BF: Acute and chronic instability of the elbow. *J Am Acad Orthop Surg* 1996;4:117-128.
O'Driscoll SW, Bell DF, Morrey BF: Posterolateral rotatory instability of the elbow. *J Bone Joint Surg Am* 1991;73:440-446.

A-35: A 28-year-old man sustains the closed injury shown in Figures 6A through 6C after falling 8 feet while rock climbing. Management should consist of

1. open reduction and internal fixation via an anteromedial arthrotomy.
2. talectomy.
3. primary tibiotalocalcaneal arthrodesis.
4. open reduction and internal fixation via a medial malleolar osteotomy and limited anterior lateral arthrotomy.
5. closed reduction and a non-weight-bearing cast.

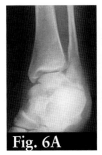
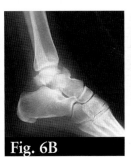
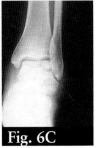

Fig. 6A   Fig. 6B   Fig. 6C

PREFERRED RESPONSE: 4

DISCUSSION: The radiographs show a comminuted talar body fracture. The goal of treatment is to minimize the risks of posttraumatic arthrosis of the ankle and subtalar joint and to maintain vascularity. Open reduction and internal fixation with an attempt at anatomic reduction will lead to improved outcomes. Attempting to repair this fracture via an arthrotomy only is extremely difficult, and the addition of a medial malleolar osteotomy is warranted. A limited anterior lateral arthrotomy with minimal soft-tissue stripping may assist with fixation of anterior-lateral and lateral fragments and allow better assessment of reduction of the major fracture line. Nonsurgical care would lead to inadequate reduction and increased risk of both ankle and hindfoot arthrosis. Talectomy and primary ankle and hindfoot arthrodesis should not be performed as primary surgical reconstructive options in this closed injury pattern.

REFERENCES: Sanders R: Fractures and fracture-dislocations of the talus, in Coughlin MJ, Mann RA (eds): *Surgery of the Foot and Ankle*, ed 7. St Louis, MO, Mosby, 1999, pp 1465-1518.
Grob D, Simpson LA, Weber BG, Bray T: Operative treatment of displaced talus fractures. *Clin Orthop Relat Res* 1985;199:88-96.

Answers: Trauma

A-36: A 20-year-old man sustains the injury shown in Figures 7A and 7B in a motorcycle accident. In addition to a prompt closed reduction, his outcome might be optimized by

1. a subtalar arthrodesis.
2. screw fixation of the talar neck.
3. repair of the medial subtalar capsule.
4. temporary transarticular pin fixation.
5. evaluation for and excision or fixation of osteochondral fractures.

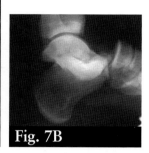

Fig. 7A   Fig. 7B

PREFERRED RESPONSE: 5

DISCUSSION: Lateral subtalar dislocations, which are less common than medial subtalar dislocations, are high-energy injuries that are frequently associated with small osteochondral fractures. It is generally recommended that large fragments be internally fixed, and small fragments entrapped within the joint be excised. Although arthrosis frequently occurs after this injury and is the most common long-term complication, primary subtalar arthrodesis is not indicated. A talar neck fracture is not evident on the radiographs, and lateral subtalar dislocation usually does not lead to instability.

REFERENCE: Saltzman C, Marsh JL: Hindfoot dislocations: When are they not benign? *J Am Acad Orthop Surg* 1997;5:192-198.

A-37: Which of the following types of displaced posterior pelvic disruptions must undergo anatomic reduction and internal fixation to ensure the best clinical outcome?

1. Sacral fracture through the foramen
2. Sacral fracture through the ala
3. Sacroiliac joint dislocation
4. Reverse fracture-dislocation of the sacroiliac joint through the ilium
5. Iliac wing fracture

PREFERRED RESPONSE: 3

DISCUSSION: Although all of the above displaced injuries require reduction, the sacroiliac joint dislocation is a ligamentous injury. Without fixation, healing is unlikely and the result will be a painful dislocation. Both Holdsworth and Tile showed that the sacroiliac joint must be reduced anatomically and stabilized. The injuries through bone will unite fairly rapidly and, if reduced and stabilized with traction or external fixation, will generally result in an acceptable outcome unless modified by other associated problems such as neurologic injury.

REFERENCES: Tile M: *Fractures of the Pelvis and the Acetabulum.* Baltimore, MD, Williams and Wilkins, 1995.
Holdsworth F W: Dislocation and fracture dislocation of the pelvis. *J Bone Joint Surg Br* 1948;30:461-465.
Henderson RC: The long-term results of nonoperatively treated major pelvic disruptions. *J Orthop Trauma* 1989;3:41-47.

A-38: A 28-year-old woman who is training for the New York Marathon reports pain in the postero-medial aspect of her right ankle. Examination reveals tenderness just posterior to the medial malleolus. Radiographs are normal. An MRI scan is shown in Figure 8. What is the most likely diagnosis?

1. Posterior tibial tendinitis
2. Osteoid osteoma
3. Posterior ankle impingement
4. Tibial stress fracture
5. Flexor hallucis longus tendinitis

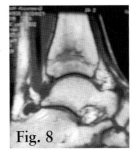

Fig. 8

PREFERRED RESPONSE: 4

DISCUSSION: Any of the above conditions is credible with a limited history. The MRI scan unequivo-cally shows the stress fracture in the distal tibia. Most tibial stress fractures can be managed with rest and immobilization.

REFERENCES: Boden BP, Osbahr DC: High risk stress fractures: Evaluation and treatment. *J Am Acad Orthop Surg* 2000;8:344-353.
Lee JK, Yao L: Stress fractures: MR imaging. *Radiology* 1988;169:217-220.

A-39: A 10-year-old boy has a painful, swollen knee after falling off his bicycle. Examination reveals that the knee is held in 45° of flexion, and any attempt to actively or passively extend the knee produces pain and muscle spasms. A lateral radiograph is shown in Figure 9. What is the most likely diagnosis?

1. Patellar sleeve fracture
2. Avulsion of the tibial tubercle
3. Avulsion of the anterior tibial spine
4. Osteochondral fracture of the femoral condyle
5. Osteochondral fracture of the patella

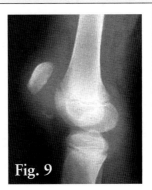

Fig. 9

PREFERRED RESPONSE: 1

DISCUSSION: This is a typical patellar sleeve fracture. The patellar tendon avulses a portion of the distal bony patella, along with the retinaculum and articular cartilage from the inferior pole of the patella. It is common in children between ages 8 and 10 years. Anatomic reduction and repair of the extensor mechanism are mandatory to reestablish full knee extension.

REFERENCES: Houghton GR, Ackroyd CE: Sleeve fractures of the patella in children: A report of three cases. *J Bone Joint Surg Br* 1979;61:165-168.
Wu CD, Huang SC, Liu TK: Sleeve fracture of the patella in children: A report of five cases. *Am J Sports Med* 1991;19:525-528.

Answers: Trauma

A-40: Which of the following factors is considered most important when assessing an ankle fracture for surgical treatment?

1. Level of the fibular fracture
2. Displacement of the fibular fracture
3. Size of the posterior malleolus
4. Position of the talus in the mortise
5. Rupture of the deltoid ligament

PREFERRED RESPONSE: 4

DISCUSSION: Although all of these factors may influence the decision to perform surgery, the most important is the position of the talus in the mortise. The goal of treatment of ankle fractures is to maintain the talus centered in the mortise. If it is in this position, the other factors do not enter into the decision to intervene surgically.

REFERENCES: Stover MD, Kellam JF: Articular fractures: Principles, in Ruedi TP, Murphy WM (eds): *AO Principles of Fracture Management*. Stuttgart, Thieme, 2000, pp 105-119.
Hahn DM, Colton CL: Malleolar fractures, in Ruedi TP, Murphy WM (eds): *AO Principles of Fracture Management*. Stuttgart, Thieme, 2000, pp 559-581.
Tile M: Fractures of the ankle, in Schatzker J, Tile M (eds): *Rationale of Operative Fracture Care*, ed 2. Berlin, Springer-Verlag, 1998, pp 523-561.

A-41: A 35-year-old woman who underwent open reduction and internal fixation of a calcaneal fracture 14 months ago reports pain that has failed to respond to nonsurgical management. Examination reveals limited painful subtalar motion but no hindfoot deformity. A lateral radiograph is shown in Figure 10. Surgical reconstruction is best accomplished with

1. calcaneal osteotomy.
2. subtalar joint arthrodesis.
3. triple arthrodesis.
4. pantalar arthrodesis.
5. distraction bone block arthrodesis.

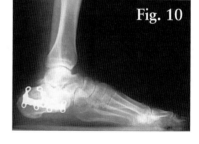

Fig. 10

PREFERRED RESPONSE: 2

DISCUSSION: The patient has posttraumatic subtalar joint arthrosis that developed following a calcaneal fracture. Because there is no hindfoot deformity, in situ subtalar joint arthrodesis is the treatment of choice. Calcaneal osteotomy or distraction bone block arthrodesis is beneficial in patients with severe talar dorsiflexion or malunion of the calcaneal body. Triple arthrodesis is not warranted without changes at the transverse tarsal joint, and typically even with injury into the calcaneocuboid joint, this joint is often asymptomatic. Pantalar arthrodesis is not indicated because the pathology is occurring at the subtalar joint and not in the ankle joint.

(continued on next page)

(A-41: *continued*)

REFERENCES: Sanders R: Fractures and fracture-dislocations of the calcaneus, in Coughlin MJ, Mann RA (eds): *Surgery of the Foot and Ankle,* ed 7. St Louis, MO, Mosby, 1999, pp 1422-1464.
Juliano TJ, Myerson MS: Fractures of the hindfoot, in Myerson MS (ed): *Foot and Ankle Disorders.* Philadelphia, PA, WB Saunders, 2000, pp 1297-1340.
Chandler JT, Bonar SK, Anderson RB, Davis WH: Results of in situ subtalar arthrodesis for late sequelae of calcaneus fractures. *Foot Ankle Int* 1999;20:18-24.

A-42: After stabilizing a bimalleolar ankle fracture with a plate and lag screws for the fibula and two interfragmental compression screws for the medial malleolus, a syndesmosis screw is indicated in which of the following situations?

1. In all suprasyndesmotic fibular fractures
2. In all transsyndesmotic fibular fractures
3. When there is increased medial clear space with external rotation stress
4. If the deltoid ligament is ruptured
5. If the posterior malleolus is fractured

PREFERRED RESPONSE: 3

DISCUSSION: It is imperative to recognize the need for a position screw (syndesmosis screw) to hold the syndesmosis in proper alignment when surgically stabilizing an ankle fracture. Although many different fracture patterns are suspicious for a disrupted syndesmosis, the only sure way to assess the syndesmosis is to stress it with abduction and external rotation of the talus and attempt to displace the fibula from the incisura fibularis. Under fluoroscopy, the talus will move laterally and displace the fibula, show a valgus talar tilt, or show an increase in the medial clear space. If any or all of these signs occur, a syndesmosis screw is inserted after making sure that the fibula is reduced into the incisura fibularis. This screw may traverse three or four cortices but must not act as a lag screw. It usually is inserted with the ankle in maximal dorsiflexion, although this is probably not necessary because it is almost impossible to over-compress the syndesmosis. The diameter of the screw does not make any difference. It may or may not be removed, but not before 3 months.

REFERENCES: Tornetta P III, Spoo JE, Reynolds FA, Lee C: Overtightening of the ankle syndesmosis: Is it really possible? *J Bone Joint Surg Am* 2001;83:489-492.
Stover MD, Kellam JF: Articular fractures: Principles, in Ruedi TP, Murphy WM (eds): *AO Principles of Fracture Management.* Stuttgart, Thieme, 2000, pp 105-119.
Hahn DM, Colton CL: Malleolar fractures, in Ruedi TP, Murphy WM (eds): *AO Principles of Fracture Management.* Stuttgart, Thieme, 2000, pp 559-581.
Tile M: Fractures of the ankle, in Schatzker J, Tile M (eds): *Rationale of Operative Fracture Care,* ed 2. Berlin, Springer-Verlag, 1998, pp 523-561.

Answers: Trauma

A-43: The primary stabilizer to valgus stress in the elbow is the

1. radiocapitellar joint.
2. anterior oblique band of the medial collateral ligament.
3. transverse band of the medial collateral ligament.
4. posterior oblique band of the medial collateral ligament.
5. ulnar trochlear articulation.

PREFERRED RESPONSE: 2

DISCUSSION: The anterior oblique band of the medial collateral ligament is the primary stabilizer to valgus stress, whereas the radiocapitellar joint provides secondary stability.

REFERENCE: Bennett JB: Articular injuries in the athlete, in Morrey BF (ed): *The Elbow and Its Disorders*, ed 2. Philadelphia, PA, WB Saunders, 1993, p 581.

A-44: A 32-year-old man sustains an iliac wing fracture and a contralateral femur fracture. Twelve hours later he has shortness of breath with tachypnea, hypoxia, and confusion. A chest radiograph is normal. What is the most likely diagnosis?

1. Fat emboli syndrome
2. Adult respiratory distress syndrome
3. Pulmonary embolus
4. Tension pneumothorax
5. Sepsis

PREFERRED RESPONSE: 1

DISCUSSION: A normal radiograph rules out a pneumothorax and adult respiratory distress syndrome. Sepsis usually does not occur during the first several days after nonpenetrating trauma. A pulmonary embolus is possible, but usually does not occur so early in a patient's course. The most likely diagnosis is fat emboli syndrome. The clinical picture includes the most common findings after fat emboli, and the patient has a pelvic fracture and a femur fracture, both of which have been associated with fat emboli. Symptoms of fat emboli have been found in up to 10% of patients with multiple fractures. The incidence of clinically significant fat emboli has been significantly decreased with the use of early skeletal fixation.

REFERENCES: Bone L, Bucholz R: The management of fractures in the patient with multiple trauma. *J Bone Joint Surg Am* 1986;68:945-949.
Chan KM, Tham KT, Chiu HS, et al: Post-traumatic fat embolism: Its clinical and subclinical presentations. *J Trauma* 1984;24:45-49.

Answers: Trauma

A-45: The nerve that traverses the triangular interval (bounded by the teres major superiorly, the long head of the triceps medially, and the humeral shaft laterally) supplies which of the following muscles?

1. Brachioradialis
2. Flexor pollicis longus
3. Deltoid
4. Teres major
5. Pronator teres

PREFERRED RESPONSE: 1

DISCUSSION: The radial nerve and profunda brachii artery gain access to the posterior aspect of the arm through the triangular interval. The radial nerve supplies the brachioradialis.

REFERENCE: Netter FH: *Atlas of Human Anatomy*. Summit, NJ, Ciba-Geigy Corp, 1989, plate 401.

A-46: A 24-year-old woman has a spleen laceration and hypotension. Radiographs reveal a pulmonary contusion and a displaced mid-diaphyseal fracture of the femur. The trauma surgeon clears the patient for stabilization of the femoral fracture. What technique will offer the least potential for initial complications?

1. External fixation
2. Plate fixation
3. Unreamed unlocked intramedullary nailing
4. Reamed statically locked intramedullary nailing
5. Reamed unlocked nailing

PREFERRED RESPONSE: 1

DISCUSSION: A concern in the multiply injured patient who has a pulmonary contusion is the potential for further pulmonary compromise because of embolization of marrow, blood clot, or fat during manipulation of the medullary canal. Recent evidence has shown that the presence of a lung injury is the most important determining factor in future deterioration. However, despite the lung injury and its potential consequences, this patient's femur fracture needs stabilization. Because damage control in the multiply injured patient requires a technique that can be performed rapidly and consistently, the treatment of choice is application of an external fixator. By placing two pins above and below the fracture and with longitudinal traction, the fracture is quickly realigned and stabilized. This allows the patient to be resuscitated and treated at a later date when definitive management of the fracture can be carried out. There is little difference between plate fixation and intramedullary nailing.

(continued on next page)

Answers: Trauma

(A-46: *continued*)

REFERENCES: Bosse MJ, MacKenzie EJ, Riemer BL, et al: Adult respiratory distress syndrome, pneumonia, and mortality following thoracic injury and a femoral fracture treated with either intramedullary nailing with reaming or with a plate: A comparative study. *J Bone Joint Surg Am* 1997;79:799-809.
Scalea TM, Boswell SA, Scott JD, Mitchell KA, Kramer ME, Pollak AN: External fixation as a bridge to intramedullary nailing for patients with multiple injuries and with femur fractures: Damage control orthopedics. *J Trauma* 2000;48:613-623.
Pape HC, Auf'm'Kolk M, Puffrath T, et al: Primary intramedullary femur fixation in multiple trauma patients with associated lung contusion: A cause of posttraumatic ARDS? *J Trauma* 1993;34:540-548.

A-47: The use of nasotracheal intubation for airway management is contraindicated in the acute multiply injured patient when the patient has

1. suspected cervical spine trauma.
2. head injuries and spontaneous respirations.
3. respiratory arrest.
4. a need for prolonged ventilatory support.
5. a hemopneumothorax.

PREFERRED RESPONSE: 3

DISCUSSION: The use of nasotracheal intubation is less desirable in patients with respiratory arrest because placement of the tube is most reliable when the patient is breathing. Nasotracheal intubation is advantageous in patients with suspected cervical spine trauma because it does not require hyperextension of the neck. A nasotracheal tube may be more comfortable than an orally placed tube because it is fixed at several points and moves less freely within the larynx, subglottic area, and trachea. The presence of a hemothorax or pneumothorax does not affect the choice of airway control but does require placement of a chest tube.

REFERENCES: Colice GL: Prolonged intubation versus tracheostomy in the adult. *J Intern Care Med* 1987;2:85.
Shackford S: Spine injury in the polytrauma patient: General surgical and orthopaedic considerations, in Levine AM, Eismont FJ, Garfin S, Zigler JE (eds): *Spine Trauma.* Philadelphia, PA, WB Saunders, 1998, pp 9-15.

A-48: A 26-year-old man is brought to the emergency department unresponsive and intubated after being found lying on the side of the road. He has a Glasgow Coma Scale score of 6. A chest tube has been inserted on the right side of the chest for a pneumothorax. An abdominal CT scan reveals a small liver laceration and minimal intraperitoneal hematoma. A pneumatic antishock garment (PASG) is on but not inflated. He has bilateral tibia fractures. A pelvic CT scan shows an anterior minimally displaced left sacral ala fracture and left superior and inferior rami fractures. He has received 2 L of saline solution and 4 units of blood but remains hemodynamically unstable. What is the next most appropriate step in management?

1. Inflation of the abdominal portion of the PASG
2. Application of a pelvic clamp
3. Application of a pelvic external fixator
4. Rapid infusion of 4 more units of blood
5. Angiography and embolization

PREFERRED RESPONSE: 5

DISCUSSION: There is no identifiable thoracic, abdominal, or long bone source of ongoing bleeding. The patient has a lateral compression Burgess-Young type I pelvic ring injury. This injury does not increase the pelvic volume because it is not unstable in external rotation. Application of a PASG, a pelvic clamp, or an external fixator may be helpful if the patient has a pelvic injury that is unstable in external rotation or translation but would be of little use in this injury pattern. Persistent hemodynamic instability after administration of 4 units of blood is the decision point where most authors would recommend angiography and embolization. If the pelvis is unstable in external rotation or translation, inflation of the PASG trousers or application of an external fixator is recommended before angiography. Attributing the hemodynamic instability to the head injury before ruling out the pelvis as a source is not indicated.

REFERENCES: Burgess AR, Eastridge BJ, Young JW, et al: Pelvic ring disruptions: Effective classification system and treatment protocols. *J Trauma* 1990;30:848-856.
Evers BM, Cryer HM, Miller FB: Pelvic fracture hemorrhage: Priorities in management. *Arch Surg* 1989;124:422-424.
Flint L, Babikian G, Anders M, Rodriguez J, Steinberg S: Definitive control of mortality from severe pelvic fracture. *Ann Surg* 1990;211:703-707.

Answers: Trauma

A-49: Figure 11 shows the radiograph of a 23-year-old man who has severe right shoulder pain after his motorcyle hit a bridge guardrail. He is neurologically intact. Nonsurgical management will most likely result in

1. nonunion of the clavicle or glenoid.
2. thoracic outlet syndrome.
3. less than 50% range of motion compared with the contralateral shoulder.
4. less than 50% strength compared with the contralateral shoulder.
5. high patient satisfaction and good shoulder function.

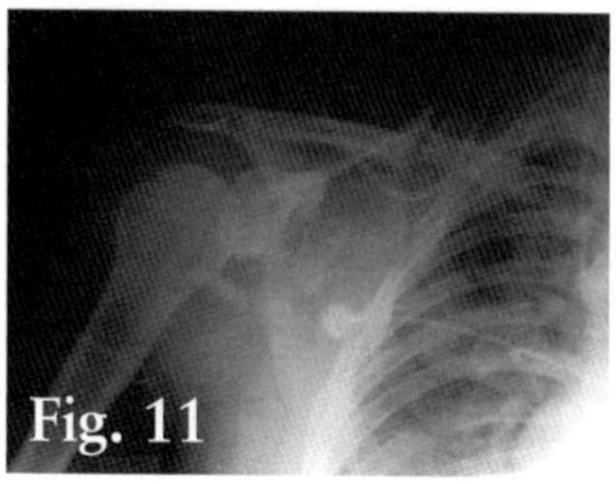

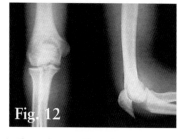
Fig. 11

PREFERRED RESPONSE: 5

DISCUSSION: Internal fixation of the clavicle, glenoid, or both has been recommended for fractures of the clavicle and glenoid neck (floating shoulders). Recently, the inherent instability of these dual fractures has been questioned in a biomechanical model without further disruption of the coracoclavicular or acromioclavicular ligamentous structures. Nonsurgical management of the majority of combined scapular/glenoid fractures in patients with less than 10 mm of displacement has resulted in excellent shoulder function and will most likely achieve an excellent result in this patient.

REFERENCES: Egol KA, Connor PM, Karunakar MA, Sims SH, Bosse MJ, Kellam JF: The floating shoulder: Clinical and functional results. *J Bone Joint Surg Am* 2001;83:1188-1194.
Williams GR Jr, Naranja J, Klimkiewicz J, et al: The floating shoulder: A biomechanical basis for classification and management. *J Bone Joint Surg Am* 2001;83:1182-1187.
Edwards SG, Whittle AP, Wood GW: Nonoperative treatment of ipsilateral fractures of the scapular and clavicle. *J Bone Joint Surg Am* 2000;82:774-779.

A-50: A left-handed 23-year-old man who fell 5 feet from a ladder onto his left elbow sustained the closed injury shown in Figure 12. Management should consist of

1. percutaneous pin fixation.
2. a percutaneous 6.5-mm screw.
3. long arm casting in flexion.
4. open reduction and internal fixation with a tension band plate.
5. closed reduction and long arm casting in extension.

Fig. 12

PREFERRED RESPONSE: 4

DISCUSSION: The radiographs reveal a displaced olecranon fracture. To maximize joint congruity of this intra-articular injury, open reduction and internal fixation is the treatment of choice. A tension band plate will assist with maintenance of the reduction and may aid in early range of motion because injuries to the elbow are prone to stiffness. The oblique fracture line is particularly well suited to plate fixation. Percutaneous pin fixation is unlikely to achieve anatomic joint reduction that can be obtained with open means. External immobilization will not accomplish joint reduction and will most likely lead to a non-union.

(continued on next page)

(A-50: *continued*)

REFERENCES: Hotchkiss RN: Fractures and dislocations of the elbow, in Rockwood CA Jr, Green DP, Bucholz RW, Heckman JD (eds): *Rockwood and Green's Fractures in Adults*, ed 4. Philadelphia, PA, Lippincott-Raven, 1996, pp 929-1024.
Murphy DF, Greene WB, Gilbert JA, Dameron TB Jr: Displaced olecranon fractures in adults: Biomechanical analysis of fixation methods. *Clin Orthop Relat Res* 1987;224:210-214.
Hume MC, Wiss DA: Olecranon fractures: A clinical and radiographic comparison of tension band wiring and plate fixation. *Clin Orthop Relat Res* 1992;285:229-235.

A-51: Which of the following is a long-term complication of ankle arthrodesis for posttraumatic arthritis?

1. Progressive limb-length discrepancy
2. Contralateral ankle arthritis
3. Ipsilateral hindfoot and midfoot arthritis
4. Ipsilateral knee arthritis
5. Talar osteonecrosis

PREFERRED RESPONSE: 3

DISCUSSION: Ankle arthrodesis for posttraumatic ankle arthrosis provides reliable pain relief. However, the long-term sequela of joint arthrodesis is the development of arthrosis in the surrounding joints. Over time, following ankle arthrodesis, the ipsilateral hindfoot and midfoot joints show signs of joint space wear, and this may be symptomatic. With a stable ankle arthrodesis, progressive limb-length discrepancy or talar osteonecrosis is not expected. Ankle arthrodesis has not been definitively linked to ipsilateral knee arthritis or contralateral ankle arthritis.

REFERENCES: Coester LM, Saltzman CL, Leupold J, Pontarelli W: Long-term results following ankle arthrodesis for post-traumatic arthritis. *J Bone Joint Surg Am* 2001;83:219-228.
Mazur JM, Schwartz E, Simon SR: Ankle arthrodesis: Long-term follow-up with gait analysis. *J Bone Joint Surg Am* 1979;61:964-975.

A-52: In displaced calcaneal fractures, what fragment is the only one that remains in its anatomic position?

1. Posterior tubercle
2. Posterior articular facet
3. Anterior process
4. Sustentaculum tali
5. Lateral wall

PREFERRED RESPONSE: 4

(continued on next page)

(A-52: *continued*)

DISCUSSION: The sustentaculum tali remains in its anatomic position because of its supporting ligamentous structures. This provides the key to the reconstruction of the calcaneus. The posterior facet is reduced to the sustentaculum tali and then fixed to it for stability. All of the other components of the calcaneus are then reduced to this complex.

REFERENCES: Sanders R: Displaced intra-articular fractures of the calcaneus. *J Bone Joint Surg Am* 2000;82:225-250.
Eastwood DM, Gregg PJ, Atkins RM: Intra-articular fractures of the calcaneum: Part I. Pathological anatomy and classification. *J Bone Joint Surg Br* 1993;75:183-188.
Eastwood DM, Langkamer VG, Atkins RM: Intra-articular fractures of the calcaneum: Part II. Open reduction and internal fixation by the extended lateral transcalcaneal approach. *J Bone Joint Surg Br* 1993;75:189-195.

A-53: What is the most common clinically significant preventable complication secondary to the treatment of a displaced talar neck fracture?

1. Osteonecrosis
2. Nonunion
3. Malunion
4. Infection
5. Osteoarthritis of the ankle joint

PREFERRED RESPONSE: 3

DISCUSSION: The most important consequence of a displaced talar neck fracture after closed or open treatment is malunion. Because displacement of the talar neck is associated with displacement of the subtalar joint, any malunion leads to intra-articular incongruity or malalignment of the subtalar joint. Varus malunion is common when there is comminution of the medial talar neck. This results in pain, osteoarthritis, and hindfoot deformity that requires further treatment. Because of these complications, it is imperative that all displaced talar neck fractures are reduced anatomically; fragmented fractures may require bone grafting to maintain the length and rotation of the neck.

REFERENCES: Tile M: Fractures of the talus, in Schatzker J, Tile M (eds): *Rationale of Operative Fracture Care*, ed 2. Berlin, Springer-Verlag, 1996, pp 563-588.
Daniels TR, Smith JW, Ross TI: Varus malalignment of the talar neck: Its effect on the position of the foot and on subtalar motion. *J Bone Joint Surg Am* 1996;78:1559-1567.
Raaymakers EL: Complications of talar fractures, in Tscherne H, Schatzker J (eds): *Major Fractures of the Pilon, the Talus, and Calcaneus: Current Concepts of Treatment.* Berlin, Springer-Verlag, 1993, pp 137-142.

Answers: Trauma

A-54: Figure 13 shows the radiograph of an 8-year-old boy who has a swollen forearm after falling out of a tree. Examination reveals that all three nerves are functionally intact, and there is no evidence of circulatory embarrassment. Management should consist of

1. open reduction of both the radius and ulna with plate and screw fixation.
2. closed reduction and a long arm cast, with the elbow in 90° of flexion and the forearm in neutral rotation.
3. closed reduction and a long arm cast, with the elbow in 120° of flexion and the forearm in full supination.
4. closed reduction and a long arm cast, with the elbow extended and the forearm pronated.
5. closed reduction and intramedullary pin fixation of both the radius and ulna.

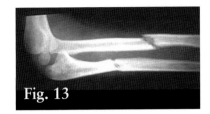

Fig. 13

PREFERRED RESPONSE: 5

DISCUSSION: The patient has a Bado type IV Monteggia lesion. It involves dislocation of the radial head and fractures of both the radial and ulnar shafts. These fractures are very difficult to manage by closed reduction alone. The radial and ulnar shafts first have to be stabilized surgically to give a lever arm to reduce the radial head. In this age group, intramedullary pins are easy to insert percutaneously and cause less tissue trauma than plates and screws. In these types of injuries, the focus is often on the forearm fracture; the radial head dislocation may not be appreciated, as was the case with this patient.

REFERENCES: Gibson WK, Timperlake RW: Operative treatment of a type IV Monteggia fracture-dislocation in a child. *J Bone Joint Surg Br* 1992;74:780-781.
Stanley EA, DeLaGarza JF: Part IV: Monteggia fracture. Dislocations in children, in Rockwood CA Jr, Wilkins KE, Beaty JH (eds): *Fractures in Children*, ed 4. Philadelphia, PA, Lippincott-Raven, 1996, vol 3, pp 576-577.

A-55: An 18-year-old man has a simple oblique fracture of the humeral shaft that requires surgical stabilization to maintain reduction and facilitate mobilization. Which of the following methods will provide the best outcome?

1. Unreamed intramedullary nail
2. Reamed statically locked intramedullary nail
3. External fixation
4. Plate fixation and interfragmentary compression
5. Bridge plate stabilization

PREFERRED RESPONSE: 4

(continued on next page)

Answers: Trauma

(A-55: *continued*)

DISCUSSION: The patient has a simple fracture pattern that can be reduced anatomically and stabilized with absolute stability by interfragmental compression and protection plating. This will guarantee a 95% to 98% union rate with no radial nerve palsy. Intramedullary nailing does not equal these results in a simple fracture pattern in the humerus. Bridge plating is indicated for multifragmented fracture patterns when anatomic reduction and absolute stability cannot be achieved. External fixation is reserved for severe open fractures.

REFERENCES: Chapman JR, Henley MP, Agel J, Benca PJ: Randomized prospective study of humeral shaft fracture fixation: Intramedullary nails versus plates. *J Orthop Trauma* 2000;14:162-166.
Farragos AF, Schemitsch EH, McKee MD: Complications of intramedullary nailing for fractures of the humeral shaft: A review. *J Orthop Trauma* 1999;13:258-267.
Modabber M, Jupiter JB: Operative management of diaphyseal fractures of the humerus: Plate versus nail. *Clin Orthop Relat Res* 1998;347:93-104.

A-56: Injury to which of the following structures has been reported following iliac crest bone graft harvest?

1. Superior gluteal artery from an anterior crest harvest
2. Superior cluneal nerve from an anterior crest harvest
3. Inferior gluteal artery from a posterior crest harvest
4. Ilioinguinal nerve from a posterior crest harvest
5. Lateral femoral cutaneous nerve from an anterior crest harvest

PREFERRED RESPONSE: 5

DISCUSSION: Injury to the lateral femoral cutaneous nerve and the ilioinguinal nerve have both been described with an anterior iliac crest bone graft harvest. The lateral femoral cutaneous nerve may be injured from retraction after elevating the iliacus muscle or from direct injury when the nerve actually courses over the crest. A posterior crest harvest can injure the superior gluteal artery if a surgical instrument violates the sciatic notch. Injury to the inferior gluteal artery has not been described; it leaves the pelvis below the piriformis muscle belly and should not be at risk even with a violation of the sciatic notch. Injury to the ilioinguinal nerve has been reported from vigorous retraction of the iliacus muscle after exposing the inner table of the anterior ilium. Cluneal nerve injury may occur with posterior crest harvest, particularly if the skin incision is horizontal or extends more than 8 cm superolateral from the posterior superior iliac spine.

REFERENCES: Kurz LT, Garfin SR, Booth RE Jr: Iliac bone grafting: Techniques and complications of harvesting, in Garfin SR (ed): *Complications of Spine Surgery.* Baltimore, MD, Williams and Wilkins, 1989, pp 323-341.
Anderson JE: *Grant's Atlas of Anatomy,* ed 7. Baltimore, MD, Williams and Wilkins, 1978, pp 4-33 to 4-34.

Answers: Trauma

A-57: A 17-year-old patient sustains a supracondylar/intercondylar humerus fracture and examination reveals a complete motor and sensory ulnar nerve palsy. At surgery for internal fixation, the nerve is found to be contused but in continuity. In the early postoperative period, examination reveals a mild flexion deformity of the ulnar two digits "clawing." At 10 weeks after surgery, the patient's mother reports that the clawing deformity is progressively worsening. What is the next most appropriate step in management?

1. Surgical exploration of the ulnar nerve
2. Hardware removal
3. Emergent office evaluation
4. Reassurance of the mother and patient
5. Tendon transfers to restore intrinsic function

PREFERRED RESPONSE: 4

DISCUSSION: In children and adults, the ulnar nerve is not infrequently injured with supracondylar fractures and subsequent treatment. A "claw" hand results from tendon imbalance, which is the result of an ulnar nerve deficit. A "high" ulnar nerve palsy shows a lesser "claw" deformity because the long flexor digitorum pollicis (FDP) to the little finger and to a lesser extent the ring finger is weak. A "low" ulnar nerve palsy shows more deformity because the FDP action is unopposed and the relative deformity is worse. The primary extensors of the interphalangeal joints and flexors of the metacarpophalangeal joints (the sites of the deformity) are the ulnar nerve-innervated intrinsic muscles. Paradoxically, as a high ulnar nerve palsy re-innervates, the "clawing" worsens as the FDP recovers before the intrinsics. Neither surgery nor emergent evaluation is indicated.

REFERENCES: Smith RJ: Balance and kinetics of the fingers under normal and pathological conditions. *Clin Orthop Relat Res* 1974;104:92-111.
Ring D, Jupiter JB, Gulotta L: Articular fractures of the distal part of the humerus. *J Bone Joint Surg Am* 2003;85:232-238.

A-58: A 23-year-old man is seen in your office after crashing his bicycle in a regional semipro race 2 days ago. Immediately after the crash, he was taken to the emergency department where he was diagnosed with a right clavicle fracture and placed in a sling. He is right hand dominant. Examination reveals no shortness of breath and he is neurovascularly intact. He has an obvious deformity of the clavicle, but the skin is intact and there is no evidence of an open fracture. A radiograph is shown in Figure 14. What should he be told about his treatment options?

1. Surgical and nonsurgical treatment programs have similar rates of nonunion.
2. Surgical treatment does not reduce the time to radiographic union.
3. Patients who are age 18 to 25 years have an increased risk of nonunion.
4. Fracture displacement is not a risk factor in developing a nonunion.
5. The most common complication of surgical treatment is related to the hardware.

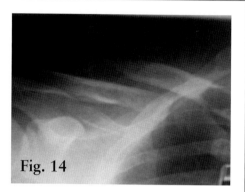
Fig. 14

PREFERRED RESPONSE: 5

DISCUSSION: The patient sustained a displaced, midshaft clavicular fracture. The radiograph reveals displacement and no opposition of the fracture fragments. Surgical stabilization of this fracture pattern has been shown to reduce the occurrence of nonunion and reduce radiographic healing time. Risk factors for developing a nonunion include advancing age, displacement of the fracture, and the presence of comminution. The most common complication of surgical stabilization is hardware related.

REFERENCES: Robinson CM, Court-Brown CM, McQueen MM, Wakefield AE: Estimating the risk of nonunion following nonoperative treatment of a clavicular fracture. *J Bone Joint Surg Am* 2005;87:676-677.

Canadian Orthopaedic Trauma Society: Nonoperative treatment compared with plate fixation of displaced midshaft clavicular fractures. *J Bone Joint Surg Am* 2007;89:1-10.

A-59: A 13-year-old hockey player reports a 1-week history of left medial clavicle pain and dysphagia. A chest radiograph obtained at the emergency department on the day of injury was negative. Examination reveals swelling and tenderness along the medial edge of the left clavicle. The upper extremity neurologic examination is normal. What is the next most appropriate test to best define the patient's injury?

1. CT of the sternoclavicular joint
2. Barium swallowing study
3. Electromyography of the upper extremity
4. MRI of the glenohumeral joint
5. Bone scan

PREFERRED RESPONSE: 1

DISCUSSION: The patient has a posterior sternoclavicular fracture-dislocation. These injuries can go unrecognized at the time of initial presentation because of difficulty in interpreting radiographs. Posterior sternoclavicular fracture-dislocations can be associated with potentially serious complications, such as pneumothorax respiratory distress, brachial plexus injury, and vascular compromise. Patients often report dysphagia and hoarseness. Accurate diagnosis and prompt treatment are essential for good functional outcomes and prevention of complications. Adolescent patients can have a posterior sternoclavicular dislocation, but usually they are a fracture through the medial physis. Axial CT scans are the most reliable radiographic modality for assessment of these injuries. Treatment consists of nonsurgical management, closed reduction, or open reduction. Most authors recommend open reduction if the patient is symptomatic with dysphagia or hoarseness. Furthermore, these patients will present late and open reduction may be the only successful treatment. The use of nonabsorbable sutures passed through drill holes in the sternum and/or the clavicular fracture fragments is recommended. Internal fixation is not recommended for this particular fracture because of concerns about hardware failure and/or migration.

REFERENCES: Waters PM, Bae DS, Kadiyala RK: Short-term outcomes after surgical treatment of traumatic posterior sternoclavicular fracture-dislocations in children and adolescents. *J Pediatr Orthop* 2003;23:464-469.
Yang J, al-Etani H, Letts M: Diagnosis and treatment of posterior sternoclavicular joint dislocations in children. *Am J Orthop* 1996;25:565-569.

Spine

Section Editor

Jeffrey C. Wang, MD

Q-1: A 40-year-old woman has local back pain and intense burning pain in her perianal region after being shot twice in the back. Motor and sensory examination of her lower extremities reveals no apparent deficit. She has present but decreased sensation in her perianal region, an intact anal wink, good rectal tone, and an intact bulbocavernosus reflex. Radiographs and CT scans are shown in Figures 1A through 1D. What is the next most appropriate step in management?

1. Initiation of spinal cord injury steroid protocol
2. MRI of the lumbar spine
3. Immobilization in a thoracolumbosacral orthosis
4. Removal of the metallic fragments via laminectomy
5. Removal of the metallic fragments and posterior fusion with instrumentation

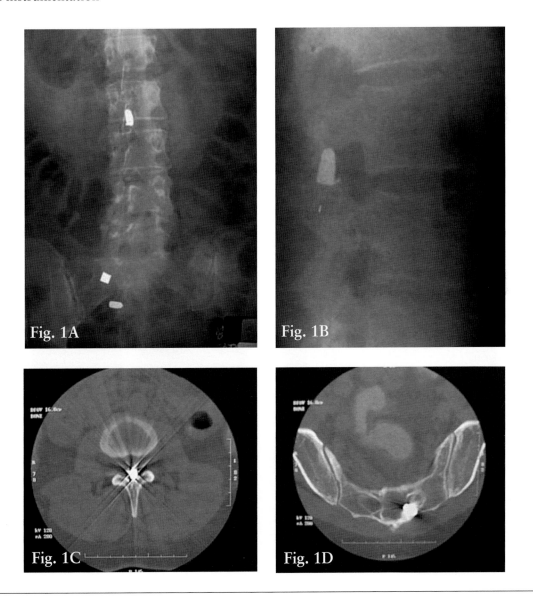

Fig. 1A

Fig. 1B

Fig. 1C

Fig. 1D

Q-2: The longus colli muscles are directly anterior to which of the following structures?

1. Prevertebral fascia
2. Pretracheal fascia
3. Esophagus
4. Vertebral arteries
5. Cervical nerve roots

Q-3: According to the Third National Acute Spinal Cord Injury Study (NASCIS 3), what is the recommended protocol for a patient who sustained a spinal cord injury 7 hours ago?

1. Methylprednisolone 30 mg/kg initial bolus, followed by 5.4 mg/kg/h for 23 hours
2. Methylprednisolone 30 mg/kg initial bolus, followed by 5.4 mg/kg/h for 48 hours
3. Dexamethasone 10 mg bolus, followed by 6 mg every 6 hours for 24 hours
4. Dexamethasone 10 mg bolus, followed by 6 mg every 6 hours for 48 hours
5. No treatment

Q-4: A 22-year-old college basketball player who was hit from behind while going up for a rebound is rendered immediately quadraparetic for approximately 10 minutes, followed by complete resolution of motor loss and return of full sensation. The radiograph and MRI scan of the cervical spine shown in Figures 2A and 2B reveal a canal diameter of 13 mm, loss of cerebrospinal fluid space about the spinal cord, and no signal change within the cord. What is the best course of action?

1. Cease participation in all sports.
2. Allow a return to noncontact sports after surgical decompression and stabilization.
3. Allow a return to basketball 1 week after resolution of all symptoms.
4. Discuss the relative risks with the player, parents, and coach regarding participation in the athlete's sport of choice.
5. Advise participation in noncontact sports only.

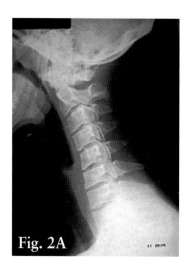

Fig. 2A

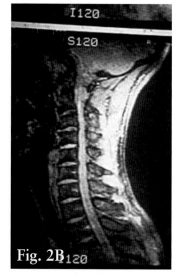

Fig. 2B

Q-5: Injury to which of the following structures has been reported following iliac crest bone graft harvest?

1. Superior gluteal artery from an anterior crest harvest
2. Superior cluneal nerve from an anterior crest harvest
3. Inferior gluteal artery from a posterior crest harvest
4. Ilioinguinal nerve from a posterior crest harvest
5. Lateral femoral cutaneous nerve from an anterior crest harvest

Q-6: A patient who sustained injuries in a motorcycle accident 30 minutes ago has significant motor and sensory deficits corresponding to a C6 level of injury. A lateral radiograph obtained during the initial on-scene evaluation reveals bilateral jumped facets at C5-C6; this appears to be an isolated injury. The patient is awake and alert. The next step in management of the dislocation should consist of

1. immediate posterior surgical reduction and stabilization.
2. immediate anterior diskectomy and fusion.
3. MRI.
4. reduction in Gardner-Wells tongs with serial traction.
5. rigid collar immobilization until spinal shock resolves.

Q-7: A 64-year-old man who underwent an L4-5 decompression approximately 1 year ago reported relief of his claudicatory leg pain initially, but he now has increasing low back pain and recurrent neurogenic claudication despite nonsurgical management. Radiographs show new asymmetric collapse and spondylolisthesis at the decompressed segment, and MRI scans show lateral recess stenosis. The next most appropriate step in management should consist of

1. L4-5 diskectomy.
2. L4-5 diskectomy and lateral recess decompression.
3. revision posterior decompression.
4. revision posterior decompression and posterolateral fusion.
5. anterior lumbar interbody fusion with cages.

Q-8: A patient who has had neck pain radiating down the arm for the past 4 weeks reports that the pain was excruciating during the first week. Management consisting of anti-inflammatory drugs and physical therapy has decreased the neck and arm symptoms from 10/10 to 3/10. He remains neurologically intact. MRI and CT scans are shown in Figures 3A and 3B. The best course of action should be

1. immediate hospital admission and surgery because of the risk of paralysis.
2. surgery within 24 hours.
3. surgery within the next several days.
4. elective surgery at the next available surgical date.
5. additional nonsurgical management.

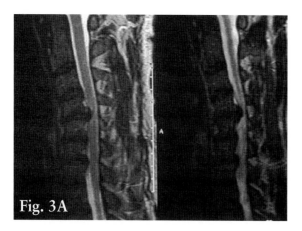
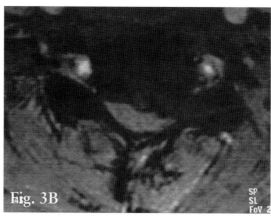

Fig. 3A   Fig. 3B

Q-9: An elderly patient falls and sustains an extension injury to the neck that results in upper extremity weakness, spared perianal sensation, and lower extremity spasticity. These findings best describe what syndrome?

1. Brown-Séquard
2. Cauda equina
3. Anterior cord
4. Posterior cord
5. Central cord

Q-10: In the upright standing position, approximately what percent of the vertical load is borne by the lumbar spine facet joints?

1. 0%
2. 20%
3. 40%
4. 60%
5. 80%

Q-11: What is the prognosis for ambulation, from best to worst, for patients with an incomplete spinal cord injury?

1. Central cord syndrome, anterior cord syndrome, Brown-Séquard syndrome
2. Central cord syndrome, Brown-Séquard syndrome, anterior cord syndrome
3. Brown-Séquard syndrome, anterior cord syndrome, central cord syndrome
4. Brown-Séquard syndrome, central cord syndrome, anterior cord syndrome
5. Anterior cord syndrome, central cord syndrome, Brown-Séquard syndrome

Q-12: A 26-year-old woman who noted right-sided lumbosacral pain 10 days ago while vacuuming now reports that the pain has intensified. She denies any history of back problems. No radicular component is present, and her neurologic examination is normal. The next most appropriate step in management should consist of

1. a brief (2 to 3 days) period of bed rest and nonsteroidal anti-inflammatory drugs.
2. bed rest for 2 weeks and nonsteroidal anti-inflamatory drugs, followed by physical therapy.
3. epidural steroid injections.
4. lumbar radiographs and MRI of the lumbar spine.
5. electromyography.

Q-13: A 32-year-old man notes increasing back pain and progressive paraparesis over the past few weeks. He is febrile, and laboratory studies show a WBC of 12,500/mm³. MRI scans are shown in Figures 4A and 4B. Management should consist of

1. CT-guided needle aspiration and organism-appropriate antibiotics.
2. laminectomy and postoperative bracing.
3. posterior fusion with instrumentation and IV antibiotics.
4. anterior debridement and strut graft, with possible posterior instrumentation.
5. posterior extracavitary decompression alone.

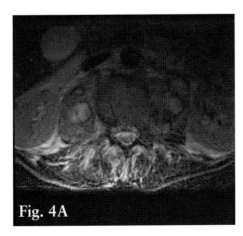

Fig. 4A

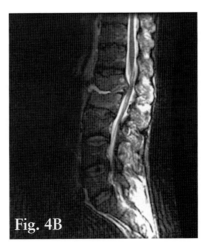

Fig. 4B

Q-14: An otherwise healthy 16-year-old boy who has had thoracolumbar pain with an increasingly worse deformity for the past 2 years now reports that the pain is worse at night. He responded well to nonsteroidal anti-inflammatory drugs initially, but they have become less effective. He denies any neurologic or constitutional symptoms. Examination is consistent with a mild thoracolumbar scoliosis and is otherwise normal. Laboratory studies show a normal CBC, erythrocyte sedimentation rate, and C-reactive protein. Standing radiographs show a 20° left thoracolumbar scoliosis, and he has a Risser stage of 4. A bone scan shows increased uptake at L2; a CT scan through this level is shown in Figure 5. Management should now consist of

1. percutaneous aspiration and appropriate antibiotic therapy.
2. an underarm Boston brace for 23 hours per day.
3. a referral for radiation therapy.
4. posterior instrumented arthrodesis from one level above to one level below the deformity.
5. removal of the lesion and local arthrodesis if necessary.

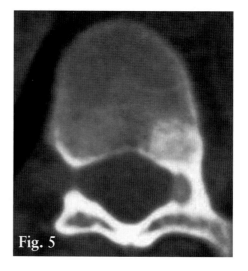

Fig. 5

Q-15: A 19-year-old man who sustained a spinal cord injury in a motor vehicle accident 3 days ago has 5/5 full strength in the deltoids and biceps bilaterally, 4/5 strength in wrist extension bilaterally, 1/5 triceps function on the right side, and 2/5 triceps function on the left side. The patient has no detectable lower extremity motor function. Based on the American Spinal Injury Association's classification, what is the patient's functional level?

1. C4
2. C5
3. C6
4. C7
5. C8

Q-16: A 44-year-old farmer involved in a rollover accident on his tractor sustained an L1 burst fracture with a 20% loss of anterior vertebral body height, 30% canal compromise, and 15° of kyphosis. He remains neurologically intact. The preferred initial course of action should consist of

1. posterior spinal fusion with instrumentation.
2. a thoracolumbosacral orthosis (TLSO) extension brace and early mobilization.
3. bed rest for 6 weeks followed by mobilization in a cast.
4. anterior L1 corpectomy and fusion with instrumentation.
5. anterior corpectomy followed by posterior fusion with instrumentation.

Q-17: A type 2A hangman's fracture, which has the potential to overdistract with traction, has which of the following hallmark findings?

1. Anterior translation of greater than 3 mm
2. Severe angulation with minimal translation
3. Extension at the fracture site
4. Associated C1 ring fracture
5. Associated C2-3 facet dislocation

Q-18: Which of the following are considered characteristic features of degeneration of a disk?

1. Reduced water and glycosaminoglycan content and increased noncollagen glycoprotein
2. Reduced water and glycosaminoglycan content and reduced noncollagen glycoprotein
3. Reduced water content, increased glycosaminoglycan content, and increased noncollagen glycoprotein
4. Increased water and glycosaminoglycan content and increased noncollagen glycoprotein
5. Increased water and glycosaminoglycan content and reduced noncollagen glycoprotein

Q-19: Figures 6A and 6B show the radiographs of a 22-year-old man who was shot through the abdomen the previous evening. An exploratory laparotomy performed at the time of admission revealed a colon injury. Current examination reveals no neurologic deficits. Management for the spinal injury should include

1. oral antibiotics for *Staphylococcus* for 48 hours.
2. oral broad-spectrum antibiotics for 7 days.
3. IV antibiotics for *Staphylococcus* for 48 hours.
4. IV broad-spectrum antibiotics for 48 hours.
5. IV broad-spectrum antibiotics for 7 days.

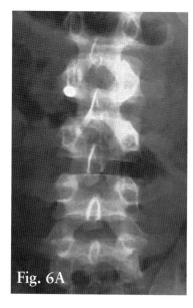

Fig. 6A

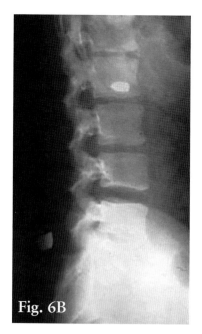

Fig. 6B

Q-20: What spinal nerves in the cauda equina are primarily responsible for innervation of the bladder?

1. L1, L2, and L3
2. L4 and L5
3. L5 and S1
4. S2, S3, and S4
5. Filum terminale

Q-21: A 23-year-old man sustains a unilateral jumped facet with an isolated cervical root injury in a motor vehicle accident. Acute reduction results in some initial improvement of his motor weakness. Over the next 48 hours, examination reveals ipsilateral loss of pain and temperature sensation in his face, limbs, and trunk, as well as nystagmus, tinnitus, and diplopia. What is the most likely etiology for these changes?

1. Intracranial hemorrhage
2. Epidural hematoma
3. Unrecognized disk extrusion
4. Delayed spinal cord hemorrhage
5. Vertebral artery injury

Q-22: A 54-year-old man undergoes uneventful anterior cervical diskectomy and interbody fusion at C4-5 for focal disk herniation and C5 radiculopathy. At the 3-week follow-up examination, the patient reports a persistent cough. Pulmonary evaluation reveals a mild but persistent aspiration. Laryngoscopy reveals partial paralysis of the left vocal cord, most likely caused by

1. entrapment of the superior laryngeal nerve during ligation of the superior thyroid artery.
2. stretch of the recurrent laryngeal as it enters the esophageal-tracheal groove.
3. injury to the vocal cord during endotracheal intubation.
4. displacement of the larynx against the endotracheal tube by retraction.
5. retractor pressure on the laryngeal nerve in the esophageal groove.

Q-23: In a patient with a C5-6 herniation, the most likely sensory deficit will be in the

1. lateral shoulder.
2. radial forearm, thumb, and index finger.
3. dorsal forearm and middle finger.
4. ulnar forearm, ring finger, and little finger.
5. volar forearm and palm.

Q-24: An otherwise healthy 32-year-old man who underwent an uneventful L5-S1 lumbar microdiskectomy 6 weeks ago now reports increasing and severe back pain that awakens him from sleep. Examination reveals a benign-appearing wound, and the neurologic examination is normal. Laboratory studies show an erythrocyte sedimentation rate (ESR) of 90 mm/h and a WBC of 9,000/mm³. Plain radiographs are normal. What is the next most appropriate step in management?

1. Oral antibiotics for *Staphylococcus*
2. Repeat laboratory studies in 1 week to recheck the ESR
3. MRI with gadolinium
4. Biopsy of the surgical disk space
5. Irrigation and débridement of the surgical wound in the operating room

Q-25: The artery of Adamkiewicz (arteria radicularis, arteria magna) is most commonly found on the

1. right side between T5 and T7.
2. right side between T9 and T11.
3. left side between T5 and T7.
4. left side between T9 and T11.
5. left side between L1 and L3.

Q-26: An otherwise healthy 45-year-old woman reports the onset of severe right leg pain. Figure 7A shows an axial MRI scan of the L4-5 level, and Figure 7B shows a sagittal view with the arrow at the L4-5 level. What nerve root is the most likely source of her pain?

1. L3
2. L4
3. L5
4. S1
5. S2

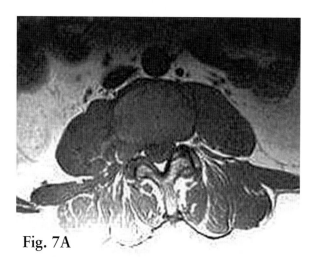

Fig. 7A

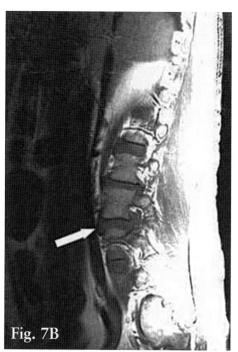

Fig. 7B

Q-27: A patient with myelopathy underwent a one-level corpectomy 1 day ago and is now home. In the middle of the night he calls to report markedly increased difficulty in swallowing, diaphoresis, a change in his voice, and difficulty lying flat. What is the best course of action?

1. Reassure the patient that the symptoms should subside gradually and that he should remain as upright as possible and loosen his cervical collar.

2. Prescribe methylprednisolone and diazepam.

3. Admit the patient for observation.

4. Advise the patient to come to the office first thing in the morning for a lateral radiograph of the cervical spine.

5. Advise immediate transport to the emergency department for evaluation of the airway, possible intubation, and possible cricothyroidotomy.

Q-28: Figure 8 shows a cross-sectional view of the spinal cord at the lower cervical level. Injury to the structure indicated by the black arrow will lead to what neurologic deficit?

1. Complete paraplegia
2. Contralateral weakness below the level of the injury
3. Ipsilateral weakness below the level of the injury
4. Unilateral loss of position sense, proprioception, and vibratory sense below the level of the injury
5. Loss of pain and temperature sensation below the level of the injury

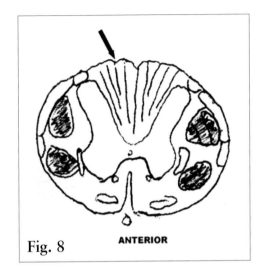

Fig. 8   ANTERIOR

Q-29: The postoperative neurologic prognosis of a patient who has a tumor that is compressing the spinal cord and causing a neurologic deficit depends primarily on the

1. pretreatment neurologic status.
2. extent of spinal cord compression.
3. extent of bony deformity.
4. MRI findings.
5. dimension of the spinal canal.

Q-30: Contraindications to cervical laminectomy as a treatment for cervical spondylotic myelopathy include which of the following findings?

1. Multilevel disease with spinal cord compression
2. Anterior spinal cord compression
3. Posterior spinal cord compression
4. Cervical kyphosis
5. Ossification of the posterior longitudinal ligament

Q-31: The transverse diameter of the pedicle is most narrow at which of the following levels?

1. T1
2. T5
3. T9
4. T12
5. L5

Q-32: Subluxation caused by rheumatoid arthritis is most commonly seen at what level of the cervical spine?

1. Occiput-C1
2. C1-C2
3. C2-C3
4. C3-C4
5. C4-C5

Q-33: A 44-year-old woman has had lower extremity dysesthesias and urinary incontinence and has been unable to walk for the past 2 days. She reports no pain or history of trauma. She notes that 3 weeks ago she missed work for 2 days because of back pain, but it resolved with rest. Examination shows decreased or absent sensation below the knees, no motor function below the knees, and decreased rectal tone. Catheterization results in a postvoid residual of 2,000 mL. Plain radiographs and MRI scans without contrast are shown in Figures 9A through 9D. What is the next most appropriate step in management?

1. Physical therapy for functional rehabilitation
2. CT/myelography of the spinal axis
3. MRI with gadolinium
4. Psychiatric consultation for possible malingering
5. Lumbar puncture for analysis of cerebrospinal fluid

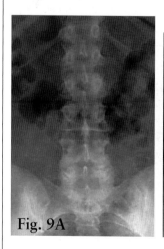
Fig. 9A

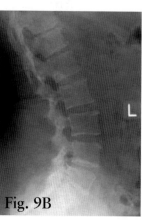
Fig. 9B

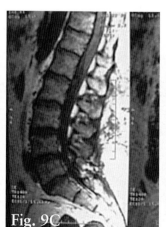
Fig. 9C

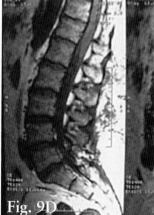
Fig. 9D

Q-34: During a transperitoneal approach to the L5-S1 interspace, care must be taken to protect the superior hypogastric plexus from injury. Which of the following techniques reduces the risk of neurologic injury?

1. Transverse incision across the posterior peritoneum and disk space, reflecting the tissues toward the sacral promontory
2. Transverse incision across the posterior peritoneum and disk space, reflecting the tissues toward the confluence of the iliac veins
3. Vertical midline incision of the posterior peritoneum, reflecting the prevertebral tissues beginning at the margin of the left iliac vein and extending toward the right iliac vein
4. Vertical midline incision of the posterior peritoneum, reflecting the prevertebral tissues beginning at the margin of the right iliac vein extending toward the left iliac vein
5. Vertical midline incision of the posterior peritoneum, reflecting the prevertebral tissues bilaterally away from the midline

Q-35: Which of the following factors has the most effect on the pullout strength of lumbar transpedicular screw fixation?

1. Depth of vertebral body penetration
2. Screw diameter
3. Percentage of pedicle filled by the screw
4. Presence of osteopenia
5. Tapping of the pedicle

Q-36: A 33-year-old woman sustains a C6 burst fracture diving into a swimming pool, resulting in a complete spinal cord injury. The canal compromise is shown in Figures 10A and 10B. Functional recovery would be maximized with

1. anterior corpectomy followed by strut grafting and instrumentation.
2. halo vest immobilization.
3. laminectomy and posterior wiring.
4. laminectomy followed by halo vest immobilization.
5. posterior lateral mass plating and fusion.

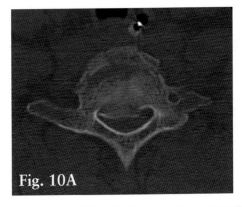

Fig. 10A

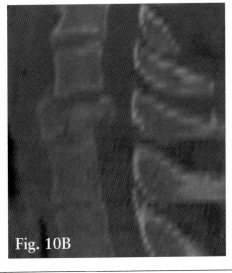

Fig. 10B

Q-37: An Asian 45-year-old man has bilateral upper extremity dysfunction. Figure 11A shows a T2-weighted sagittal MRI scan of the cervical spine, and Figure 11B shows a T2-weighted axial MRI scan at the level of the C3 vertebral body. What is the most likely pathologic process?

1. Cervical spondylosis

2. Diffuse idiopathic skeletal hyperostosis (DISH)

3. Ossification of the posterior longitudinal ligament (OPLL)

4. Ankylosing spondylitis

5. Neurofibromatosis

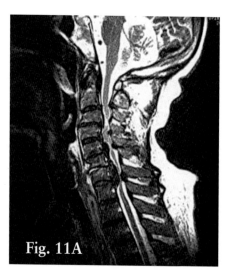

Fig. 11A

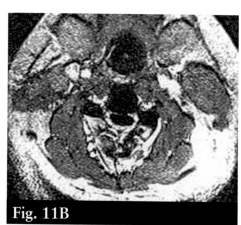

Fig. 11B

Q-38: What is the anatomic relationship of the inferior vena cava to the aorta at T-12?

1. Anterior to the aorta

2. Posterior to the aorta

3. To the right of the aorta

4. To the left of the aorta

5. Posterior and to the left of the aorta

Q-39: During anterior surgery on the cervical spine, at what level would the lateral dissection of the longus colli muscle most likely cause Horner syndrome?

1. C3

2. C4

3. C5

4. C6

5. C7

A-1: A 40-year-old woman has local back pain and intense burning pain in her perianal region after being shot twice in the back. Motor and sensory examination of her lower extremities reveals no apparent deficit. She has present but decreased sensation in her perianal region, an intact anal wink, good rectal tone, and an intact bulbocavernosus reflex. Radiographs and CT scans are shown in Figures 1A through 1D. What is the next most appropriate step in management?

1. Initiation of spinal cord injury steroid protocol
2. MRI of the lumbar spine
3. Immobilization in a thoracolumbosacral orthosis
4. Removal of the metallic fragments via laminectomy
5. Removal of the metallic fragments and posterior fusion with instrumentation

PREFERRED RESPONSE: 4

DISCUSSION: Because the patient has an apparent compressive neuropathy secondary to the metallic fragments, removal of the fragments in this incomplete lesion at the cauda equina level can be expected to improve her sensory dysesthesias and pain. Steroids are not indicated in a root lesion secondary to a penetrating injury. MRI will have significant artifact effect and will not provide much additional information. The posterior bony elements are not significantly injured; therefore, stabilization is not indicated.

REFERENCES: Bracken MB, Shepard MJ, Holford TR, et al: Administration of methylprednisolone for 24 or 48 hours or tirilazad mesylate for 48 hours in the treatment of acute spinal cord injury: Results of the Third National Acute Spinal Cord Injury Randomized Controlled Trial. National Acute Spinal Cord Injury Study. *JAMA* 1997;277:1597-1604.

Waters RL, Adkins RH: The effects of removal of bullet fragments retained in the spinal canal: A collaborative study by the National Spinal Cord Injury Model Systems. *Spine* 1991;16:934-939.

Stauffer ES, Wood RW, Kelly EG: Gunshot wounds of the spine: The effects of laminectomy. *J Bone Joint Surg Am* 1979;61:389-392.

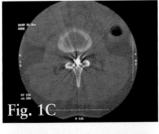

Fig. 1C

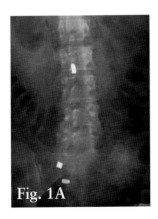

Fig. 1A

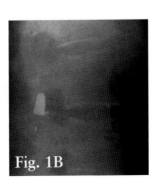

Fig. 1B

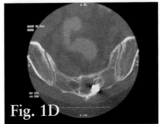

Fig. 1D

A-2: The longus colli muscles are directly anterior to which of the following structures?

1. Prevertebral fascia
2. Pretracheal fascia
3. Esophagus
4. Vertebral arteries
5. Cervical nerve roots

PREFERRED RESPONSE: 4

DISCUSSION: The longus colli muscles are posterior to the prevertebral fascia, pretracheal fascia, and esophagus. They are anterior to both the vertebral arteries and cervical nerve roots, but the latter are posterior to the vertebral arteries.

REFERENCE: Parke WW, Sherk HH: Anatomy: Normal adult anatomy, in The Cervical Spine Research Society Editorial Committee (ed): *The Cervical Spine*, ed 2. Philadelphia, PA, JB Lippincott, 1989, p 30.

A-3: According to the Third National Acute Spinal Cord Injury Study (NASCIS 3), what is the recommended protocol for a patient who sustained a spinal cord injury 7 hours ago?

1. Methylprednisolone 30 mg/kg initial bolus, followed by 5.4 mg/kg/h for 23 hours
2. Methylprednisolone 30 mg/kg initial bolus, followed by 5.4 mg/kg/h for 48 hours
3. Dexamethasone 10 mg bolus, followed by 6 mg every 6 hours for 24 hours
4. Dexamethasone 10 mg bolus, followed by 6 mg every 6 hours for 48 hours
5. No treatment

PREFERRED RESPONSE: 2

DISCUSSION: NASCIS 2 established the recommended doses of methylprednisolone for spinal cord injury. This included an initial bolus of 30 mg/kg over 1 hour, followed by an infusion of 5.4 mg/kg/h for an additional 23 hours. If the injury was more than 8 hours old, the methylprednisolone was not recommended. NASCIS 3 changed the dosing schedule based on the time from injury. If the time from injury to treatment was less than 3 hours, the standard protocol was followed (30 mg/kg bolus followed by 5.4 mg/kg/h for 23 hours). If the time from injury to treatment was between 3 and 8 hours, the infusion was continued at 5.4 mg/kg for an additional 23 hours (48 hours total). In this situation with a time of injury 7 hours ago, treatment should consist of a bolus and further steroid therapy for 48 hours.

REFERENCES: Bracken MB, Shepard MJ, Holford TR, et al: Administration of methylprednisolone for 24 or 48 hours or tirilazad mesylate for 48 hours in the treatment of acute spinal cord injury: Results of the Third National Acute Spinal Cord Injury Randomized Controlled Trial. National Acute Spinal Cord Injury Study. *JAMA* 1997;277:1597-1604.
Bracken MB, Shepard MJ, Collins WF, et al: A randomized, controlled trial of methylprednisolone or naloxone in the treatment of acute spinal-cord injury: Results of the Second National Acute Spinal Cord Injury Study. *N Engl J Med* 1990;322:1405-1411.

A-4: A 22-year-old college basketball player who was hit from behind while going up for a rebound is rendered immediately quadraparetic for approximately 10 minutes, followed by complete resolution of motor loss and return of full sensation. The radiograph and MRI scan of the cervical spine shown in Figures 2A and 2B reveal a canal diameter of 13 mm, loss of cerebrospinal fluid space about the spinal cord, and no signal change within the cord. What is the best course of action?

1. Cease participation in all sports.
2. Allow a return to noncontact sports after surgical decompression and stabilization.
3. Allow a return to basketball 1 week after resolution of all symptoms.
4. Discuss the relative risks with the player, parents, and coach regarding participation in the athlete's sport of choice.
5. Advise participation in noncontact sports only.

PREFERRED RESPONSE: 4

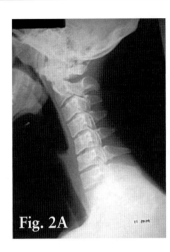
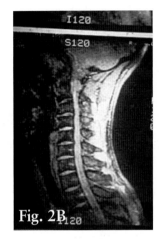

Fig. 2A   Fig. 2B

DISCUSSION: The correct decision on return to sports participation after episodes of transient quadra-paresis is controversial. Cantu and Mueller feel strongly that the loss of cerebrospinal fluid space about the spinal cord signifies an unacceptable risk for future spinal cord injury if the athlete returns to sports. However, Watkins and Torg and Lasgow have reported no evidence of increased spinal cord injury in athletes with narrow spinal canals, even in football. These authors suggest judgment be used in advising return to contact or high-energy sports and that the physician's responsibility is to give accurate and relevant information, allowing the athlete to make his or her own choice regarding return to sports participation.

REFERENCES: Cantu R, Mueller FO: Catastrophic spine injuries in football (1977-1989). *J Spinal Disord* 1990;3:227-231.
Watkins RG: Neck injuries in football players. *Clin Sports Med* 1986;5:215-246.
Torg JS, Lasgow SG: Criteria for return to contact activities following cervical spine injury. *Clin Sports Med* 1991;1:12-26.
Morganti C, Sweeney CA, Albanese SA, Burak C, Hosea T, Connolly PJ: Return to play after cervical spine injury. *Spine* 2001;26:1131-1136.

A-5: Injury to which of the following structures has been reported following iliac crest bone graft harvest?

1. Superior gluteal artery from an anterior crest harvest
2. Superior cluneal nerve from an anterior crest harvest
3. Inferior gluteal artery from a posterior crest harvest
4. Ilioinguinal nerve from a posterior crest harvest
5. Lateral femoral cutaneous nerve from an anterior crest harvest

PREFERRED RESPONSE: 5

(continued on next page)

(A-5: *continued*)

DISCUSSION: Injury to the lateral femoral cutaneous nerve and the ilioinguinal nerve have both been described with an anterior iliac crest bone graft harvest. The lateral femoral cutaneous nerve may be injured from retraction after elevating the iliacus muscle or from direct injury when the nerve actually courses over the crest. A posterior crest harvest can injure the superior gluteal artery if a surgical instrument violates the sciatic notch. Injury to the inferior gluteal artery has not been described; it leaves the pelvis below the piriformis muscle belly and should not be at risk even with a violation of the sciatic notch. Injury to the ilioinguinal nerve has been reported from vigorous retraction of the iliacus muscle after exposing the inner table of the anterior ilium. Cluneal nerve injury may occur with posterior crest harvest, particularly if the skin incision is horizontal or extends more than 8 cm superolateral from the posterior superior iliac spine.

REFERENCES: Kurz LT, Garfin SR, Booth RE Jr: Iliac bone grafting: Techniques and complications of harvesting, in Garfin SR (ed): *Complications of Spine Surgery*. Baltimore, MD, Williams and Wilkins, 1989, pp 323-341.

Anderson JE: *Grant's Atlas of Anatomy*, ed 7. Baltimore, MD, Williams and Wilkins, 1978, pp 4-33 to 4-34.

A-6: A patient who sustained injuries in a motorcycle accident 30 minutes ago has significant motor and sensory deficits corresponding to a C6 level of injury. A lateral radiograph obtained during the initial on-scene evaluation reveals bilateral jumped facets at C5-C6; this appears to be an isolated injury. The patient is awake and alert. The next step in management of the dislocation should consist of

1. immediate posterior surgical reduction and stabilization.
2. immediate anterior diskectomy and fusion.
3. MRI.
4. reduction in Gardner-Wells tongs with serial traction.
5. rigid collar immobilization until spinal shock resolves.

PREFERRED RESPONSE: 4

DISCUSSION: Surgical open reduction may increase the neurologic deficit if a disk herniation exists. Evidence from animal studies suggests that rapid decompression of the spinal cord may improve recovery. Serially increasing traction weight to reduce the dislocation has been shown to be safe when used in patients who are awake. Indications for MRI include patients who are unable to cooperate with serial examinations, the need for open reduction, and progression of deficit during awake reduction.

REFERENCES: Delamarter RB, Sherman J, Carr JB: Pathophysiology of spinal cord injury: Recovery after immediate and delayed decompression. *J Bone Joint Surg Am* 1995;77:1042-1049.

Star AM, Jones AA, Cotler JM, Balderston RA, Sinha R: Immediate closed reduction of cervical spine dislocations using traction. *Spine* 1990;15:1068-1072.

Eismont FJ, Arena MJ, Green BA: Extrusion of an intervertebral disc associated with traumatic subluxation or dislocation of cervical facets: Case report. *J Bone Joint Surg Am* 1991;73:1555-1560.

A-7: A 64-year-old man who underwent an L4-5 decompression approximately 1 year ago reported relief of his claudicatory leg pain initially, but he now has increasing low back pain and recurrent neurogenic claudication despite nonsurgical management. Radiographs show new asymmetric collapse and spondylolisthesis at the decompressed segment, and MRI scans show lateral recess stenosis. The next most appropriate step in management should consist of

1. L4-5 diskectomy.
2. L4-5 diskectomy and lateral recess decompression.
3. revision posterior decompression.
4. revision posterior decompression and posterolateral fusion. *with instrumentation*
5. anterior lumbar interbody fusion with cages.

PREFERRED RESPONSE: 4

DISCUSSION: When radiographic findings reveal postlaminectomy instability, procedures that do not include some type of fusion will fail to solve the problem. In fact, wider decompression or diskectomy alone will only further destabilize the segment. Because there is radiographic evidence of recurrent lateral recess stenosis and symptomatic neurogenic claudication, a revision decompression should be included. Since access to the canal involves a posterior approach, the stabilization should be performed through that same approach.

REFERENCES: Herkowitz HN, Kurz LT: Degenerative lumbar spondylolisthesis with spinal stenosis: A prospective study comparing decompression with decompression and intertransverse process arthrodesis. *J Bone Joint Surg Am* 1991;73:802-808.
Hansraj KK, O'Leary PF, Cammisa FP Jr, et al: Decompression, fusion, and instrumentation surgery for complex lumbar spinal stenosis. *Clin Orthop Relat Res* 2001;384:18-25.

A-8: A patient who has had neck pain radiating down the arm for the past 4 weeks reports that the pain was excruciating during the first week. Management consisting of anti-inflammatory drugs and physical therapy has decreased the neck and arm symptoms from 10/10 to 3/10. He remains neurologically intact. MRI and CT scans are shown in Figures 3A and 3B. The best course of action should be

1. immediate hospital admission and surgery because of the risk of paralysis.
2. surgery within 24 hours.
3. surgery within the next several days.
4. elective surgery at the next available surgical date.
5. additional nonsurgical management.

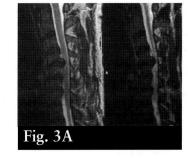

Fig. 3A

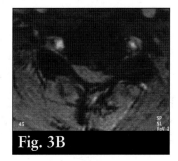

Fig. 3B

PREFERRED RESPONSE: 5

(continued on next page)

Answers: Spine

(A-8: *continued*)

DISCUSSION: Although the patient has a large herniated nucleus pulposus, the pain has decreased from 10/10 to 3/10 over a 4-week period and the patient is now free of any neurologic symptoms. It is quite likely that further nonsurgical management will continue to resolve his symptoms. In the absence of any neurologic deficits, there is no evidence that the patient is at significant risk for paralysis.

REFERENCES: Saal JS, Saal JA, Yurth EF: Nonoperative management of herniated cervical intervertebral disc with radiculopathy. *Spine* 1996;21:1877-1883.
Komori H, Shinomiya K, Nakai O, Yamaura I, Takeda S, Furuya K: The natural history of herniated nucleus pulposus with radiculopathy. *Spine* 1996;21:225-229.

A-9: An elderly patient falls and sustains an extension injury to the neck that results in upper extremity weakness, spared perianal sensation, and lower extremity spasticity. These findings best describe what syndrome?

1. Brown-Séquard
2. Cauda equina
3. Anterior cord
4. Posterior cord
5. Central cord

PREFERRED RESPONSE: 5

DISCUSSION: These findings indicate central cord syndrome, an injury that is more common in the older population who have some degree of spondylosis. The physiologic insult can be a central spinal hematoma with resultant hematomyelia. Bowel and bladder functional return has a good prognosis, unlike the upper extremity motor loss. Cauda equina syndrome generally involves injury at the lumbar levels, with some degree of lower extremity motor loss. Posterior cord syndrome is characterized by preservation of motor function below the level of injury and position/vibratory sensory loss. Brown-Séquard syndrome, which is often produced by a penetrating injury, results in contralateral hypalgesia and ipsilateral weakness. Anterior cord syndrome has a poor prognosis for functional return; lower extremity findings include loss of light touch, sharp/dull, and temperature sensations below the level of injury, as well as motor function.

REFERENCES: Apple DF Jr: Spinal cord injury rehabilitation, in Rothman RH, Simeone FA (eds): *The Spine*, ed 3. Philadelphia, PA, WB Saunders, 1992: chap 31.
Leventhal MR: Fractures, dislocations and fracture-dislocations of spine, in Crenshaw AH (ed): *Campbell's Operative Orthopaedics*, ed 8. St. Louis, MO, Mosby, 1992.

A-10: In the upright standing position, approximately what percent of the vertical load is borne by the lumbar spine facet joints?

1. 0%
2. 20%
3. 40%
4. 60%
5. 80%

PREFERRED RESPONSE: 2

DISCUSSION: Direct measurement and finite element modeling results show that approximately 20% of the vertical load is borne by the posterior structures of the lumbar spine in the upright position.

REFERENCES: Adams MA, Hutton WC: The effect of posture on the role of the apophyseal joints in resisting intervertebral compressive forces. *J Bone Joint Surg Br* 1980;62:358-362.
Goel VK, Kong W, Han JS, Weinstein JN, Gilbertson LG: A combined finite element and optimization investigation of lumbar spine mechanics with and without muscles. *Spine* 1993;18:1531-1541.

A-11: What is the prognosis for ambulation, from best to worst, for patients with an incomplete spinal cord injury?

1. Central cord syndrome, anterior cord syndrome, Brown-Séquard syndrome
2. Central cord syndrome, Brown-Séquard syndrome, anterior cord syndrome
3. Brown-Séquard syndrome, anterior cord syndrome, central cord syndrome
4. Brown-Séquard syndrome, central cord syndrome, anterior cord syndrome
5. Anterior cord syndrome, central cord syndrome, Brown-Séquard syndrome

PREFERRED RESPONSE: 4

DISCUSSION: Of the incomplete spinal cord injuries, Brown-Sequard syndrome has the best prognosis for ambulation. Central cord syndrome has a variable recovery. Anterior cord syndrome has the worst prognosis, with motor recovery rare below the level of the injury.

REFERENCES: Apple DF: Spinal cord injury rehabilitation, in Herkowitz HN, Garfin SR, Balderston RA, Eismont FJ, Bell GR, Wiesel SW (eds): *Rothman-Simeone The Spine*, ed 4. Philadelphia, PA, WB Saunders, 1999, pp 1130-1131.
Northrup BE: Evaluation and early treatment of acute injuries to the spine and spinal cord, in Clark CR (ed): *The Cervical Spine*, ed 3. Philadelphia, PA, Lippincott Raven, 1998, pp 544-545.

Answers: Spine

A-12: A 26-year-old woman who noted right-sided lumbosacral pain 10 days ago while vacuuming now reports that the pain has intensified. She denies any history of back problems. No radicular component is present, and her neurologic examination is normal. The next most appropriate step in management should consist of

1. a brief (2 to 3 days) period of bed rest and nonsteroidal anti-inflammatory drugs.
2. bed rest for 2 weeks and nonsteroidal anti-inflamatory drugs, followed by physical therapy.
3. epidural steroid injections.
4. lumbar radiographs and MRI of the lumbar spine.
5. electromyography.

PREFERRED RESPONSE: 1

DISCUSSION: The initial management of a lumbar strain should consist of 2 to 3 days of bed rest when symptoms are severe, activity restrictions, and nonsteroidal anti-inflammatory drugs. It has been estimated that 60% to 80% of the adult population experiences back pain, with 2% to 5% affected yearly. Spontaneous improvement generally will occur within 4 weeks. Further study is indicated by the presence of radiculopathy, weakness, trauma, or suspicion of malignancy.

REFERENCES: Bigos S, Boyer O, Braen GR, et al: Acute low back pain in adults: Clinical practice guideline No. 14. AHCPR Publication No. 95.0642. Rockville, MD, Agency for Health Care Policy and Research, Public Health Service, US Department of Health and Human Services, December, 1994.
Deyo RA: Conservative therapy for low back pain: Distinguishing useful from useless therapy. *JAMA* 1983;250:1057-1062.

A-13: A 32-year-old man notes increasing back pain and progressive paraparesis over the past few weeks. He is febrile, and laboratory studies show a WBC of 12,500/mm³. MRI scans are shown in Figures 4A and 4B. Management should consist of

1. CT-guided needle aspiration and organism-appropriate antibiotics.
2. laminectomy and postoperative bracing.
3. posterior fusion with instrumentation and IV antibiotics.
4. anterior debridement and strut graft, with possible posterior instrumentation.
5. posterior extracavitary decompression alone.

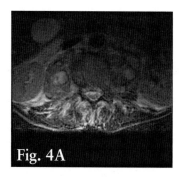
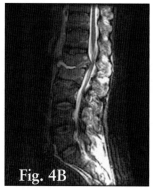

Fig. 4A   Fig. 4B

PREFERRED RESPONSE: 4

DISCUSSION: Indications for surgery in spinal infections include progressive destruction despite antibiotic treatment, an abscess requiring drainage, neurologic deficit, need for diagnosis, and/or instability.

(continued on next page)

(A-13: *continued*)

This patient has a progressive neurologic deficit. Débridement performed at the site of the abscess should effect canal decompression. Once the débridement is complete back to viable bone, the defect can be reconstructed with a strut graft. Additional posterior stabilization is used as deemed necessary by the degree of anterior destruction. CT-guided needle aspiration, while occasionally useful in the earliest phases of an infection, produces frequent false-negative results and would provide little useful information in the management of this patient.

REFERENCES: Emery SE, Chan DP, Woodward HR: Treatment of hematogenous pyogenic vertebral osteomyelitis with anterior debridement and primary bone grafting. *Spine* 1989;14:284-291.
Lifeso RM: Pyogenic spinal sepsis in adults. *Spine* 1990;15:1265-1271.
Andreshak JL, Currier BL: Spinal infections, in Beaty JH (ed): *Orthopaedic Knowledge Update 6*. Rosemont, IL, American Academy of Orthopaedic Surgeons, 1999, pp 713-721.

A-14: An otherwise healthy 16-year-old boy who has had thoracolumbar pain with an increasingly worse deformity for the past 2 years now reports that the pain is worse at night. He responded well to nonsteroidal anti-inflammatory drugs initially, but they have become less effective. He denies any neurologic or constitutional symptoms. Examination is consistent with a mild thoracolumbar scoliosis and is otherwise normal. Laboratory studies show a normal CBC, erythrocyte sedimentation rate, and C-reactive protein. Standing radiographs show a 20° left thoracolumbar scoliosis, and he has a Risser stage of 4. A bone scan shows increased uptake at L2; a CT scan through this level is shown in Figure 5. Management should now consist of

1. percutaneous aspiration and appropriate antibiotic therapy.
2. an underarm Boston brace for 23 hours per day.
3. a referral for radiation therapy.
4. posterior instrumented arthrodesis from one level above to one level below the deformity.
5. removal of the lesion and local arthrodesis if necessary.

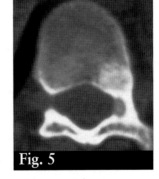

Fig. 5

PREFERRED RESPONSE: 5

DISCUSSION: The findings and radiographic appearance are most consistent with osteoid osteoma involving the medial pedicle. Scoliosis is commonly seen with this lesion and usually does not need surgical intervention. Excellent results have been reported with surgical excision as well as with percutaneous thermocoagulation. Nonsurgical treatment also has been described in peripheral osteoid osteoma but is not well described for lesions within the spine.

REFERENCES: Cove JA, Taminiau AH, Obermann WR, Vanderschueren GM: Osteoid osteoma of the spine treated with percutaneous computed tomography-guided thermocoagulation. *Spine* 2000;25:1283-1286.
Kneisl JS, Simon MA: Medical management compared with operative treatment for osteoid osteoma. *J Bone Joint Surg Am* 1992;74:179-185.
Pettine KA, Klassen RA: Osteoid osteoma and osteoblastoma of the spine. *J Bone Joint Surg Am* 1986;68:354-361.

A-15: A 19-year-old man who sustained a spinal cord injury in a motor vehicle accident 3 days ago has 5/5 full strength in the deltoids and biceps bilaterally, 4/5 strength in wrist extension bilaterally, 1/5 triceps function on the right side, and 2/5 triceps function on the left side. The patient has no detectable lower extremity motor function. Based on the American Spinal Injury Association's classification, what is the patient's functional level?

1. C4
2. C5
3. C6
4. C7
5. C8

PREFERRED RESPONSE: 3

DISCUSSION: By convention, when determining the motor level, the key muscle must be at least 3/5. The next most rostral level must be 4/5. Therefore, this patient's functional level is C6.

REFERENCE: *International Standards for Neurological and Functional Classification of Spinal Cord Injury.* Chicago, IL, American Spinal Injury Association, 1996.

A-16: A 44-year-old farmer involved in a rollover accident on his tractor sustained an L1 burst fracture with a 20% loss of anterior vertebral body height, 30% canal compromise, and 15° of kyphosis. He remains neurologically intact. The preferred initial course of action should consist of

1. posterior spinal fusion with instrumentation.
2. a thoracolumbosacral orthosis (TLSO) extension brace and early mobilization.
3. bed rest for 6 weeks followed by mobilization in a cast.
4. anterior L1 corpectomy and fusion with instrumentation.
5. anterior corpectomy followed by posterior fusion with instrumentation.

PREFERRED RESPONSE: 2

DISCUSSION: Surgical decompression is unnecessary in a patient with no neurologic deficit and canal compromise of less than 50%. A compression deformity of less than 50% and kyphosis of less than 30° may be successfully treated with a TLSO extension brace. Deformity in this range will reliably heal with minimal risk for late deformity or residual pain. Although some studies suggest 6 weeks of bed rest as treatment, early mobilization and bracing is preferred.

REFERENCES: Hartman MB, Chrin AM, Rechtine GR: Nonoperative treatment of thoracolumbar fractures. *Paraplegia* 1995;33:73-76.
Chow GH, Nelson BJ, Gebhard JS, Brugman JL, Brown CW, Donaldson DH: Functional outcome of thoracolumbar burst fractures managed with hyperextension casting or bracing and early mobilization. *Spine* 1996;21:2170-2175.
Kraemer WJ, Schemitsch EH, Lever J, McBroom RJ, McKee MD, Waddel JP: Functional outcome of thoracolumbar burst fractures without neurological deficit. *J Orthop Trauma* 1996;10:541-544.

Answers: Spine

A-17: A type 2A hangman's fracture, which has the potential to overdistract with traction, has which of the following hallmark findings?

1. Anterior translation of greater than 3 mm
2. Severe angulation with minimal translation
3. Extension at the fracture site
4. Associated C1 ring fracture
5. Associated C2-3 facet dislocation

PREFERRED RESPONSE: 2

DISCUSSION: Type 2A hangman's fractures are thought to have a flexion mechanism rather than extension and axial loading. This allows them to rotate around the anterior longitudinal ligament into flexion. Anterior translation of greater than 3 mm and angulation distinguish type 2 fractures from type 1 fractures. Although there is an association between C1 ring fractures and C2 fractures, this does not factor into the classification. If a C2-3 facet dislocation exists in combination with a C2 pars fracture, it is considered a type 3 fracture.

REFERENCES: Connolly PJ, Abitol J-J, Martin RJ, Yuan HA: Spine: trauma, in Garfin SR, Vaccaro AR (eds): *Orthopaedic Knowledge Update: Spine.* Rosemont, IL, American Academy of Orthopaedic Surgeons, 1997, pp 197-217.
Levine AM, Edwards CC: The management of traumatic spondylolisthesis of the axis. *J Bone Joint Surg Am* 1985;67:217-226.

A-18: Which of the following are considered characteristic features of degeneration of a disk?

1. Reduced water and glycosaminoglycan content and increased noncollagen glycoprotein
2. Reduced water and glycosaminoglycan content and reduced noncollagen glycoprotein
3. Reduced water content, increased glycosaminoglycan content, and increased noncollagen glycoprotein
4. Increased water and glycosaminoglycan content and increased noncollagen glycoprotein
5. Increased water and glycosaminoglycan content and reduced noncollagen glycoprotein

PREFERRED RESPONSE: 1

DISCUSSION: Gradual dessication of the disk begins in the third decade as glycosaminoglycan levels within the nucleus begin to decline. The original water content of 88% decreases to 70% in the sixth decade and beyond. As glycosaminoglycan content decreases, there is a corresponding increase in non-collagen glycoprotein.

REFERENCES: Happey F, Weissman A, Naylor A: Polysaccharide content of the prolapsed nucleus pulposus of the human intervertebral disc. *Nature* 1961;192:868.
Naylor A, Shentall R: Biomechanical aspects of intervertebral discs in aging and disease, in Jayson M (ed): *The Lumbar Spine and Back Pain.* New York, NY, Grune and Stratton Inc, 1976, pp 317-326.
Watkins RG, Collis JS: *Lumbar Discectomy and Laminectomy.* Rockville, MD, Aspen, 1987, pp 2-3.

Answers: Spine

A-19: Figures 6A and 6B show the radiographs of a 22-year-old man who was shot through the abdomen the previous evening. An exploratory laparotomy performed at the time of admission revealed a colon injury. Current examination reveals no neurologic deficits. Management for the spinal injury should include

1. oral antibiotics for *Staphylococcus* for 48 hours.
2. oral broad-spectrum antibiotics for 7 days.
3. IV antibiotics for *Staphylococcus* for 48 hours.
4. IV broad-spectrum antibiotics for 48 hours.
5. IV broad-spectrum antibiotics for 7 days.

PREFERRED RESPONSE: 5

DISCUSSION: IV broad-spectrum antibiotics should be administered for 7 days. This regimen, when compared to fragment removal or other antibiotic regimens, has been shown to reduce the incidence of spinal infections and reduce the need for metallic fragment removal with perforation of a viscus.

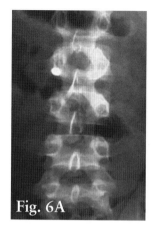 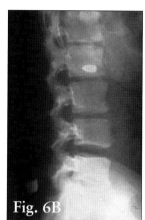
Fig. 6A Fig. 6B

REFERENCES: Roffi RP, Waters RL, Adkins RH: Gunshot wounds to the spine associated with a perforated viscus. *Spine* 1989;14:808-811.
Velmahoos GC, Demetriades D: Gunshot wounds of the spine: Should retained bullets be removed to prevent infection? *Ann R Coll Surg Engl* 1976;94:85-87.

A-20: What spinal nerves in the cauda equina are primarily responsible for innervation of the bladder?

1. L1, L2, and L3
2. L4 and L5
3. L5 and S1
4. S2, S3, and S4
5. Filum terminale

PREFERRED RESPONSE: 4

DISCUSSION: The spinal nerves primarily responsible for bladder function are the S2, S3, and S4 nerve roots. With significant compression of the cauda equina by either disk herniation, tumor, or degenerative stenosis, bladder dysfunction may result.

REFERENCES: Hoppenfeld S: *Physical Examination of the Spine and Extremities.* Norwalk, CT, Appleton-Century-Crofts, 1976, p 254.
Pick TP, Howden R (eds): *Gray's Anatomy.* New York, NY, Bounty Books, 1977, p 1004.

A-21: A 23-year-old man sustains a unilateral jumped facet with an isolated cervical root injury in a motor vehicle accident. Acute reduction results in some initial improvement of his motor weakness. Over the next 48 hours, examination reveals ipsilateral loss of pain and temperature sensation in his face, limbs, and trunk, as well as nystagmus, tinnitus, and diplopia. What is the most likely etiology for these changes?

1. Intracranial hemorrhage
2. Epidural hematoma
3. Unrecognized disk extrusion
4. Delayed spinal cord hemorrhage
5. Vertebral artery injury

PREFERRED RESPONSE: 5

DISCUSSION: The patient is showing signs of vertebral artery stroke. The signs of Wallenberg syndrome include those listed above, as well as contralateral loss of pain and temperature sensation throughout the body, an ipsilateral Horner syndrome, dysphagia, and ataxia. Vertebral artery injuries are not unusual in significant cervical facet injuries. A lesion in the cervical spinal cord is not associated with these symptoms, and an intracranial hemorrhage from trauma is unlikely to present in this manner.

REFERENCES: Young PA, Young PH: *Basic Clinical Neuroanatomy.* Baltimore, MD, Williams and Wilkins, 1997, pp 242-243.
Harrop JS, Sharan AD, Vaccaro AR, Przybylski GJ: The cause of neurologic deterioration after acute cervical spinal cord injury. *Spine* 2001;26:340-346.
Veras LM, Pedraza Gutierrez S, Castellanos J, Capellades J, Casamitjana J, Rovira-Canellas A: Vertebral artery occlusion after acute cervical spine trauma. *Spine* 2000;25:1171-1177.

A-22: A 54-year-old man undergoes uneventful anterior cervical diskectomy and interbody fusion at C4-5 for focal disk herniation and C5 radiculopathy. At the 3-week follow-up examination, the patient reports a persistent cough. Pulmonary evaluation reveals a mild but persistent aspiration. Laryngoscopy reveals partial paralysis of the left vocal cord, most likely caused by

1. entrapment of the superior laryngeal nerve during ligation of the superior thyroid artery.
2. stretch of the recurrent laryngeal as it enters the esophageal-tracheal groove.
3. injury to the vocal cord during endotracheal intubation.
4. displacement of the larynx against the endotracheal tube by retraction.
5. retractor pressure on the laryngeal nerve in the esophageal groove.

PREFERRED RESPONSE: 4

(continued on next page)

Answers: Spine

(A-22: *continued*)

DISCUSSION: The exact anatomic event responsible for vocal cord paralysis associated with anterior cervical surgery remains a question. Apfelbaum and associates, in an excellent review of 900 anterior cervical surgeries, identified 30 patients with vocal cord paralysis, 3 of which were permanent. They showed that retractors placed under the longus colli for anterior cervical exposures can compress the laryngeal-tracheal branches within the larynx against the tented endotracheal tube rather than the recurrent laryngeal nerve, which is extrinsic to the larynx. By releasing the endotracheal cuff and allowing the tube to recenter itself after placement of the retractors, they were able to decrease vocal cord injury from 6.4% to 1.7%. Jewett and associates suggested that a left-sided approach may result in a lower incidence of injury. Endotracheal intubation is the second most common cause of vocal cord injury, with an incidence of approximately 2%.

REFERENCES: Apfelbaum RI, Kriskovich MD, Haller JR: On the incidence, cause, and prevention of recurrent laryngeal nerve paralysis during anterior cervical spine surgery. *Spine* 2000;25:2906-2912. Jewett BA, Menico GA, Spengler DM, Coleman SC, Netterville JL: Vocal Cord Paralysis Following Anterior Cervical Spine Surgery. Paper presented at: Annual meeting of the Cervical Spine Research Society; December 2000; Charleston SC. Paper 7.

A-23: In a patient with a C5-6 herniation, the most likely sensory deficit will be in the

1. lateral shoulder.
2. radial forearm, thumb, and index finger.
3. dorsal forearm and middle finger.
4. ulnar forearm, ring finger, and little finger.
5. volar forearm and palm.

PREFERRED RESPONSE: 2

DISCUSSION: A C5-6 herniation compresses the C6 root, which innervates the radial forearm, thumb, and index finger. The lateral shoulder is innervated by C5. The dorsal forearm and the middle finger typically are innervated by C7. The ulnar forearm, ring finger, and little finger are innervated by C8. There is no specific nerve associated with the volar forearm and palm.

REFERENCE: Hoppenfeld S: Evaluation of nerve root lesions involving the upper extremity, in *Orthopaedic Neurology*. Philadelphia, PA, JB Lippincott, 1977, pp 7-23.

A-24: An otherwise healthy 32-year-old man who underwent an uneventful L5-S1 lumbar microdiskectomy 6 weeks ago now reports increasing and severe back pain that awakens him from sleep. Examination reveals a benign-appearing wound, and the neurologic examination is normal. Laboratory studies show an erythrocyte sedimentation rate (ESR) of 90 mm/h and a WBC of 9,000/mm^3. Plain radiographs are normal. What is the next most appropriate step in management?

1. Oral antibiotics for *Staphylococcus*
2. Repeat laboratory studies in 1 week to recheck the ESR
3. MRI with gadolinium
4. Biopsy of the surgical disk space
5. Irrigation and débridement of the surgical wound in the operating room

PREFERRED RESPONSE: 3

DISCUSSION: The patient's history and laboratory studies are very suspicious for a postoperative diskitis. The predominant symptom often is back pain. An ESR of 90 mm/h is considered significantly elevated and normally would be expected to return to near baseline by 2 weeks postoperatively. A normal WBC result is not unusual with postoperative diskitis. Management should consist of an MRI with gadolinium to confirm the diagnosis, followed by a biopsy percutaneously to obtain tissues for pathology and microbiology. Surgical débridement is reserved for patients whose percutaneous biopsy results are negative and a high index of suspicion for diskitis remains, or when management consisting of IV antibiotics, bed rest, and spinal immobilization fails to provide relief.

REFERENCES: Levine MJ, Heller JG: Spinal infections, in Garfin SR, Vaccaro AR (eds): *Orthopaedic Knowledge Update: Spine*. Rosemont, IL, American Academy of Orthopaedic Surgeons, 1997, pp 257-271. Andreshak JL, Currier BL: Spinal infections, in Beaty JH (ed): *Orthopaedic Knowledge Update 6*. Rosemont, IL, American Academy of Orthopaedic Surgeons, 1999, pp 713-721.

A-25: The artery of Adamkiewicz (arteria radicularis, arteria magna) is most commonly found on the

1. right side between T5 and T7.
2. right side between T9 and T11.
3. left side between T5 and T7.
4. left side between T9 and T11.
5. left side between L1 and L3.

PREFERRED RESPONSE: 4

DISCUSSION: Approximately 75% of people have the artery on the left side between T9 and T11. Its relevance to iatrogenic spinal cord problems is still uncertain.

REFERENCES: Stambaugh J, Simeone F: Vascular complication in spine surgery, in Herkowitz HH (ed): *The Spine*, ed 4. Philadelphia, PA, WB Saunders, 1992, p 1715. Lazorthes G: Arterial vascularization of the spinal cord. *J Neurosurg* 1971;35:253-262.

A-26: An otherwise healthy 45-year-old woman reports the onset of severe right leg pain. Figure 7A shows an axial MRI scan of the L4-5 level, and Figure 7B shows a sagittal view with the arrow at the L4-5 level. What nerve root is the most likely source of her pain?

1. L3
2. L4
3. L5
4. S1
5. S2

PREFERRED RESPONSE: 2

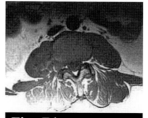

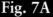
Fig. 7A

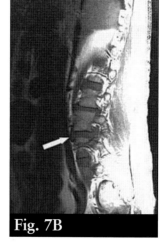
Fig. 7B

DISCUSSION: The scans show a disk herniation in the far lateral region of the disk. In particular, the sagittal view shows the herniation adjacent to the exiting L4 nerve root. Disk herniations in this area that cause symptoms are more likely to compress the nerve exiting at the same level rather than the next most caudal level.

REFERENCES: McCulloch JA: Microdiscectomy, in Frymoyer JW (ed): *The Adult Spine: Principles and Practice.* New York, NY, Raven Press, 1991, vol 2, pp 1765-1783.
Hodges SD, Humphreys SC, Eck JC, Covington LA: The surgical treatment of far lateral L3-L4 and L4-L5 disc herniations: A modified technique and outcomes analysis of 25 patients. *Spine* 1999;24:1243-1246.

A-27: A patient with myelopathy underwent a one-level corpectomy 1 day ago and is now home. In the middle of the night he calls to report markedly increased difficulty in swallowing, diaphoresis, a change in his voice, and difficulty lying flat. What is the best course of action?

1. Reassure the patient that the symptoms should subside gradually and that he should remain as upright as possible and loosen his cervical collar.
2. Prescribe methylprednisolone and diazepam.
3. Admit the patient for observation.
4. Advise the patient to come to the office first thing in the morning for a lateral radiograph of the cervical spine.
5. Advise immediate transport to the emergency department for evaluation of the airway, possible intubation, and possible cricothyroidotomy.

PREFERRED RESPONSE: 5

DISCUSSION: The patient has respiratory distress as manifested by his difficulty in lying flat. In addition, the diaphoresis and the change in his voice indicate retropharyngeal edema or hematoma that is compressing his larynx. The only appropriate treatment is hospital admission and elective intubation. During intubation it is possible to cause laryngospasm in a patient with a hyperacute airway; therefore, the surgeon should be prepared to perform a cricothyroidotomy. Often a fiberoptically guided intubation is the only way to find the airway in the presence of retropharyngeal edema or hematoma.

(continued on next page)

(A-27: *continued*)

REFERENCES: Emery SE, Smith MD, Bohlman HH: Upper-airway obstruction after multilevel cervical corpectomy for myelopathy. *J Bone Joint Surg Am* 1991;73:544-551.
McAfee PC, Bohlman HH, Riley LH Jr, Robinson RA, Southwick WO, Nachlas NE: The anterior retropharyngeal approach to the upper part of the cervical spine. *J Bone Joint Surg Am* 1987;69:1371-1383.

A-28: Figure 8 shows a cross-sectional view of the spinal cord at the lower cervical level. Injury to the structure indicated by the black arrow will lead to what neurologic deficit?

1. Complete paraplegia
2. Contralateral weakness below the level of the injury
3. Ipsilateral weakness below the level of the injury
4. Unilateral loss of position sense, proprioception, and vibratory sense below the level of the injury
5. Loss of pain and temperature sensation below the level of the injury

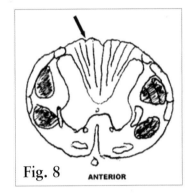

Fig. 8   ANTERIOR

PREFERRED RESPONSE: 4

DISCUSSION: The arrow is pointing to the posterior columns of the spinal cord that transmit position sense, vibratory sense, and proprioception. There are no motor tracts in the posterior columns.

REFERENCES: Bohlman H, Ducker T, Levine A: Spine trauma in adults, in Herkowitz HH (ed): *The Spine*, ed 4. Philadelphia, PA, WB Saunders, 1992, p 911.
Northrup B: Evaluation and early treatment of acute injuries to the spine and spinal cord, in Clark CR (ed): *The Cervical Spine*, ed 3. Philadelphia, PA, Lippincott Raven, 1998, p 545.

A-29: The postoperative neurologic prognosis of a patient who has a tumor that is compressing the spinal cord and causing a neurologic deficit depends primarily on the

1. pretreatment neurologic status.
2. extent of spinal cord compression.
3. extent of bony deformity.
4. MRI findings.
5. dimension of the spinal canal.

PREFERRED RESPONSE: 1

(continued on next page)

Answers: Spine

(A-29: *continued)*

DISCUSSION: The tumor biology, location, and pretreatment neurologic status are the best predictors of a patient's postoperative neurologic prognosis. Between 60% to 90% of patients who are ambulatory at the time of diagnosis will retain this ability after treatment. Location is important in that less space is available for the cord in the thoracic spine. Lesions located in vascular watershed regions may disrupt the vascular supply of the cord.

REFERENCES: Weinstein JN: Differential diagnosis and surgical treatment of primary benign and malignant neoplasms, in Frymoyer JW (ed): *The Adult Spine: Principles and Practice*. New York, NY, Raven Press, 1991, vol 1, pp 829-860.
Siegal T, Siegal T: Current considerations in the management of neoplastic spinal cord compression. *Spine* 1989;14:223-228.

A-30: Contraindications to cervical laminectomy as a treatment for cervical spondylotic myelopathy include which of the following findings?

1. Multilevel disease with spinal cord compression
2. Anterior spinal cord compression
3. Posterior spinal cord compression
4. Cervical kyphosis
5. Ossification of the posterior longitudinal ligament

PREFERRED RESPONSE: 4

DISCUSSION: Cervical laminectomy is an accepted treatment for multilevel cervical spondylotic myelopathy. When the compression is posterior, laminectomy addresses it directly; when the compression is anterior, it is addressed indirectly (the spinal cord floats posteriorly away from the anterior compression). Preexisting kyphosis is a contraindication to laminectomy because the cord is unable to float posteriorly away from the anterior compression, and the risk for increasing kyphosis is significant. Kyphosis after laminectomy is more likely to develop in younger patients who have fewer degenerative changes to stabilize the spine.

REFERENCES: Malone DG, Benzyl EC: Laminotomy and laminectomy for spinal stenosis causing radiculopathy or myelopathy, in Clark CR (ed.): *The Cervical Spine*, ed 3. Philadelphia, PA, Lippincott Raven, 1998, pp 817-825.
Emery SE: Cervical denerative disk disorders, in Beaty JH (ed): *Orthopaedic Knowledge Update 6*. Rosemont, IL, American Academy of Orthopaedic Surgeons, 1999, pp 673-680.

A-31: The transverse diameter of the pedicle is most narrow at which of the following levels?

1. T1
2. T5
3. T9
4. T12
5. L5

PREFERRED RESPONSE: 2

DISCUSSION: Of the levels given, T5 has the most narrow pedicle in anatomic studies. One study in patients with scoliosis did note that T7 on the concave side was more narrow than T5, but T7 is not listed here as a possible answer.

REFERENCES: O'Brien MF, Lenke LG, Mardjetko S, et al: Pedicle morphology in thoracic adolescent idiopathic scoliosis: Is pedicle fixation an anatomically viable technique? *Spine* 2000;25:2285-2293.
Vaccaro AR, Rizzolo SJ, Allardyce TJ, et al: Placement of pedicle screws in the thoracic spine: Part I. Morphometric analysis of the thoracic vertebrae. *J Bone Joint Surg Am* 1995;77:1193-1199.

A-32: Subluxation caused by rheumatoid arthritis is most commonly seen at what level of the cervical spine?

1. Occiput-C1
2. C1-C2
3. C2-C3
4. C3-C4
5. C4-C5

PREFERRED RESPONSE: 2

DISCUSSION: Approximately 65% of cervical subluxations occur at C1-C2. Of these, 50% are anterior, with the remainder being lateral and posterior. The second most common type is basilar invagination, occurring in 40% of patients. The third most common type is subaxial, occurring in 20% of patients with rheumatoid arthritis. Subluxation at more than one level is common.

REFERENCES: Boden S, Clark CR: Rheumatoid arthritis of the cervical spine, in Clark CR (ed): *The Cervical Spine*, ed 3. Philadelphia, PA, Lippincott Raven, 1998, p 693.
Boden SD, Dodge LD, Bohlman HH, Rechtine GR: Rheumatoid arthritis of the cervical spine: A long-term analysis with predictors of paralysis and recovery. *J Bone Joint Surg Am* 1993;75:1282-1297.
Oxner WM, Kang JD: Inflammatory arthritis of the spine, in Koval KJ (ed): *Orthopaedic Knowledge Update 7*. Rosemont, IL, American Academy of Orthopaedic Surgeons, 2002, pp 689-701.

Answers: Spine

A-33: A 44-year-old woman has had lower extremity dysesthesias and urinary incontinence and has been unable to walk for the past 2 days. She reports no pain or history of trauma. She notes that 3 weeks ago she missed work for 2 days because of back pain, but it resolved with rest. Examination shows decreased or absent sensation below the knees, no motor function below the knees, and decreased rectal tone. Catheterization results in a postvoid residual of 2,000 mL. Plain radiographs and MRI scans without contrast are shown in Figures 9A through 9D. What is the next most appropriate step in management?

1. Physical therapy for functional rehabilitation
2. CT/myelography of the spinal axis
3. MRI with gadolinium
4. Psychiatric consultation for possible malingering
5. Lumbar puncture for analysis of cerebrospinal fluid

PREFERRED RESPONSE: 3

DISCUSSION: The patient has had a clear and sudden onset of a profound neurologic deficit. The radiographic studies suggest a lesion in the conus medullaris that appears to be intradural and intramedullary. MRI, with and without contrast, will best evaluate this mass further. The addition of gadolinium allows further evaluation of vascularity and the extent of the lesion.

REFERENCES: Eichler ME, Dacey RG: Intramedullary spinal cord tumors, in Bridwell KH, Dewald RL (eds): *The Textbook of Spine Surgery*, ed 2. Philadelphia, PA, Lippincott.Raven, 1997, vol 2, pp 2089-2116.
Potter HG: Imaging beyond conventional radiology, in Beaty JH (ed): *Orthopaedic Knowledge Update 6*. Rosemont, IL, American Academy of Orthopaedic Surgeons, 1999, pp 81-87.

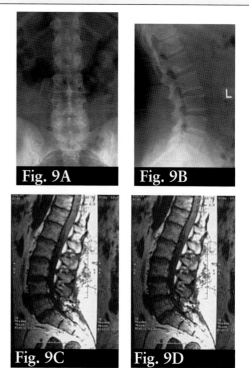

Fig. 9A   Fig. 9B
Fig. 9C   Fig. 9D

A-34: During a transperitoneal approach to the L5-S1 interspace, care must be taken to protect the superior hypogastric plexus from injury. Which of the following techniques reduces the risk of neurologic injury?

1. Transverse incision across the posterior peritoneum and disk space, reflecting the tissues toward the sacral promontory
2. Transverse incision across the posterior peritoneum and disk space, reflecting the tissues toward the confluence of the iliac veins
3. Vertical midline incision of the posterior peritoneum, reflecting the prevertebral tissues beginning at the margin of the left iliac vein and extending toward the right iliac vein
4. Vertical midline incision of the posterior peritoneum, reflecting the prevertebral tissues beginning at the margin of the right iliac vein extending toward the left iliac vein
5. Vertical midline incision of the posterior peritoneum, reflecting the prevertebral tissues bilaterally away from the midline

PREFERRED RESPONSE: 3

(continued on next page)

(A-34: *continued*)

DISCUSSION: Retrograde ejaculation is the sequela of superior hypogastric plexus injury. This structure needs protection, especially during anterior exposure of the L5-S1 disk space. Only blunt dissection should be used, and use of monopolar electrocautery should be avoided. If possible, preserve and retract the middle sacral artery. Once the iliac veins are isolated, blunt dissection is begun along the course of the medial edge of the left iliac vein, reflecting the prevertebral tissues toward the patient's right side. The dissection goes from left to right because the parasympathetic plexus is more adherent on the right side.

REFERENCE: Transperitoneal midline approach to L4-S1, in Watkins RG (ed): *Surgical Approaches to the Spine*, ed 1. New York, NY, Springer Verlag, 1983, pp 123-129.

A-35: Which of the following factors has the most effect on the pullout strength of lumbar transpedicular screw fixation?

1. Depth of vertebral body penetration
2. Screw diameter
3. Percentage of pedicle filled by the screw
4. Presence of osteopenia
5. Tapping of the pedicle

PREFERRED RESPONSE: 4

DISCUSSION: Although all of the factors listed contribute to the pullout strength of transpedicular  screw fixation, low bone density generally is felt to be the most influential.

REFERENCES: Wittenberg RH, Shea M, Swartz DE, Lee KS, White AA III, Hayes WC: Importance of bone mineral density in instrumented spine fusions. *Spine* 1991;16:647-652.
Zindrick MR, Wiltse LL, Widell EH, et al: A biomechanical study of intrapeduncular screw fixation in the lumbosacral spine. *Clin Orthop Relat Res* 1986;203:99-112.

A-36: A 33-year-old woman sustains a C6 burst fracture diving into a swimming pool, resulting in a complete spinal cord injury. The canal compromise is shown in Figures 10A and 10B. Functional recovery would be maximized with

1. anterior corpectomy followed by strut grafting and instrumentation.
2. halo vest immobilization.
3. laminectomy and posterior wiring.
4. laminectomy followed by halo vest immobilization.
5. posterior lateral mass plating and fusion.

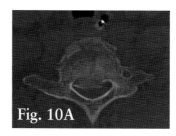
Fig. 10A

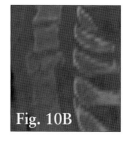
Fig. 10B

PREFERRED RESPONSE: 1

DISCUSSION: Although the patient has sustained a complete spinal cord injury, an anterior decompression, even performed late, can gain an additional level of root function. In the quadriplegic patient, this can mean the difference between dependent and independent function. Posterior procedures do not afford adequate access to the retropulsed bony fragments compromising the canal.

REFERENCES: Bohlman HH, Anderson PA: Anterior decompression and arthrodesis of the cervical spine: Long.term motor improvement. Part I: Improvement in incomplete traumatic quadriparesis. *J Bone Joint Surg Am* 1992;74:671-682.
Benz R, Abitbol JJ, Ozanne S, Garfin SR: Cervical burst fractures, in Levine AM, Eismont FJ, Garfin SR, Zigler JE (eds): *Spine Trauma*. Philadelphia, PA, WB Saunders, 1998, pp 300-330.

A-37: An Asian 45-year-old man has bilateral upper extremity dysfunction. Figure 11A shows a T2-weighted sagittal MRI scan of the cervical spine, and Figure 11B shows a T2-weighted axial MRI scan at the level of the C3 vertebral body. What is the most likely pathologic process?

1. Cervical spondylosis
2. Diffuse idiopathic skeletal hyperostosis (DISH)
3. Ossification of the posterior longitudinal ligament (OPLL)
4. Ankylosing spondylitis
5. Neurofibromatosis

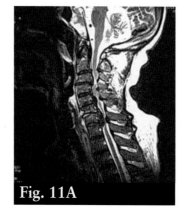

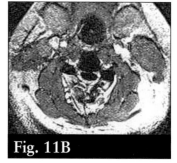
Fig. 11A   **Fig. 11B**

PREFERRED RESPONSE: 3

DISCUSSION: Although relatively common in people of Asian origin, OPLL has been reported in other races as well. The radiographic appearance can be variable as there are different types described, but some of the discerning characteristics are seen in these images.

(continued on next page)

(A-37: *continued*)

On the sagittal view, the bone posterior to the vertebral body extends along the entire length of C2 and C3. This is characteristic of OPLL, whereas cervical spondylosis and DISH more commonly are not confluent. Ankylosing spondylitis more commonly extends significantly into the spinal canal, and neurofibromatosis generally does not cause any bony growth. The axial view shows a large, oval bony projection into the spinal canal, a typical finding of OPLL.

REFERENCES: McAfee PC, Regan JJ, Bohlman HH: Cervical cord compression from ossification of the posterior longitudinal ligament in non-orientals. *J Bone Joint Surg Br* 1987;69:569-575.
Kricun R, Kricun ME: *MRI and CT of the Spine.* New York, NY, Raven Press, 1994, pp 126-130.

A-38: What is the anatomic relationship of the inferior vena cava to the aorta at T-12?

1. Anterior to the aorta
2. Posterior to the aorta
3. To the right of the aorta
4. To the left of the aorta
5. Posterior and to the left of the aorta

PREFERRED RESPONSE: 3

DISCUSSION: The inferior vena cava returns blood from all parts below the diaphragm to the heart. It is formed by the junction of two common iliac veins on the right side of the fifth lumbar vertebra. It passes upward along the front of the spine on the right side of the aorta.

REFERENCES: Pick TP, Howden R (eds): *Anatomy, Descriptive and Surgical*, ed 15. New York, NY, Gramercy Books, 1977, p 617.
Hoppenfeld S, deBoer P, (eds): *Surgical Exposures in Orthopaedics: The Anatomic Approach.* Philadelphia, PA, JB Lippincott, 1984, pp 230-233.

A-39: During anterior surgery on the cervical spine, at what level would the lateral dissection of the longus colli muscle most likely cause Horner syndrome?

1. C3
2. C4
3. C5
4. C6
5. C7

PREFERRED RESPONSE: 4

DISCUSSION: The sympathetic chain approaches the lateral border of the longus colli muscle at C6 and is more vulnerable to injury at this level. Injury to the chain will cause Horner syndrome, usually seen as unilateral ptosis.

REFERENCE: Ebraheim NA, Lu J, Yang H, Heck BE, Yeasting RA: Vulnerability of the sympathetic trunk during the anterior approach to the lower cervical spine. *Spine* 2000;25:1603-1606.

Shoulder and Elbow

Section Editor

Leesa M. Galatz, MD

Q-1: What structure(s) course(s) through the quadrangular (quadrilateral) space?

1. Circumflex scapular artery

2. Radial nerve, posterior humeral circumflex artery

3. Axillary nerve, posterior humeral circumflex artery

4. Radial nerve, circumflex scapular artery

5. Axillary nerve, profunda brachii artery

Q-2: Proximal extension of the triceps-splitting approach to the distal humerus is limited by potential injury to what structure?

1. Posterior humeral circumflex artery

2. Anterior humeral circumflex artery

3. Ulnar nerve

4. Posterior interosseous nerve

5. Radial nerve

Q-3: The primary stabilizer to valgus stress in the elbow is the

1. radiocapitellar joint.

2. anterior oblique band of the medial collateral ligament.

3. transverse band of the medial collateral ligament.

4. posterior oblique band of the medial collateral ligament.

5. ulnar trochlear articulation.

Q-4: Which of the following structures can cause nerve compression that decreases forearm supination strength?

1. Transverse carpal ligament

2. Ligament of Struthers

3. Anconeus epitrochlearis

4. Arcade of Frohse

5. Lacertus fibrosus

Q-5: Nerve entrapment at the spinoglenoid notch can result in atrophy of which muscle(s)?

1. Infraspinatus
2. Supraspinatus
3. Teres major
4. Teres minor
5. Supraspinatus and infraspinatus

Q-6: The rotator interval capsule of the shoulder acts to limit what type of motion?

1. Shoulder extension and external rotation
2. Shoulder extension and internal rotation
3. Shoulder flexion and external rotation
4. Shoulder flexion and internal rotation
5. Shoulder extension and adduction

Q-7: The nerve that traverses the triangular interval (bounded by the teres major superiorly, the long head of the triceps medially, and the humeral shaft laterally) supplies which of the following muscles?

1. Brachioradialis
2. Flexor pollicis longus
3. Deltoid
4. Teres major
5. Pronator teres

Q-8: Which peripheral nerve is most likely to be affected by a brachial plexus injury associated with a medial clavicle fracture?

1. Ulnar
2. Median
3. Thoracodorsal
4. Musculocutaneous
5. Radial

Q-9: Which of the following structures is the primary constraint to posterolateral rotatory instability of the elbow?

1. Radial head
2. Annular ligament
3. Anconeus muscle
4. Ulnar part of the lateral collateral ligament
5. Radial part of the lateral collateral ligament

Q-10: In the straight lateral approach to the humeral shaft, in contrast to the anterolateral approach, the plane of dissection is between what structures?

1. Biceps and brachialis
2. Biceps and lateral head of the triceps
3. Brachialis and brachioradialis
4. Brachialis and lateral head of the triceps
5. Lateral third of the brachialis and medial two thirds of the brachialis

Q-11: An abnormal lift-off sign, noted as an inability to lift the dorsum of the hand and wrist away from the body when it is placed just above the ipsilateral buttock, indicates injury to which of the following anatomic structures?

1. Infraspinatus
2. Supraspinatus
3. Subscapularis
4. Coracohumeral ligament
5. Biceps tendon

Q-12: The posterolateral approach to the radial head utilizes the internervous plane between which of the following muscles?

1. Brachioradialis and the anconeus
2. Extensor carpi ulnaris and the anconeus
3. Extensor carpi radialis longus and the anconeus
4. Extensor carpi radialis brevis and the anconeus
5. Extensor carpi radialis brevis and extensor carpi radialis longus

Q-13: Which of the following anatomic structures is often difficult to visualize during elbow arthroscopy?

1. Ulnar collateral ligament
2. Olecranon fossa
3. Radial head
4. Coronoid process
5. Anterior superior capsular attachment to the humerus

Q-14: The quadrilateral space in the shoulder contains which of the following structures?

1. Axillary nerve and posterior humeral circumflex artery
2. Axillary artery and radial nerve
3. Axillary artery and axillary nerve
4. Recurrent suprascapular nerve and artery
5. Profunda brachii artery

Q-15: The dorsal (Thompson) approach to the proximal forearm uses which of the following intermuscular intervals?

1. Extensor carpi radialis longus and the extensor carpi radialis brevis
2. Extensor pollicis longus and the extensor pollicis brevis
3. Extensor digitorum communis and the extensor carpi radialis brevis
4. Extensor carpi ulnaris and the extensor carpi radialis brevis
5. Abductor pollicis longus and the extensor carpi radialis brevis

Q-16: Which of the following muscles attaches to the coracoid process of the scapula?

1. Subscapularis
2. Supraspinatus
3. Pectoralis minor
4. Long head of the biceps brachii
5. Serratus anterior

Q-17: The artery located within the substance of the coracoacromial ligament is a branch of what artery?

1. Thoracoacromial
2. Anterior circumflex humeral
3. Posterior circumflex humeral
4. Subscapular
5. Thyrocervical

Q-18: The main arterial supply to the humeral head is provided by which of the following arteries?

1. Anterior humeral circumflex
2. Posterior humeral circumflex
3. Thoracoacromial
4. Subscapular
5. Deep (profunda) brachial

Q-19: Which of the following statements best describes why the ulnar nerve is most prone to neuropathy at the elbow?

1. It has the least longitudinal excursion required to accommodate elbow range of motion.
2. It is subjected to both compression and traction during elbow motion.
3. It passes between two muscle heads as it enters the forearm.
4. The dimensions of the entrance of the cubital tunnel do not change with elbow motion.
5. The vascular supply leaves a watershed area of diminished arterial supply.

Q-20: The MRI scan of the shoulder shown in Figure 1 was performed with the arm in abduction and external rotation. The image reveals what condition?

1. Contact between the rotator cuff and the posterior superior labrum
2. Anterior instability
3. A ganglion cyst of the spinoglenoid notch
4. Osteonecrosis of the humeral head
5. Posterior subluxation

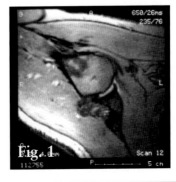

Q-21: A 38-year-old man has winging of the ipsilateral scapula after undergoing a transaxillary resection of the first rib 3 weeks ago. What is the most likely cause of this finding?

1. Persistent thoracic outlet syndrome
2. Injury to the upper trunk of the brachial plexus
3. Injury to the long thoracic nerve
4. Injury to the lower trunk of the brachial plexus
5. Injury to the spinal accessory nerve

Q-22: A 45-year-old woman has had progressive right shoulder pain for the past 6 months. She notes that the pain disrupts her sleep, she has pain at rest that requires the use of narcotic analgesics, and she has limited use of her left shoulder for most activities of daily living. History reveals the use of corticosteroids for systemic lupus erythematosus. Examination shows diminished range of motion. Radiographs of the right shoulder are shown in Figures 2A and 2B. Treatment should consist of

1. core decompression of the humeral head.
2. humeral arthroplasty.
3. total shoulder arthroplasty.
4. glenohumeral arthrodesis.
5. vascularized fibular allograft.

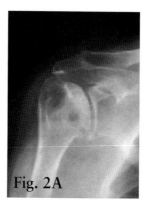
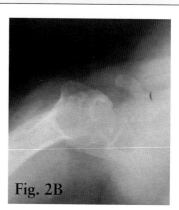

Fig. 2A   Fig. 2B

Q-23: A 16-year-old high school pitcher notes acute pain on the medial side of his elbow during a pitch. Examination that day reveals medial elbow tenderness, pain with valgus stress, mild swelling, and loss of extension. Plain radiographs show closed physes and no fracture. Which of the following diagnostic studies will best reveal his injury?

1. Technetium Tc 99m bone scan
2. Contrast-enhanced MRI
3. CT
4. Electromyography
5. Arthroscopy

Q-24: Figures 3A and 3B show the radiographs of a 45-year-old patient. What is the most likely diagnosis?

1. Glenoid dysplasia
2. Rheumatoid arthritis with centralization
3. Osteoarthritis with posterior glenoid wear
4. Posterior scapular fracture deformity
5. Traumatic posterior subluxation of the shoulder

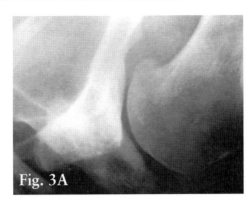
Fig. 3A

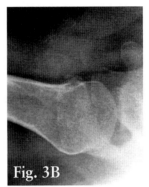
Fig. 3B

Q-25: A 23-year-old baseball pitcher who has diffuse pain along the posterior deltoid reports pain during late acceleration and follow-through. Examination of his arc of motion from external rotation to internal rotation at 90° of shoulder abduction reveals a significant deficit in internal rotation when compared to the nonthrowing shoulder. Initial management should consist of

1. a cortisone injection to the subscapular bursa.
2. posterior capsular stretching.
3. strengthening of the external rotators and scapular stabilizers.
4. continued pitching and working through the pain.
5. a sling and rest.

Q-26: A 54-year-old man has left shoulder pain and weakness after falling while skiing 4 months ago. Examination reveals full range of motion passively, but he has a positive abdominal compression test and weakness with the lift-off test. External rotation strength with the arm at the side and strength with the arm abducted and internally rotated are normal. MRI scans are shown in Figures 4A and 4B. Treatment should consist of

1. arthroscopy and labral repair.
2. arthroscopy and supraspinatus repair.
3. arthroscopy and subscapularis repair.
4. arthroscopy and supraspinatus and infraspinatus repair.
5. open repair of the pectoralis major.

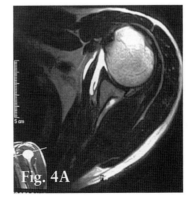
Fig. 4A

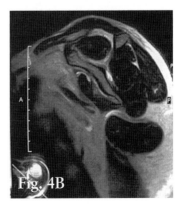
Fig. 4B

Q-27: Figure 5 shows the radiograph of a 26-year-old auto mechanic who injured his right dominant elbow in a fall during a motocross race. Examination reveals pain and catching that limits his range of motion to 45 degrees of supination and 20 degrees of pronation. The interosseous space and distal radio-ulnar joint are stable. Management should consist of

1. splinting for 3 weeks, followed by range-of-motion exercises.
2. aspiration of the hemarthrosis, followed by range-of-motion exercises the following day.
3. fragment excision.
4. open reduction and internal fixation.
5. radial head excision.

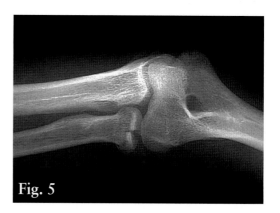

Fig. 5

Q-28: A 22-year-old swimmer underwent thermal capsulorrhaphy treatment for recurrent anterior subluxation. Following 3 weeks in a sling, the patient began an accelerated rehabilitation program that allowed him to return to swimming in 3 1/2 months. While practicing the butterfly stroke, he sustained an anterior dislocation. He now continues to have symptoms of anterior instability and has elected to have further surgery. Surgical findings may include a

1. biceps subluxation.
2. glenoid rim fracture.
3. subscapularis detachment.
4. loose body.
5. deficient anterior capsule.

Q-29: During the anterior approach for repair of a distal biceps tendon rupture, what structure, shown under the scissors in Figure 6, is at risk for injury?

1. Brachial artery
2. Median nerve
3. Posterior interosseous nerve
4. Lateral antebrachial cutaneous nerve
5. Antecubital vein

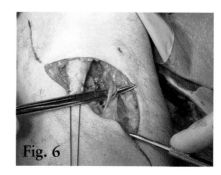

Fig. 6

Q-30: A 23-year-old man undergoes surgery for the condition shown in Figure 7. At surgery, a nerve is seen to be contused but in continuity. Postoperatively, the muscles at the elbow and below which this nerve innervates show no motor function. Which of the following muscles will first show recovery of function?

1. Flexor carpi ulnaris (FCU)

2. Extensor pollicis longus (EPL)

3. Brachioradialis (BR)

4. Extensor carpi radialis brevis (ECRB)

5. Flexor digitorum profundus (FDP) to the little finger

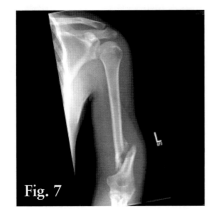

Fig. 7

Q-31: A 35-year-old woman was injured while snowboarding 2 days ago. Immediately after the injury she was taken to the emergency department and diagnosed with a clavicle fracture. Examination of the fracture reveals 2 cm of shortening with obvious bone contact between the fracture fragments. In your discussion you mention the options of surgical fixation versus nonsurgical treatment. In comparing the two options, you mention that posttreatment results are identical in

1. shoulder range of motion.

2. maximal strength testing.

3. ultimate internal and external rotation endurance.

4. satisfaction rates.

5. rates of nonunion.

Q-32: Which of the following anatomic structures is most commonly injured after an elbow dislocation?

1. Anterior band of the medial collateral ligament

2. Lateral ulnar collateral ligament

3. Radial head

4. Coronoid process

5. Olecranon

Q-33: A 62-year-old man who is right-hand dominant reports persistent pain in the left shoulder for the past 6 weeks. He denies any trauma or any prior problems with the shoulder. He states that he participated in some physical therapy to "strengthen" his shoulder but it failed to provide much relief. Examination reveals his right shoulder motion is 180, 60, and T8 (forward flexion, external rotation with arm at side, and internal rotation). His left shoulder motion, both active and passive, is 120, 30, and L1. He has minimal weakness about the left shoulder. T1- and T2-weighted MRI scans are shown in Figures 8A and 8B. What is the most appropriate treatment at this time?

1. Arthroscopic distal clavicle resection

2. Manipulation under anesthesia

3. Arthroscopic acromioplasty and, if needed, rotator cuff repair

4. Supervised and home-based physical therapy for motion exercises

5. Physical therapy for rotator cuff strengthening and scapula stabilization

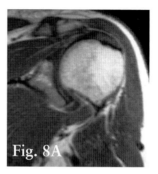
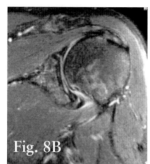

Fig. 8A   Fig. 8B

Q-34: Arthroscopic rotator cuff repair, when compared with mini-open rotator cuff repair, has shown which of the following results?

1. Increased failure rate

2. Increased postoperative pain

3. Increased postoperative motion

4. Better clinical outcome

5. Lower infection rate

Q-35: A healthy 52-year-old man has right shoulder pain and weakness of internal rotation after sustaining an injury 4 months ago. Examination reveals passive external rotation of 100 degrees on the right compared with 60 degrees on the left. At the time of arthroscopy, the long head of the biceps tendon is found to be dislocated from the intertubercular groove. What is the most appropriate management at this time?

1. Anterior shoulder stabilization

2. Acromioplasty

3. Subscapularis repair

4. Superior labral anterior to posterior (SLAP) repair

5. Posterior labral repair

Q-36: A 32-year-old man reports a history of pain and restricted range of motion in his left shoulder after injuring his shoulder skiing 3 months ago. He was diagnosed with a soft-tissue injury at the time of his original injury and treated with physiotherapy. Figures 9A through 9C show a current radiograph, CT scan, and 3-D CT reconstruction. What is the most appropriate management at this time?

1. Closed reduction under conscious sedation
2. Nonsurgical management with continued physiotherapy
3. Closed reduction under general anesthesia followed by arthroscopic anterior stabilization
4. Shoulder hemiarthroplasty
5. Open reduction and bone grafting of the humeral head

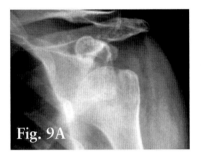
Fig. 9A

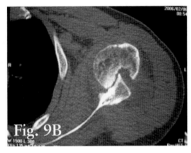
Fig. 9B

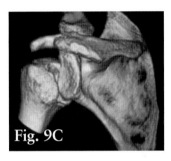
Fig. 9C

Q-37: A 13-year-old hockey player reports a 1-week history of left medial clavicle pain and dysphagia. A chest radiograph obtained at the emergency department on the day of injury was negative. Examination reveals swelling and tenderness along the medial edge of the left clavicle. The upper extremity neurologic examination is normal. What is the next most appropriate test to best define the patient's injury?

1. CT of the sternoclavicular joint
2. Barium swallowing study
3. Electromyography of the upper extremity
4. MRI of the glenohumeral joint
5. Bone scan

Q-38: Figures 10A and 10B show the radiographs of a 72-year-old woman who sustained a right shoulder injury 1 week ago. What is the most appropriate management?

1. Sling
2. Closed reduction and a sling and swath
3. Shoulder hemiarthroplasty
4. Total shoulder hemiarthroplasty
5. Neurologic consultation with electromyography

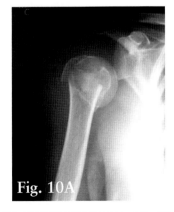
Fig. 10A

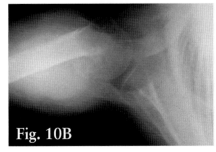
Fig. 10B

A-1: What structure(s) course(s) through the quadrangular (quadrilateral) space?

1. Circumflex scapular artery
2. Radial nerve, posterior humeral circumflex artery
3. Axillary nerve, posterior humeral circumflex artery
4. Radial nerve, circumflex scapular artery
5. Axillary nerve, profunda brachii artery

PREFERRED RESPONSE: 3

DISCUSSION: The quadrangular space is bordered longitudinally by the long head of the triceps medially and humeral shaft laterally. Superiorly it is bordered by the teres minor and inferiorly by the teres major. Through this roughly square outline pass the posterior humeral circumflex artery and axillary nerve en route to the posterior aspect of the shoulder.

REFERENCE: Netter FH (ed): *Atlas of Human Anatomy*. Summit, NJ, Ciba-Geigy Corp, 1989, plate 401.

A-2: Proximal extension of the triceps-splitting approach to the distal humerus is limited by potential injury to what structure?

1. Posterior humeral circumflex artery
2. Anterior humeral circumflex artery
3. Ulnar nerve
4. Posterior interosseous nerve
5. Radial nerve

PREFERRED RESPONSE: 5

DISCUSSION: The triceps-splitting approach to the distal humerus may be extended proximally only as far as the radial nerve.

REFERENCE: Rhoades LE: Elbow, in Reckling FW, Reckling JB, Mohn MP, et al (eds): *Orthopaedic Anatomy and Surgical Approaches*. St Louis, Mosby-Year Book, 1990, p 71.

A-3: The primary stabilizer to valgus stress in the elbow is the

1. radiocapitellar joint.
2. anterior oblique band of the medial collateral ligament.
3. transverse band of the medial collateral ligament.
4. posterior oblique band of the medial collateral ligament.
5. ulnar trochlear articulation.

PREFERRED RESPONSE: 2

DISCUSSION: The anterior oblique band of the medial collateral ligament is the primary stabilizer to valgus stress, whereas the radiocapitellar joint provides secondary stability.

REFERENCE: Bennett JB: Articular injuries in the athlete, in Morrey BF (ed): *The Elbow and Its Disorders*, ed 2. Philadelphia, WB Saunders, 1993, p 581.

A-4: Which of the following structures can cause nerve compression that decreases forearm supination strength?

1. Transverse carpal ligament
2. Ligament of Struthers
3. Anconeus epitrochlearis
4. Arcade of Frohse
5. Lacertus fibrosus

PREFERRED RESPONSE: 4

DISCUSSION: The arcade of Frohse is a tendinous proximal edge of the superficial head of the supinator muscle in the proximal forearm. The deep branch of the radial nerve passes beneath this arcade to enter the supinator en route to the posterior aspect of the forearm. Compression of the nerve at this site generally causes aching. On its way through, the deep branch of the radial nerve innervates the supinator, but any supinator weakness would generally be masked by the powerful supination of the biceps.

REFERENCE: Netter FH: *Atlas of Human Anatomy*. Summit, NJ, Ciba-Geigy Corp, 1989, plate 451.

A-5: Nerve entrapment at the spinoglenoid notch can result in atrophy of which muscle(s)?

1. Infraspinatus
2. Supraspinatus
3. Teres major
4. Teres minor
5. Supraspinatus and infraspinatus

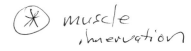
(*) muscle innervation

supraspinatus & infraspinatus

PREFERRED RESPONSE: 1

DISCUSSION: The suprascapular nerve passes through the suprascapular notch and innervates the supraspinatus muscle before passing around the spinoglenoid notch and innervating the infraspinatus muscle. Injury at the spinoglenoid notch will produce denervation and atrophy to the infraspinatus muscle. The teres major is innervated by the subscapular nerve. The teres minor is innervated by the axillary nerve.

REFERENCE: Shoulder: Reconstruction, in Frymoyer JW (ed): *Orthopaedic Knowledge Update 4: Home Study Syllabus*. Rosemont, IL, American Academy of Orthopaedic Surgeons, 1993, p 313.

A-6: The rotator interval capsule of the shoulder acts to limit what type of motion?

1. Shoulder extension and external rotation
2. Shoulder extension and internal rotation
3. Shoulder flexion and external rotation
4. Shoulder flexion and internal rotation
5. Shoulder extension and adduction

PREFERRED RESPONSE: 3

DISCUSSION: Recent cadaver studies of the rotator interval capsule have demonstrated its importance in the management of instability of the shoulder. The rotator interval capsule limits flexion and external rotation.

REFERENCE: Harryman DT II, Sidles JA, Harris SL, et al: The role of the rotator interval capsule in passive motion and stability of the shoulder. *J Bone Joint Surg Am* 1992;74:53-66.

Answers: Shoulder and Elbow

A-7: The nerve that traverses the triangular interval (bounded by the teres major superiorly, the long head of the triceps medially, and the humeral shaft laterally) supplies which of the following muscles?

1. Brachioradialis

2. Flexor pollicis longus

3. Deltoid

4. Teres major

5. Pronator teres

PREFERRED RESPONSE: 1

DISCUSSION: The radial nerve and profunda brachii artery gain access to the posterior aspect of the arm through the triangular interval. The radial nerve supplies the brachioradialis.

REFERENCE: Netter FH: *Atlas of Human Anatomy.* Summit, NJ, Ciba-Geigy Corp, 1989, plate 401.

A-8: Which peripheral nerve is most likely to be affected by a brachial plexus injury associated with a medial clavicle fracture?

1. Ulnar

2. Median

3. Thoracodorsal

4. Musculocutaneous

5. Radial

PREFERRED RESPONSE: 1

DISCUSSION: The space between the medial clavicle and the first rib is called the costoclavicular. Space compression of neurovascular structures in this area associated with medial clavicle fractures or thoracic outlet syndrome usually causes symptoms in the distribution of the ulnar nerve. The subclavian and axillary arteries are also at increased risk for injury.

REFERENCE: Craig EV: Fractures of the clavicle, in Rockwood CA Jr, Matsen FA III (eds): *The Shoulder.* Philadelphia, WB Saunders, 1990, vol 1, p 369.

A-9: Which of the following structures is the primary constraint to posterolateral rotatory instability of the elbow?

1. Radial head
2. Annular ligament
3. Anconeus muscle
4. Ulnar part of the lateral collateral ligament
5. Radial part of the lateral collateral ligament

PREFERRED RESPONSE: 4

DISCUSSION: Posterolateral instability is associated with injury to the ulnar part of the lateral collateral ligament. The anterior band of the medial collateral ligament is the primary constraint to valgus instability. The other structures are secondary restraints.

REFERENCES: O'Driscoll SW, Bell DF, Morrey BF: Posterolateral rotatory instability of the elbow. *J Bone Joint Surg Am* 1991;73:440-446.
Kasser JR: *Orthopaedic Knowledge Update 5*. Rosemont, IL, American Academy of Orthopaedic Surgeons, 1996, pp 283-294.

A-10: In the straight lateral approach to the humeral shaft, in contrast to the anterolateral approach, the plane of dissection is between what structures?

1. Biceps and brachialis
2. Biceps and lateral head of the triceps
3. Brachialis and brachioradialis
4. Brachialis and lateral head of the triceps
5. Lateral third of the brachialis and medial two thirds of the brachialis

PREFERRED RESPONSE: 4

DISCUSSION: The straight lateral approach to the humerus is between the brachialis and lateral head of the triceps. It is an intermuscular plane, but may denervate part of the brachialis supplied by the radial nerve. The radial nerve can be exposed and the patient can be positioned supine in contrast to the posterior approach. The anterolateral approach consists of muscle splitting through the lateral portion of the brachialis and produces less denervation.

REFERENCES: Hoppenfeld S, deBoer P: *Surgical Exposures in Orthopedics: The Anatomic Approach*, ed 2. Philadelphia, PA, JB Lippincott, 1994, pp 79-80.
Mills WJ, Hanel DP, Smith DG: Lateral approach to the humerus shaft: An alternative approach for fracture treatment. *J Orthop Trauma* 1996;10:81-86.

Answers: Shoulder and Elbow

A-11: An abnormal lift-off sign, noted as an inability to lift the dorsum of the hand and wrist away from the body when it is placed just above the ipsilateral buttock, indicates injury to which of the following anatomic structures?

1. Infraspinatus
2. Supraspinatus
3. Subscapularis
4. Coracohumeral ligament
5. Biceps tendon

PREFERRED RESPONSE: 3

DISCUSSION: The subscapularis is the primary internal rotator of the shoulder with the arm in this position. Injuries of the subscapularis tendon are being recognized with more frequency, and an abnormal lift-off sign is a reliable indicator of injury to this structure. Patients with injury to the other structures have normal lift-off signs.

REFERENCE: Wirth MA, Rockwood CA Jr: Operative treatment of irreparable rupture of the subscapularis. *J Bone Joint Surg Am* 1997;79:722-731.

A-12: The posterolateral approach to the radial head utilizes the internervous plane between which of the following muscles?

1. Brachioradialis and the anconeus
2. Extensor carpi ulnaris and the anconeus
3. Extensor carpi radialis longus and the anconeus
4. Extensor carpi radialis brevis and the anconeus
5. Extensor carpi radialis brevis and extensor carpi radialis longus

PREFERRED RESPONSE: 2

DISCUSSION: The posterolateral approach to the elbow is performed between the extensor carpi ulnaris, supplied by the posterior interosseus nerve, and the anconeus, supplied by the radial nerve proper. The brachioradialis, extensor carpi radialis brevis, and extensor carpi radialis longus are innervated by the radial nerve.

REFERENCE: Hoppenfeld S, deBoer P: *Surgical Exposures in Orthopaedics: The Anatomic Approach*. Philadelphia, PA, JB Lippincott, 1984, pp 97-101.

A-13: Which of the following anatomic structures is often difficult to visualize during elbow arthroscopy?

1. Ulnar collateral ligament
2. Olecranon fossa
3. Radial head
4. Coronoid process
5. Anterior superior capsular attachment to the humerus

PREFERRED RESPONSE: 1

DISCUSSION: The ulnar collateral ligament is often difficult to visualize during elbow arthroscopy. It can be seen clearly in only 10% to 30% of elbow arthroscopies. All of the other structures should be easily and thoroughly seen and palpated during elbow arthroscopy.

REFERENCES: Johnson LL: *Arthroscopic Surgery: Principles and Practice*. St Louis, MO, CV Mosby, 1988.
Morrey BF: Arthroscopy of the elbow. *Instr Course Lect* 1986;35:102-107.

A-14: The quadrilateral space in the shoulder contains which of the following structures?

1. Axillary nerve and posterior humeral circumflex artery
2. Axillary artery and radial nerve
3. Axillary artery and axillary nerve
4. Recurrent suprascapular nerve and artery
5. Profunda brachii artery

PREFERRED RESPONSE: 1

DISCUSSION: The quadrilateral or quadrangular space of the shoulder is formed laterally by the humerus, proximally by the subscapularis (and teres minor viewed from posterior), distally by the teres major, and medially by the long head of the triceps. The posterior humeral circumflex artery and axillary nerve pass through it. The axillary artery is more proximal. The radial nerve and profunda brachii pass through a triangular space more inferior. The circumflex scapular artery passes through a triangular space more medial.

REFERENCES: Hollinshead WH: *Textbook of Anatomy*, ed 3. Hagerstown, MD, Harper and Row, 1974, pp 205-206.
Last RJ: *Anatomy: Regional and Applied*, ed 6. London, England, Churchill Livingstone, 1978, pp 61-62.

A-15: The dorsal (Thompson) approach to the proximal forearm uses which of the following intermuscular intervals?

1. Extensor carpi radialis longus and the extensor carpi radialis brevis
2. Extensor pollicis longus and the extensor pollicis brevis
3. Extensor digitorum communis and the extensor carpi radialis brevis
4. Extensor carpi ulnaris and the extensor carpi radialis brevis
5. Abductor pollicis longus and the extensor carpi radialis brevis

PREFERRED RESPONSE: 3

DISCUSSION: The Thompson posterior approach is used in treatment of fractures of the proximal radius. Dissection is carried out through the interval between the extensor carpi radialis brevis (radial nerve) and the extensor digitorum communis (posterior interosseous nerve). To identify this interval, the forearm is pronated and the mobile lateral wad of muscles (the ulnar-most belly is the extensor carpi radialis brevis) is grasped with the thumb and finger and pulled from the much less mobile mass of the extensor digitorum communis. The furrow created is marked with a skin marker for subsequent skin incision. The skin incision follows a line from the lateral epicondyle of the humerus to a point corresponding to the middle of the posterior aspect of the wrist. Distally, the intermuscular plane is between the extensor carpi radialis brevis and the extensor pollicis longus.

REFERENCES: Crenshaw AH Jr: Surgical techniques and approaches, in Canale ST (ed): *Campbell's Operative Orthopaedics*, ed 9. St Louis, MO, Mosby-Year Book, 1998, vol 1, pp 128-129.
Hoppenfeld S, deBoer P: Posterior approach to the radius, in *Surgical Exposures in Orthopaedics: The Anatomic Approach*, ed 2. Philadelphia, PA, Lippincott-Raven, 1992, pp 136-146.
Thompson JE: Anatomical methods of approach in operations on the long bones of the extremities. *Ann Surg* 1918;68:309-316.

A-16: Which of the following muscles attaches to the coracoid process of the scapula?

1. Subscapularis
2. Supraspinatus
3. Pectoralis minor
4. Long head of the biceps brachii
5. Serratus anterior

PREFERRED RESPONSE: 3

DISCUSSION: The insertion of the pectoralis minor is on the base of the coracoid process. The coracoid helps define the interval between the subscapularis and supraspinatus muscles but neither attaches to it. The coracobrachialis and short head of the biceps attach to the tip of the coracoid but are not listed as options. The long head of the biceps attaches to the supraglenoid tubercle. The serratus arises from the vertebral border of the scapula.

(continued on next page)

(A-16: *continued*)

REFERENCES: Jobe CM: Anatomy and surgical approaches, in Jobe FW (ed): *Operative Techniques in Upper Extremity Sports Injuries*. St Louis, MO, Mosby, 1996, pp 140-142.
Jobe CM: Gross anatomy of the shoulder, in Rockwood CA, Matsen FA III (eds): *The Shoulder*. Philadelphia, PA, WB Saunders, 1990, pp 49-66.

A-17: The artery located within the substance of the coracoacromial ligament is a branch of what artery?

1. Thoracoacromial
2. Anterior circumflex humeral
3. Posterior circumflex humeral
4. Subscapular
5. Thyrocervical

PREFERRED RESPONSE: 1

DISCUSSION: The acromial branch of the thoracoacromial artery courses along the medial aspect of the coracoacromial ligament and may be encountered when performing an open or arthroscopic subacromial decompression. Bleeding can be controlled by ligation of its branch from the thoracoacromial artery. The other arteries may be injured in other surgical exposures of the shoulder.

REFERENCES: Esch JC, Baker CL: The shoulder and elbow, in Whipple TL (ed): *Arthroscopic Surgery*. Philadelphia, PA, JB Lippincott, 1993, pp 65-66.
Woodburne RT (ed): *Essentials of Human Anatomy*, ed 2. New York, NY, Oxford University Press, 1983, pp 75-76.

A-18: The main arterial supply to the humeral head is provided by which of the following arteries?

1. Anterior humeral circumflex
2. Posterior humeral circumflex
3. Thoracoacromial
4. Subscapular
5. Deep (profunda) brachial

PREFERRED RESPONSE: 1

DISCUSSION: The main arterial supply to the humeral head is provided by the ascending branch of the anterior humeral circumflex artery and its intraosseous continuation, the arcuate artery. There are significant intraosseous anastomoses between the arcuate artery, the posterior humeral circumflex artery through vessels entering the posteromedial aspect of the proximal humerus, the metaphyseal vessels, and the vessels of the greater and lesser tuberosities. Four-part fractures and dissection during exposure affect perfusion of the humeral head.

(continued on next page)

(A-18: *continued*)

REFERENCES: Brooks CH, Revell WJ, Heatley FW: Vascularity of the humeral head after proximal humeral fractures: An anatomical cadaver study. *J Bone Joint Surg Br* 1993;75:132-136.
Gerber C, Schneeberger AG, Vinh TS: The arterial vascularization of the humeral head: An anatomical study. *J Bone Joint Surg Am* 1990;72:1486-1494.

A-19: Which of the following statements best describes why the ulnar nerve is most prone to neuropathy at the elbow?

1. It has the least longitudinal excursion required to accommodate elbow range of motion.
2. It is subjected to both compression and traction during elbow motion.
3. It passes between two muscle heads as it enters the forearm.
4. The dimensions of the entrance of the cubital tunnel do not change with elbow motion.
5. The vascular supply leaves a watershed area of diminished arterial supply.

PREFERRED RESPONSE: 2

DISCUSSION: The ulnar nerve is more prone to neuropathy than the radial or median nerves for many reasons. It has the greatest longitudinal excursion required to accommodate elbow range of motion, subjecting it to potential traction forces. The dimensions of the entrance of the cubital tunnel change with elbow motion, potentially causing compression in flexion. For these two reasons, the ulnar nerve is subjected to both compression and traction during elbow motion. Although it passes between two muscle heads as it enters the forearm, so do the median and radial nerves. Finally, the vascular supply is adequate because of the anastomoses between the superior ulnar collateral artery, the posterior ulnar recurrent artery, and the inferior ulnar collateral artery.

REFERENCES: Norris TR (ed): *Orthopaedic Knowledge Update: Shoulder and Elbow*. Rosemont, IL, American Academy of Orthopaedic Surgeons, 1997, pp 369-378.
Prevel CD, Matloub HS, Ye Z, Sanger JR, Yousif NJ: The extrinsic blood supply of the ulnar nerve at the elbow: An anatomic study. *J Hand Surg [Am]* 1993;18:433-438.
Gelberman RH, Yamaguchi K, Hollstein SB, et al: Changes in interstitial pressure and cross-sectional area of the cubital tunnel and of the ulnar nerve with flexion of the elbow. *J Bone Joint Surg Am* 1998;80:492-501.

A-20: The MRI scan of the shoulder shown in Figure 1 was performed with the arm in abduction and external rotation. The image reveals what condition?

1. Contact between the rotator cuff and the posterior.superior labrum
2. Anterior instability
3. A ganglion cyst of the spinoglenoid notch
4. Osteonecrosis of the humeral head
5. Posterior subluxation

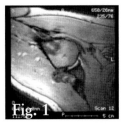

Fig. 1

PREFERRED RESPONSE: 1

DISCUSSION: Internal impingement of the shoulder is now a well-recognized cause of shoulder pain in the throwing athlete. First described by Walch and associates, it involves contact of the rotator cuff and labrum in the maximally externally rotated and abducted shoulder, such as in the late cocking phase of the throwing motion. Schickendantz and associates have shown this contact to be physiologic in most patients and becoming pathologic with repetitive overhead activity.

REFERENCES: Schickendantz MS, Ho CP, Keppler L, Shaw BD: MR imaging of the thrower's shoulder: Internal impingement, latissimus dorsi/subscapularis strains, and related injuries. *Magn Reson Imaging Clin N Am* 1999;7:39-49.
Walch G, Boileau P, Noel E, et al: Impingement of the deep surface of the supraspinatus tendon on the posterosuperior glenoid rim: An arthroscopic study. *J Shoulder Elbow Surg* 1992;1:238-245.
McFarland EG, Hsu CY, Neira C, O'Neil O: Internal impingement of the shoulder: A clinical and arthroscopic analysis. *J Shoulder Elbow Surg* 1999;8:458-460.

A-21: A 38-year-old man has winging of the ipsilateral scapula after undergoing a transaxillary resection of the first rib 3 weeks ago. What is the most likely cause of this finding?

1. Persistent thoracic outlet syndrome
2. Injury to the upper trunk of the brachial plexus
3. Injury to the long thoracic nerve
4. Injury to the lower trunk of the brachial plexus
5. Injury to the spinal accessory nerve

PREFERRED RESPONSE: 3

DISCUSSION: During transaxillary resection of the first rib, the long thoracic nerve is at risk as it passes either through or posterior to the middle scalene muscle. Injury to this nerve may occur as the result of overly aggressive retraction of the middle scalene during the procedure.

REFERENCES: Leffert RD: Thoracic outlet syndrome. *J Am Acad Orthop Surg* 1994;2:317-325.
Todd TW: The descent of the shoulder after birth: Its significance in the production of pressure-symptoms on the lowest brachial trunk. *Anat Anz* 1912;41:385-397.

A-22: A 45-year-old woman has had progressive right shoulder pain for the past 6 months. She notes that the pain disrupts her sleep, she has pain at rest that requires the use of narcotic analgesics, and she has limited use of her left shoulder for most activities of daily living. History reveals the use of corticosteroids for systemic lupus erythematosus. Examination shows diminished range of motion. Radiographs of the right shoulder are shown in Figures 2A and 2B. Treatment should consist of

1. core decompression of the humeral head.

2. humeral arthroplasty.

3. total shoulder arthroplasty.

4. glenohumeral arthrodesis.

5. vascularized fibular allograft.

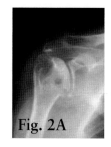 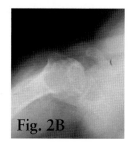
Fig. 2A   Fig. 2B

PREFERRED RESPONSE: 2

DISCUSSION: Humeral arthroplasty provides excellent pain relief and function for stage IV osteonecrosis with humeral collapse. In late disease with glenoid involvement (stage V), total shoulder arthroplasty is preferred. Some authors have reported satisfactory results with core decompression of the humeral head for early stages of osteonecrosis, but results for stage IV osteonecrosis are less satisfactory when compared with those for humeral arthroplasty.

REFERENCES: Cruess RL: Steroid-induced avascular necrosis of the head of the humerus: Natural history and management. *J Bone Joint Surg Br* 1976;58:313-317.
LePorte DM, Mont MA, Mohan V, Pierre-Jacques H, Jones LC, Hungerford DS: Osteonecrosis of the humeral head treated by core decompression. *Clin Orthop Relat Res* 1998;355:254-260.
Neer CS II (ed): *Shoulder Reconstruction*. Philadelphia, PA, WB Saunders, 1990, pp 194-202.

A-23: A 16-year-old high school pitcher notes acute pain on the medial side of his elbow during a pitch. Examination that day reveals medial elbow tenderness, pain with valgus stress, mild swelling, and loss of extension. Plain radiographs show closed physes and no fracture. Which of the following diagnostic studies will best reveal his injury?

1. Technetium Tc 99m bone scan

2. Contrast-enhanced MRI

3. CT

4. Electromyography

5. Arthroscopy

PREFERRED RESPONSE: 2

(continued on next page)

(A-23: *continued*)

DISCUSSION: The history and findings are consistent with a diagnosis of a sprain of the medial collateral ligament (MCL) of the elbow; therefore, contrast-enhanced MRI is considered the most sensitive and specific study for accurately showing this injury. Arthroscopic visualization of the MCL is limited to the most anterior portion of the anterior bundle only; complete inspection of the MCL using the arthroscope is not possible. CT without the addition of contrast is of no value in this situation. Use of a technetium Tc 99m bone scan is limited to aiding in the diagnosis of occult fracture, a highly unlikely injury in this patient. There are no clinical indications for electromyography.

REFERENCES: Timmerman LA, Andrews JR: Undersurface tear of the ulnar collateral ligament in baseball players: A newly recognized lesion. *Am J Sports Med* 1994;22:33-36.
Timmerman LA, Schwartz ML, Andrews JR: Preoperative evaluation of the ulnar collateral ligament by magnetic resonance imaging and computed tomography arthrography: Evaluation of 25 baseball players with surgical confirmation. *Am J Sports Med* 1994;22:26-32.
Fritz RC, Stoller DW: The elbow, in Stoller DW (ed): *Magnetic Resonance Imaging in Orthopedics and Sports Medicine*, ed 2. Philadelphia, PA, Lippincott Raven, 1995, pp 743-849.

A-24: Figures 3A and 3B show the radiographs of a 45-year-old patient. What is the most likely diagnosis?

1. Glenoid dysplasia
2. Rheumatoid arthritis with centralization
3. Osteoarthritis with posterior glenoid wear
4. Posterior scapular fracture deformity
5. Traumatic posterior subluxation of the shoulder

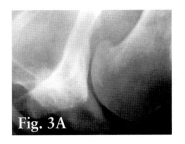
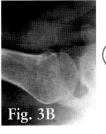

Fig. 3A   Fig. 3B

PREFERRED RESPONSE: 1

DISCUSSION: Glenoid dysplasia is an uncommon anomaly that usually has a benign course but may result in shoulder pain, arthritis, or multidirectional instability. Shoulder pain and instability often improve with shoulder strengthening exercises.

REFERENCES: Wirth MA, Lyons FR, Rockwood CA Jr: Hypoplasia of the glenoid: A review of sixteen patients. *J Bone Joint Surg Am* 1993;75:1175-1184.
Resnick D, Walter RD, Crudale AS: Bilateral dysplasia of the scapular neck. *AJR Am J Roentgenol* 1982;139:387-390.

A-25: A 23-year-old baseball pitcher who has diffuse pain along the posterior deltoid reports pain during late acceleration and follow-through. Examination of his arc of motion from external rotation to internal rotation at 90° of shoulder abduction reveals a significant deficit in internal rotation when compared to the nonthrowing shoulder. Initial management should consist of

1. a cortisone injection to the subscapular bursa.

2. posterior capsular stretching.

3. strengthening of the external rotators and scapular stabilizers.

4. continued pitching and working through the pain.

5. a sling and rest.

PREFERRED RESPONSE: 2

DISCUSSION: Loss of internal rotation is common among overhead throwers and tennis players. Posterior capsular stretching can improve symptoms when accompanied by rest and gradual resumption of throwing. To avoid a false impression of improvement, cortisone injection is not recommended. Pitching through pain can cause further damage to the labrum and capsule. A sling and external rotator strengthening will not improve internal rotation.

REFERENCES: Kibler WB: Biomechanical analysis of the shoulder during tennis activities. *Clin Sports Med* 1995;14:79-85.
Jobe FW, Tibone JE, Jobe CM, Kvitne RS: The shoulder in sports, in Rockwood CA, Matsen FA (eds): *The Shoulder*. Philadelphia, PA, WB Saunders, 1990, pp 961-990.

A-26: A 54-year-old man has left shoulder pain and weakness after falling while skiing 4 months ago. Examination reveals full range of motion passively, but he has a positive abdominal compression test and weakness with the lift-off test. External rotation strength with the arm at the side and strength with the arm abducted and internally rotated are normal. MRI scans are shown in Figures 4A and 4B. Treatment should consist of

1. arthroscopy and labral repair.

2. arthroscopy and supraspinatus repair.

3. arthroscopy and subscapularis repair.

4. arthroscopy and supraspinatus and infraspinatus repair.

5. open repair of the pectoralis major.

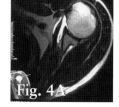 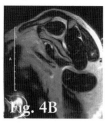

Fig. 4A   Fig. 4B

PREFERRED RESPONSE: 3

DISCUSSION: The examination findings are consistent with subscapularis muscle weakness but normal supraspinatus and infraspinatus strength. The lift-off test and abdominal compression test are specific for subscapularis function. The MRI scan reveals a chronic avulsion and retraction of the subscapularis. The transverse image reveals a normal infraspinatus muscle, and the sagittal image reveals an atrophic subscapularis. Surgical repair of the isolated subscapularis tendon is indicated.

(continued on next page)

(A-26: *continued*)

REFERENCES: Iannotti JP, Williams GR: *Disorders of the Shoulder: Diagnosis and Management*, ed 1. Philadelphia, PA, Lippincott Williams & Wilkins, 1999, pp 31-56.
Gerber C, Hersche O, Farron A: Isolated rupture of the subscapularis tendon: Results of operative treatment. *J Bone Joint Surg Am* 1996;78:1015-1023.

A-27: Figure 5 shows the radiograph of a 26-year-old auto mechanic who injured his right dominant elbow in a fall during a motocross race. Examination reveals pain and catching that limits his range of motion to 45° of supination and 20° of pronation. The interosseous space and distal radioulnar joint are stable. Management should consist of

1. splinting for 3 weeks, followed by range-of-motion exercises.
2. aspiration of the hemarthrosis, followed by range-of-motion exercises the following day.
3. fragment excision.
4. open reduction and internal fixation.
5. radial head excision.

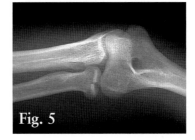

Fig. 5

PREFERRED RESPONSE: 4

DISCUSSION: The radial head is an important secondary stabilizer of the elbow, helping to resist valgus forces. There has been a movement toward open reduction and internal fixation of the radial head when technically feasible, especially in a relatively high-demand athlete or laborer. The examination and radiograph suggest that displacement of the fragment is great enough to create a mechanical block. Extended splinting would only serve to encourage arthrofibrosis. Early range of motion is appropriate if there is minimal displacement of the radial head fragment, it is stable, and there is no mechanical block to motion. Fragments larger than one third of the joint surface should be excised only if it is not possible to reduce and repair the fragment. Primary excision of the radial head should be avoided if possible. Complications after excision of the radial head include muscle weakness, wrist pain, valgus elbow instability, heterotopic ossification, and arthritis.

REFERENCES: Hotchkiss RN: Displaced fractures of the radial head: Internal fixation or excision? *J Am Acad Orthop Surg* 1997;5:1-10.
Esser RD, Davis S, Taavao T: Fractures of the radial head treated by internal fixation: Late results in 26 cases. *J Orthop Trauma* 1995;9:318-323.

Answers: Shoulder and Elbow

A-28: A 22-year-old swimmer underwent thermal capsulorrhaphy treatment for recurrent anterior subluxation. Following 3 weeks in a sling, the patient began an accelerated rehabilitation program that allowed him to return to swimming in 3 1/2 months. While practicing the butterfly stroke, he sustained an anterior dislocation. He now continues to have symptoms of anterior instability and has elected to have further surgery. Surgical findings may include a

1. biceps subluxation.

2. glenoid rim fracture.

3. subscapularis detachment.

4. loose body.

5. deficient anterior capsule.

PREFERRED RESPONSE: 5

DISCUSSION: Complications of thermal capsule shrinkage or accelerated rehabilitation include capsule ablation. Since the original surgery did not include labral reattachment, findings of a Bankart lesion or a glenoid fracture from a nontraumatic injury are unlikely. Subscapularis detachment or biceps subluxation is a postoperative complication of open repairs. Failure of early postoperative instability treatment should not produce loose bodies.

REFERENCES: Abrams JS: Thermal capsulorrhaphy for instability of the shoulder: Concerns and applications of the heat probe. *Instr Course Lect* 2001;50:29-36.

Hecht P, Hayashi K, Lu Y, et al: Monopolar radiofrequency energy effects on joint capsular tissue: Potential treatment for joint instability. An in vivo mechanical, morphological, and biochemical study using an ovine model. *Am J Sports Med* 1999;27:761-771.

A-29: During the anterior approach for repair of a distal biceps tendon rupture, what structure, shown under the scissors in Figure 6, is at risk for injury?

1. Brachial artery

2. Median nerve

3. Posterior interosseous nerve

4. Lateral antebrachial cutaneous nerve

5. Antecubital vein

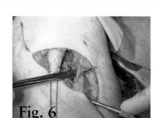

Fig. 6

PREFERRED RESPONSE: 4

DISCUSSION: The most commonly injured neurovascular structure during an anterior approach for the repair of a distal biceps tendon rupture is the lateral antebrachial cutaneous nerve. This structure is located lateral to the biceps tendon and in a superficial location just deep to the subcutaneous layer. The antecubital vein is medial and superficial with the brachial artery and median nerve also medial to the biceps tendon but deep to the common flexors. The posterior interosseous nerve is deep within the supinator muscle and can be injured in the deep dissection or through the posterior approach when using a two-incision approach.

(continued on next page)

(A-29: *continued*)

REFERENCES: Kelly EW, Morrey BF, O'Driscoll SW: Complications of repair of the distal biceps tendon with the modified two-incision technique. *J Bone Joint Surg Am* 2000;82:1575-1581.
Ramsey ML: Distal biceps tendon injuries: Diagnosis and management. *J Am Acad Orthop Surg* 1999;7:199-207.

A-30: A 23-year-old man undergoes surgery for the condition shown in Figure 7. At surgery, a nerve is seen to be contused but in continuity. Postoperatively, the muscles at the elbow and below which this nerve innervates show no motor function. Which of the following muscles will first show recovery of function?

1. Flexor carpi ulnaris (FCU)

2. Extensor pollicis longus (EPL)

3. Brachioradialis (BR)

4. Extensor carpi radialis brevis (ECRB)

5. Flexor digitorum profundus (FDP) to the little finger

PREFERRED RESPONSE: 3

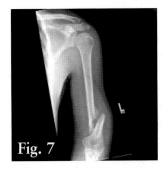

Fig. 7

DISCUSSION: Distal humerus fractures (Holstein-Lewis injuries) are notorious for radial nerve palsies. The order of innervation/reinnervation is the BR, extensor carpi radialis longus, and ECRB, followed by the supinator and the thumb and digital extensors. Brachioradialis function can be elicited by having the patient flex the elbow against resistance and the muscle belly can be palpated firing on the anterior proximal forearm/elbow. The FCU and FDP to the little finger are innervated by the ulnar nerve.

REFERENCES: Jawa A, McCarty P, Doornberg J, Harris M, Ring D: Extra-articular distal-third diaphyseal fractures of the humerus: A comparison of functional bracing and plate fixation. *J Bone Joint Surg Am* 2006;88:2343-2347.
Hoppenfeld S: *Surgical Exposures in Orthopaedics: The Anatomic Approach*, ed 2. JB Lippincott, Philadelphia, PA, 1994, p73.

A-31: A 35-year-old woman was injured while snowboarding 2 days ago. Immediately after the injury she was taken to the emergency department and diagnosed with a clavicle fracture. Examination of the fracture reveals 2 cm of shortening with obvious bone contact between the fracture fragments. In your discussion you mention the options of surgical fixation versus nonsurgical treatment. In comparing the two options, you mention that posttreatment results are identical in

1. shoulder range of motion.
2. maximal strength testing.
3. ultimate internal and external rotation endurance.
4. satisfaction rates.
5. rates of nonunion.

PREFERRED RESPONSE: 1

DISCUSSION: Despite historical reports of excellent results following nonsurgical treatment of displaced clavicle fractures, recent studies have determined multiple deficiencies when compared to surgical stabilization. Ultimate endurance and maximal strength are both statistically lower in the nonsurgical treatment group. Satisfaction rates as determined by patient questionnaires, Constant scores, and DASH scores reflect significantly worse outcomes with nonsurgical management. Rates of nonunion are significantly lower with surgical treatment. Range of motion, however, is well maintained in both groups.

REFERENCES: McKee MD, Pedersen EM, Jones C, et al: Deficits following nonoperative treatment of displaced midshaft clavicular fractures. *J Bone Joint Surg Am* 2006;88:35-40.
Canadian Orthopaedic Trauma Society: Nonoperative treatment compared with plate fixation of displaced midshaft clavicular fractures: A multicenter, randomized clinical trial. *J Bone Joint Surg Am* 2007;89:1-10.

A-32: Which of the following anatomic structures is most commonly injured after an elbow dislocation?

1. Anterior band of the medial collateral ligament
2. Lateral ulnar collateral ligament
3. Radial head
4. Coronoid process
5. Olecranon

PREFERRED RESPONSE: 2

DISCUSSION: Although all the listed structures can be injured during an elbow dislocation, the mechanism of dislocation in most individuals includes an initial rupture of the lateral ulnar collateral ligament. According to one study, all elbow dislocations and fracture-dislocations that required surgery demonstrated injury of the lateral ulnar collateral ligament.

REFERENCES: O'Driscoll SW: Elbow dislocations, in Morrey BF (ed): *The Elbow and Its Disorders*, ed. 3. Philadelphia, PA, WB Saunders, 2000, 409-420.
McKee MD, Schemitsch EH, Sala MJ, O'Driscoll SW: The pathoanatomy of lateral ligamentous disruption in complex elbow instability. *J Shoulder Elbow Surg* 2003;12(4):391-396.

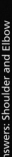

Answers: Shoulder and Elbow

A-33: A 62-year-old man who is right-hand dominant reports persistent pain in the left shoulder for the past 6 weeks. He denies any trauma or any prior problems with the shoulder. He states that he participated in some physical therapy to "strengthen" his shoulder but it failed to provide much relief. Examination reveals his right shoulder motion is 180, 60, and T8 (forward flexion, external rotation with arm at side, and internal rotation). His left shoulder motion, both active and passive, is 120, 30, and L1. He has minimal weakness about the left shoulder. T1- and T2-weighted MRI scans are shown in Figures 8A and 8B. What is the most appropriate treatment at this time?

1. Arthroscopic distal clavicle resection
2. Manipulation under anesthesia
3. Arthroscopic acromioplasty and, if needed, rotator cuff repair
4. Supervised and home-based physical therapy for motion exercises
5. Physical therapy for rotator cuff strengthening and scapula stabilization

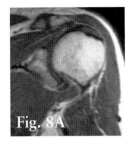
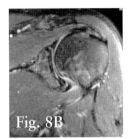

Fig. 8A   Fig. 8B

PREFERRED RESPONSE: 4

DISCUSSION: The patient lacks both active and passive motion in all planes of shoulder motion. Therefore, although the MRI scans reveal rotator cuff tendinosis and a partial-thickness tear, the primary diagnosis is adhesive capsulitis. At this relatively early stage of the disease, the most appropriate treatment is physical therapy for restoration of motion.

REFERENCE: Cuomo F, Holloway GB: Diagnosis and management of the stiff shoulder, in Iannotti JP, Williams GR(eds): *Disorders of the shoulder*, ed 2. Lippincott Williams & Wilkins, 2006, pp 541-562.

A-34: Arthroscopic rotator cuff repair, when compared with mini-open rotator cuff repair, has shown which of the following results?

1. Increased failure rate
2. Increased postoperative pain
3. Increased postoperative motion
4. Better clinical outcome
5. Lower infection rate

PREFERRED RESPONSE: 3

DISCUSSION: Arthroscopic rotator cuff repair has become popularized over the last decade. There are many articles that look at retrospective evaluation of both arthroscopic as well as mini open rotator cuff repairs. One prospective study by Severud looked at two groups with 35 patients undergoing an arthroscopic rotator cuff repair and 29 patients undergoing a mini-open repair, with a minimum follow-up of 24 months (average follow-up was 44.6 months). The UCLA score was 31.4 in the mini-open group and 32.6 in the arthroscopic group.

(continued on next page)

(A-34: *continued)*

The ASES score was 90 in the mini-open group and 91.7 in the arthroscopic group. Complications included arthrofibrosis in four patients in the open group and none in the arthroscopic group. Most studies have shown that the arthroscopic rotator cuff repair group with small to moderate size tears have similar failure rates, decreased postoperative pain, and increased postoperative motion. As can be seen by the data above, clinical outcomes are similar and to this date no study has shown a difference in infection rate between the two techniques.

REFERENCES: Severud EL, Ruotolo C, Abbott DD, Nottage WM: All-arthroscopic versus mini-open rotator cuff repair: A long-term retrospective outcome comparison. *Arthroscopy* 2003;19:234-238.
Gartsman GM, Khan M, Hammerman SM: Arthroscopic repair of full-thickness tears of the rotator cuff. *J Bone Joint Surg Am* 1998;80:832-840.

A-35: A healthy 52-year-old man has right shoulder pain and weakness of internal rotation after sustaining an injury 4 months ago. Examination reveals passive external rotation of 100° on the right compared with 60° on the left. At the time of arthroscopy, the long head of biceps tendon is found to be dislocated from the intertubercular groove. What is the most appropriate management at this time?

1. Anterior shoulder stabilization
2. Acromioplasty
3. Subscapularis repair
4. Superior labral anterior to posterior (SLAP) repair
5. Posterior labral repair

PREFERRED RESPONSE: 3

DISCUSSION: The clinical finding of excessive passive external rotation is strongly suggestive of a subscapularis tear. The intraoperative finding of dislocation of the biceps tendon from the intertubercular groove confirms the diagnosis. Arthroscopic or open repair is the most appropriate management of large subscapularis tears in active, medically fit patients. There is no history of instability or impingement requiring decompression, stabilization, or labral repair.

REFERENCES: Lyons RP, Green A: Subscapularis tendon tears. *J Am Acad Orthop Surg* 2005;13:353-363.
Norris TR (ed): *Orthopaedic Knowledge Update: Shoulder and Elbow 2*. Rosemont, IL. American Academy of Orthopaedic Surgeons, 2003, p 191.

A-36: A 32-year-old man reports a history of pain and restricted range of motion in his left shoulder after injuring his shoulder skiing 3 months ago. He was diagnosed with a soft-tissue injury at the time of his original injury and treated with physiotherapy. Figures 9A through 9C show a current radiograph, CT scan, and 3-D CT reconstruction. What is the most appropriate management at this time?

1. Closed reduction under conscious sedation
2. Nonsurgical management with continued physiotherapy
3. Closed reduction under general anesthesia followed by arthroscopic anterior stabilization
4. Shoulder hemiarthroplasty
5. Open reduction and bone grafting of the humeral head

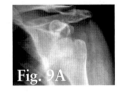
Fig. 9A

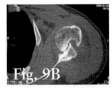
Fig. 9B

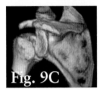
Fig. 9C

PREFERRED RESPONSE: 5

DISCUSSION: Open reduction of a chronic shoulder dislocation is most appropriate 3 to 4 weeks after injury. A gentle attempt at closed reduction under general anesthesia could be considered in patients who present within 3 to 4 weeks after injury. Closed reduction under sedation alone is contraindicated for chronic dislocations due to the risk of propagating the Hill-Sachs lesion and producing an anatomic neck fracture. Following open reduction, shoulder stability must be assessed with management guided by the size of the humeral head defect. Hill-Sachs lesions representing less than 20% of the head may be appropriate for anterior soft-tissue stabilization alone. Lesions involving between 20% to 45% of the head require management of the defect with either bone grafting, soft-tissue transfer into the defect, or rotational osteotomy of the humerus. Lesions involving greater than 45% of the head have traditionally been treated with hemiarthroplasty; however, in younger patients the indications for osteochondral grafting are expanding. This problem often presents in elderly, low demand patients, and in some cases benign neglect is appropriate. In younger, active patients, open reduction and management of the humeral head and/or glenoid defect is indicated.

REFERENCES: Loebenberg MI, Cuomo F: The treatment of chronic anterior and posterior dislocations of the glenohumeral joint and associated articular surface defects. *Clin Orthop North Am* 2000;31:23-34. Norris TR (ed): *Orthopaedic Knowledge Update: Shoulder and Elbow 2.* Rosemont, IL. American Academy of Orthopaedic Surgeons, 2003, pp 77-79.

A-37: A 13-year-old hockey player reports a 1-week history of left medial clavicle pain and dysphagia. A chest radiograph obtained at the emergency department on the day of injury was negative. Examination reveals swelling and tenderness along the medial edge of the left clavicle. The upper extremity neurologic examination is normal. What is the next most appropriate test to best define the patient's injury?

1. CT of the sternoclavicular joint
2. Barium swallowing study
3. Electromyography of the upper extremity
4. MRI of the glenohumeral joint
5. Bone scan

PREFERRED RESPONSE: 1

(continued on next page)

Answers: Shoulder and Elbow

(**A-37**: *continued*)

DISCUSSION: The patient has a posterior sternoclavicular fracture-dislocation. These injuries can go unrecognized at the time of initial presentation because of difficulty in interpreting radiographs. Posterior sternoclavicular fracture-dislocations can be associated with potentially serious complications, such as pneumothorax respiratory distress, brachial plexus injury, and vascular compromise. Patients often report dysphagia and hoarseness. Accurate diagnosis and prompt treatment are essential for good functional outcomes and prevention of complications. Adolescent patients can have a posterior sterno-clavicular dislocation, but usually they have a fracture through the medial physis. Axial CT scans are the most reliable radiographic modality for assessment of these injuries. Treatment consists of nonsurgical management, closed reduction, or open reduction. Most authors recommend open reduction if the patient is symptomatic with dysphagia or hoarseness. Furthermore, these patients will present late and open reduction may be the only successful treatment. The use of nonabsorbable sutures passed through drill holes in the sternum and/or the clavicular fracture fragments is recommended. Internal fixation is not recommended for this particular fracture because of concerns about hardware failure and/or migration.

REFERENCES: Waters PM, Bae DS, Kadiyala RK: Short-term outcomes after surgical treatment of traumatic posterior sternoclavicular fracture-dislocations in children and adolescents. *J Pediatr Orthop* 2003;23:464-469.

Yang J, al-Etani H, Letts M: Diagnosis and treatment of posterior sternoclavicular joint dislocations in children. *Am J Orthop* 1996;25:565-569.

A-38: Figures 10A and 10B show the radiographs of a 72-year-old woman who sustained a right shoulder injury 1 week ago. What is the most appropriate management?

1. Sling
2. Closed reduction and a sling and swath
3. Shoulder hemiarthroplasty
4. Total shoulder hemiarthroplasty
5. Neurologic consultation with electromyography

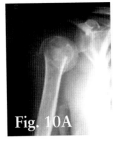
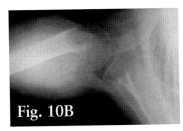

Fig. 10A   Fig. 10B

PREFERRED RESPONSE: 2

DISCUSSION: The radiographs show a minimally displaced, three-part, impacted proximal humeral fracture. The humeral head is subluxated below the glenoid. This is referred to as "pseudosubluxation." This commonly occurs after proximal humerus fractures and does not mandate any treatment or further evaluation in the weeks after the fracture. Therefore, the most appropriate management is closed reduction and a sling and swath. Axillary nerve function usually returns by the 6-week mark.

REFERENCES: Bigliani LU, Flatow EL, Pollock RG: in Rockwood CA, Green DP, Bucholz RW, Heckman JD (eds): *Fractures in Adults*. Lippincott-Raven Publishers, Philadelphia, PA, 1996.

Pritchett JW: Inferior subluxation of the humeral head after trauma or surgery. *J Shoulder Elbow Surg* 1997;6:356-359.

Hand and Wrist

Section Editor

Martin I. Boyer, MD, MSc, FRCSC

Q-1: What component (pulley) of the flexor tendon sheath is commonly involved in trigger finger?

1. A1
2. A2
3. A4
4. C1
5. C2

Q-2: The ulnar nerve innervates which of the following muscles in the hand and forearm?

1. Four lumbricals and abductor digiti minimi
2. Adductor pollicis and abductor digiti minimi
3. Extensor carpi ulnaris and flexor carpi ulnaris
4. Abductor digiti minimi and abductor pollicis brevis
5. Flexor pollicis brevis and opponens pollicis

Q-3: Which of the following structures is typically spared in ulnar impaction syndrome?

1. Ulnar head
2. Lunate
3. Triquetrum
4. Triangular fibrocartilage
5. Pisiform

Q-4: Which of the following structures form the boundaries of the anatomic snuff box of the wrist?

1. Extensor pollicis longus tendon and abductor pollicis longus tendon
2. Abductor pollicis brevis tendon and abductor pollicis longus tendon
3. Extensor pollicis longus tendon and extensor pollicis brevis tendon
4. Radial artery and extensor pollicis longus tendon
5. Abductor pollicis longus tendon and extensor pollicis brevis tendon

Q-5: Management of a patient with an acute nail bed laceration should consist of

1. soaks and oral antibiotics.
2. volar splinting.
3. removal of the nail plate.
4. repair of the nail bed with 6-0 chromic suture.
5. reconstruction of the nail with split sterile matrix grafts.

Q-6: The recurrent motor branch of the median nerve innervates which of the following muscles?

1. Abductor pollicis brevis, first dorsal interosseous, opponens pollicis
2. Abductor pollicis brevis, flexor pollicis brevis, opponens pollicis
3. Adductor pollicis, first dorsal interosseous, opponens pollicis
4. Adductor pollicis, flexor pollicis brevis (deep and superficial heads)
5. Adductor pollicis, flexor pollicis brevis, opponens pollicis

Q-7: A purulent flexor tenosynovitis of the thumb may communicate with the small finger flexor through which of the following structures?

1. Hypothenar space
2. Thenar space
3. Midpalmar space
4. Distal forearm (Parona space)
5. Lumbrical canal

Q-8: Which of the following nerves travels with the deep palmar arch?

1. Recurrent motor branch of the median nerve
2. Medial branch of the median nerve
3. Lateral branch of the median nerve
4. Superficial branch of the ulnar nerve
5. Deep motor branch of the ulnar nerve

Q-9: Pacinian corpuscles are lamellated nerve endings that are responsible for providing the perception of

1. pain.
2. light touch.
3. pressure.
4. temperature.
5. vibration.

Q-10: A positive Froment sign indicates weakness of which of the following muscles?

1. First dorsal interosseous
2. Adductor pollicis
3. Opponens pollicis
4. Flexor pollicis brevis
5. Abductor pollicis longus

Q-11: The vascularity of the digital flexor tendons is significantly richer in what cross-sectional region?

1. Volar ulnar quadrant
2. Volar radial quadrant
3. Peripheral one third
4. Dorsal one half
5. Center

Q-12: In the first dorsal compartment of the wrist, what tendon most frequently contains multiple slips?

1. Extensor pollicis longus
2. Extensor pollicis brevis
3. Extensor carpi radialis longus
4. Extensor carpi radialis brevis
5. Abductor pollicis longus

Q-13: An untreated mallet finger can progress into what type of deformity?

1. Boutonniere
2. Jersey finger
3. Swan-neck
4. Clinodactyly
5. Camptodactyly

Q-14: The strength of a repaired flexor tendon in the immediate postoperative period is most closely related to the

1. diameter of the suture used in the repair.
2. addition of a circumferential epitendinous stitch.
3. number of suture knots at the repair site.
4. number of suture strands that cross the repair site.
5. number of grasping loops on either side of the repair site.

Q-15: In the early stage of carpal tunnel syndrome, Semmes-Weinstein monofilament testing is considered more sensitive than static two-point discrimination testing in assessing median nerve dysfunction because it measures the

1. innervation density of slowly adapting fibers.
2. innervation density of quickly adapting fibers.
3. threshold of quickly adapting fibers.
4. threshold of slowly adapting fibers.
5. conduction velocity of sensory fibers.

Q-16: A 45-year-old housepainter injured his index finger holding it against the nozzle of a spray gun while painting 1 hour ago. He reports moderate pain that does not change markedly with passive motion of his fingers. Examination reveals a 0.5-cm puncture wound on the volar aspect of the finger at the level of the proximal interphalangeal joint. There is minimal swelling in his palm and distal forearm and no erythema. Management at this time should consist of

1. hospital admission for IV antibiotics.
2. injections of 10% calcium gluconate.
3. splinting and observation.
4. débridement in the operating room.
5. compartment pressure measurements.

Q-17: A 28-year-old woman has had progressive pain and loss of motion in her nondominant wrist for the past 6 months. Plain radiographs are shown in Figures 1A and 1B. Treatment should consist of

1. proximal row carpectomy.
2. total wrist arthrodesis.
3. lunate excision and silicone prosthesis replacement.
4. radial shortening osteotomy.
5. capitohamate fusion.

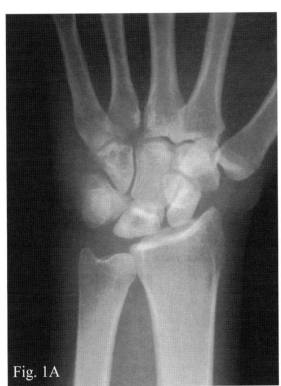

Fig. 1A

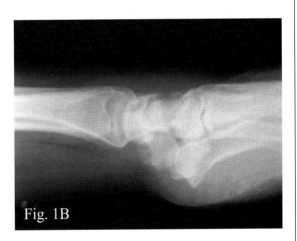

Fig. 1B

Q-18: When evaluating fractures of the distal radius, which of the following factors most likely indicates an associated injury of the triangular fibrocartilage complex and potential instability of the distal radio-ulnar joint?

1. Avulsion of the ulnar styloid
2. Greater than 5 mm of radial shortening
3. Greater than 10° of dorsal angulation
4. An open fracture
5. A fracture involving the sigmoid notch

Q-19: A 23-year-old man undergoes surgery for the condition shown in Figure 2. At surgery, a nerve is seen to be contused but in continuity. Postoperatively, the muscles at the elbow and below which this nerve innervates show no motor function. Which of the following muscles will first show recovery of function?

1. Flexor carpi ulnaris (FCU)
2. Extensor pollicis longus (EPL)
3. Brachioradialis (BR)
4. Extensor carpi radialis brevis (ECRB)
5. Flexor digitorum profundus (FDP) to the little finger

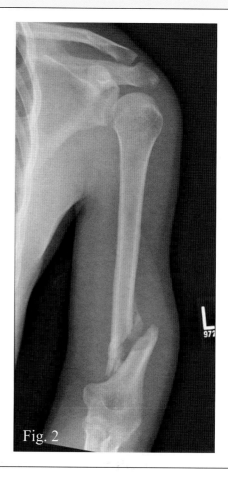

Fig. 2

A-1: What component (pulley) of the flexor tendon sheath is commonly involved in trigger finger?

1. A1
2. A2
3. A4
4. C1
5. C2

PREFERRED RESPONSE: 1

DISCUSSION: Although flexor tendons are occasionally seen to trigger anywhere within the fibro-osseous tunnel, the most common location of mechanical mismatch is at the proximal opening, A1 pulley, of the tunnel. The pulleys are named by their configuration, either annular (A) or cruciate (C), and numbered by their location, beginning proximally.

REFERENCE: Froimson AL: Tenosynovitis and tennis elbow, in Green DP (ed): *Operative Hand Surgery*, ed 3. New York, NY, Churchill Livingstone, 1993, vol 2, pp 1992-1995.

A-2: The ulnar nerve innervates which of the following muscles in the hand and forearm?

1. Four lumbricals and abductor digiti minimi
2. Adductor pollicis and abductor digiti minimi
3. Extensor carpi ulnaris and flexor carpi ulnaris
4. Abductor digiti minimi and abductor pollicis brevis
5. Flexor pollicis brevis and opponens pollicis

Muscle Innervated of Hand

PREFERRED RESPONSE: 2

DISCUSSION: The ulnar nerve innervates the abductor digiti minimi, adductor pollicis, flexor carpi ulnaris, the lumbricals to the small and ring fingers, and frequently a portion of the flexor pollicis brevis. The median nerve innervates the lumbricals to the index and long fingers, the flexor pollicis brevis, opponens pollicis, and the abductor pollicis brevis. The radial nerve innervates the extensor carpi ulnaris.

REFERENCE: Spinner M (ed): *Kaplan's Functional and Surgical Anatomy of the Hand*, ed 3. Philadelphia, PA, JB Lippincott, 1984, pp 230-233.

Answers: Hand and Wrist

A-3: Which of the following structures is typically spared in ulnar impaction syndrome?

1. Ulnar head
2. Lunate
3. Triquetrum
4. Triangular fibrocartilage
5. Pisiform

PREFERRED RESPONSE: 5

DISCUSSION: The bones of the ulnocarpal joint consist of the ulna, triquetrum, and lunate. The triangular fibrocartilage is interposed between the carpal bones and the ulnar head, and is typically the first structure to undergo degeneration. The interosseous ligament provides a continuation of the articular surface between the lunate and triquetrum, and also frequently shows early degeneration. Chondromalacia of the ulnar head, lunate, and occasionally the triquetrum is followed by cystic and sclerotic changes within these bones. The pisiform is not typically involved in this syndrome.

REFERENCE: Chun S, Palmer AK: The ulnar impaction syndrome: Follow-up of ulnar shortening osteotomy. *J Hand Surg [Am]* 1993;18:46-53.

A-4: Which of the following structures form the boundaries of the anatomic snuff box of the wrist?

1. Extensor pollicis longus tendon and abductor pollicis longus tendon
2. Abductor pollicis brevis tendon and abductor pollicis longus tendon
3. Extensor pollicis longus tendon and extensor pollicis brevis tendon
4. Radial artery and extensor pollicis longus tendon
5. Abductor pollicis longus tendon and extensor pollicis brevis tendon

PREFERRED RESPONSE: 3

DISCUSSION: In the first dorsal compartment, the extensor pollicis brevis tendon is ulnar to the abductor pollicis longus tendon. The anatomic snuff box of the wrist is bounded by the abductor pollicis longus and extensor pollicis brevis on its radial border and the extensor pollicis longus on its ulnar border. The distal half of the scaphoid and the tubercle of the trapezium form the floor. The radial artery and branches of the superficial radial nerve pass through this area. Branches of the lateral antebrachial cutaneous nerve, which is a branch of the musculocutaneous nerve, may also pass through this area.

REFERENCE: Spinner M (ed): *Kaplan's Functional and Surgical Anatomy of the Hand*, ed 3. Philadelphia, PA, JB Lippincott, 1984, pp 359-371.

A-5: Management of a patient with an acute nail bed laceration should consist of

1. soaks and oral antibiotics.
2. volar splinting.
3. removal of the nail plate.
4. repair of the nail bed with 6-0 chromic suture.
5. reconstruction of the nail with split sterile matrix grafts.

PREFERRED RESPONSE: 4

DISCUSSION: It is important to properly treat a nail bed injury acutely. As a rule, reconstruction does not provide the same results as proper early care. Using the proper suture (6-0 or 7-0 chromic) on a fine needle with magnification, 90% of patients should have good or better results. Reconstruction of the nail with split sterile matrix grafts or split germinal matrix grafts will improve nail appearance, but will most likely result in a permanent deformity.

REFERENCES: Manske PR (ed): *Hand Surgery Update*. Rosemont, IL, American Academy of Orthopaedic Surgeons, 1994, pp 289-293.
The perionychium, in Zook EG (ed): *Hand Clinics*. Chicago, IL, WB Saunders, 1990, vol 6, pp 36-43.

Thenar mustles

A-6: The recurrent motor branch of the median nerve innervates which of the following muscles?

1. Abductor pollicis brevis, first dorsal interosseous, opponens pollicis
2. Abductor pollicis brevis, flexor pollicis brevis, opponens pollicis   *Thenar muscle*
3. Adductor pollicis, first dorsal interosseous, opponens pollicis
4. Adductor pollicis, flexor pollicis brevis (deep and superficial heads)
5. Adductor pollicis, flexor pollicis brevis, opponens pollicis

PREFERRED RESPONSE: 2

DISCUSSION: The recurrent motor branch of the median nerve supplies the thenar muscles (abductor pollicis brevis, flexor pollicis brevis, and opponens pollicis) that are primarily responsible for thumb opposition. The nerve can be injured in carpal tunnel release. A branch of the nerve also supplies the first lumbrical. The adductor pollicis and the interossei are supplied by the ulnar nerve.

REFERENCES: Last RJ: *Anatomy: Regional and Applied*, ed 6. London, England, Churchill Livingstone, 1978, p 109.
Hoppenfeld S, deBoer P: *Surgical Exposures in Orthopaedics: The Anatomic Approach*. Philadelphia, PA, JB Lippincott, 1984, p 170.

Answers: Hand and Wrist

A-7: A purulent flexor tenosynovitis of the thumb may communicate with the small finger flexor through which of the following structures?

1. Hypothenar space

2. Thenar space

3. Midpalmar space

4. Distal forearm (Parona space)

5. Lumbrical canal

PREFERRED RESPONSE: 4

DISCUSSION: Only the flexor sheaths of the thumb and small finger are continuous from the digit through the carpal canal and into the distal forearm. If one of the sheaths ruptures from synovitis, it may contaminate the other sheath through the Parona space in the distal forearm. This potential space lies superficial to the pronator quadratus and deep to the flexor tendons.

REFERENCES: Green DP, Hotchkiss RN, Pederson WC (eds): *Operative Hand Surgery*, ed 4. New York, NY, Churchill Livingstone, 1999, pp 1044-1045.
Burkhalter WE: Deep space infections. *Hand Clin* 1989;5:553-559.

A-8: Which of the following nerves travels with the deep palmar arch?

1. Recurrent motor branch of the median nerve

2. Medial branch of the median nerve

3. Lateral branch of the median nerve

4. Superficial branch of the ulnar nerve

5. Deep motor branch of the ulnar nerve

PREFERRED RESPONSE: 5

DISCUSSION: The ulnar nerve divides alongside the pisiform, and the deep branch supplies the three hypothenar muscles and crosses the palm with the deep palmar arch to supply the two ulnar lumbricals, all interossei, and finally the adductor pollicis. The superficial branch supplies the ulnar digital branches to the small and ring fingers. The median nerve branches are more superficial in the palm near the superficial palmar arch.

REFERENCES: Last RJ: *Anatomy: Regional and Applied*, ed 6. London, England, Churchill Livingstone, 1978, p 109.
Hoppenfeld S, deBoer P: *Surgical Exposures in Orthopaedics: The Anatomic Approach*. Philadelphia, PA, JB Lippincott, 1984, pp 166-169.

A-9: Pacinian corpuscles are lamellated nerve endings that are responsible for providing the perception of

1. pain.
2. light touch.
3. pressure.
4. temperature.
5. vibration.

PREFERRED RESPONSE: 3

DISCUSSION: Pacinian corpuscles are nerve endings that provide the perception of pressure.

REFERENCE: Sunderland SS: *Nerves and Nerve Injuries*, ed 2. New York, NY, Churchill Livingstone, 1978, pp 343-347.

A-10: A positive Froment sign indicates weakness of which of the following muscles?

1. First dorsal interosseous
2. Adductor pollicis   — *Ulnar nerve*
3. Opponens pollicis
4. Flexor pollicis brevis
5. Abductor pollicis longus

PREFERRED RESPONSE: 2

DISCUSSION: Thumb adduction is powered by the adductor pollicis (ulnar nerve). Testing involves having the patient forcibly hold a piece of paper between the thumb and radial side of the index proximal phalanx. When this muscle is weak or nonfunctioning, the thumb interphalangeal joint flexes with this maneuver, resulting in a positive Froment sign. The paper is held by action of the thumb flexion (flexor pollicis longus and flexor pollicis brevis; median innervated).

REFERENCE: Burton RI: *The Hand: Examination and Diagnosis*. Chicago, IL, American Society for Surgery of the Hand, 1978, pp 26-27.

A-11: The vascularity of the digital flexor tendons is significantly richer in what cross-sectional region?

1. Volar ulnar quadrant
2. Volar radial quadrant
3. Peripheral one third
4. Dorsal one half
5. Center

PREFERRED RESPONSE: 4

DISCUSSION: The vascularity of the dorsal portion of the digital flexor tendons is considerably richer than the volar portion. The other regions are not preferentially more vascular.

REFERENCES: Hunter JM, Scheider LH, Makin EJ (eds): *Tendon Surgery in the Hand.* St Louis, MO, Mosby, 1987, pp 91-99.

Gelberman RH, Khabie V, Cahill CJ: The revascularization on healing flexor tendons in the digital sheath: A vascular injection study in dogs. *J Bone Joint Surg Am* 1991;73:868-881.

A-12: In the first dorsal compartment of the wrist, what tendon most frequently contains multiple slips?

1. Extensor pollicis longus
2. Extensor pollicis brevis
3. Extensor carpi radialis longus
4. Extensor carpi radialis brevis
5. Abductor pollicis longus

PREFERRED RESPONSE: 5

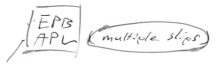

DISCUSSION: The first extensor compartment of the wrist typically contains a single extensor pollicis brevis tendon and the abductor pollicis longus tendon that nearly always has multiple tendon slips. The extensor pollicis brevis tendon is frequently found to be separated from the slips of the abductor pollicis longus tendon by an intracompartmental septum. During surgery, this septum must be divided to complete the release of the compartment.

REFERENCES: Jackson WT, Viegas SF, Coon TM, Stimpson KD, Frogameni AD, Simpson JM: Anatomical variations in the first extensor compartment of the wrist: A clinical and anatomical study. *J Bone Joint Surg Am* 1986;68:923-926.

Minamikawa Y, Peimer CA, Cox WL, Sherwin FS: DeQuervain's syndrome: Surgical and anatomical studies of the fibro-osseous canal. *Orthopedics* 1991;14:545-549.

A-13: An untreated mallet finger can progress into what type of deformity?

1. Boutonniere
2. Jersey finger
3. Swan-neck
4. Clinodactyly
5. Camptodactyly

PREFERRED RESPONSE: 3

DISCUSSION: The loss of the extensor insertion at the distal phalanx results in a mallet finger deformity that permits the extension mechanism to shift proximally, thereby increasing the extensor tone at the proximal interphalangeal (PIP) joint relative to the distal interphalangeal joint. If the volar plate of the PIP joint is lax, the joint will hyperextend as a secondary deformity. As the PIP joint hyperextends, the extensor mechanism will migrate dorsally to the axis of rotation of the PIP joint and a swan-neck deformity will result.

REFERENCES: Littler JW: The digital extensor-flexor system, in Converse JM (ed): *Reconstructive Plastic Surgery*. Philadelphia, PA, WB Saunders, 1977, vol 6, pp 3166-3214.
Burton RI: Extensor tendon—late reconstruction, in Green DP (ed): *Operative Hand Surgery*. New York, NY, Churchill Livingstone, 1993, pp 1955-1988.

A-14: The strength of a repaired flexor tendon in the immediate postoperative period is most closely related to the

1. diameter of the suture used in the repair.
2. addition of a circumferential epitendinous stitch.
3. number of suture knots at the repair site.
4. number of suture strands that cross the repair site.
5. number of grasping loops on either side of the repair site.

PREFERRED RESPONSE: 4

DISCUSSION: Numerous in vitro studies have demonstrated that the strength of a flexor tendon repair is directly proportional to the number of core suture strands that cross the repair site. Four-strand repairs have twice the strength of two-strand repairs, and complex six-strand repairs are up to three times stronger. Repair strength has never been shown to be significantly affected by the diameter of the suture employed or by the addition of multiple grasping loops that have been shown to contribute to gap formation in one experimental model. The addition of a circumferential epitendinous stitch has been shown to increase the strength of the repair by 10% to 50%; therefore, it is recommended but is not considered essential. While most repairs rupture at the suture knot, the number of knots employed has not been shown to be a factor in the initial repair strength.

(Continued on next page)

(A-14: *continued*)

REFERENCES: Boyer MI, Strickland JW, Engles D, Sachar K, Leversedge FJ: Flexor tendon repair and rehabilitation: State of the art in 2002. *Instr Course Lect* 2003;52:137-161.
Winters SC, Gelberman RH, Woo SL, Chan SS, Grewal R, Seiler JG III: The effects of multiple-strand suture methods on the strength and excursion of repaired intrasynovial flexor tendons: A biomechanical study in dogs. *J Hand Surg [Am]* 1998;23:97-104.

A-15: In the early stage of carpal tunnel syndrome, Semmes-Weinstein monofilament testing is considered more sensitive than static two-point discrimination testing in assessing median nerve dysfunction because it measures the

1. innervation density of slowly adapting fibers.
2. innervation density of quickly adapting fibers.
3. threshold of quickly adapting fibers.
4. threshold of slowly adapting fibers.
5. conduction velocity of sensory fibers.

PREFERRED RESPONSE: 4

DISCUSSION: A threshold test measures the function of a single nerve fiber innervating a group of receptors, whereas an innervation density test measures numerous overlapping receptor fields. Therefore, threshold tests such as Semmes-Weinstein monofilament testing and vibration testing are more likely to show a gradual change in nerve function. Semmes-Weinstein monofilament testing reflects the function of slowly adapting touch fibers (Group-A beta), and vibration testing measures the quickly adapting fibers. Static and moving two-point discrimination testing both measure innervation density and are more a reflection of complex cortical organization. Therefore, they are most useful in assessing functional nerve regeneration after nerve repair. Conduction velocity is a useful measure of nerve dysfunction in compressive neuropathies but can be measured only with electrodiagnostic equipment.

REFERENCES: Gelberman RH: *Operative Nerve Repair and Reconstruction.* Philadelphia, PA, JB Lippincott, 1991, pp 158-162.
MacKinnon SE, Dellon AL: *Surgery of the Peripheral Nerve.* New York, NY, Thieme, 1988, pp 217-219.

A-16: A 45-year-old housepainter injured his index finger holding it against the nozzle of a spray gun while painting 1 hour ago. He reports moderate pain that does not change markedly with passive motion of his fingers. Examination reveals a 0.5-cm puncture wound on the volar aspect of the finger at the level of the proximal interphalangeal joint. There is minimal swelling in his palm and distal forearm and no erythema. Management at this time should consist of

1. hospital admission for IV antibiotics.

2. injections of 10% calcium gluconate.

3. splinting and observation.

4. débridement in the operating room.

5. compartment pressure measurements.

PREFERRED RESPONSE: 4

DISCUSSION: High-pressure injection injuries are often innocuous in appearance because a small entry site is often all that is seen. However, they are considered surgical emergencies because oil-based agents like paint can cause rapid tissue necrosis and fibrosis. Thorough débridement of all involved compartments is mandatory, although poor outcomes are still not unexpected. Antibiotics are of no value initially because tissue destruction occurs from chemical irritation. Calcium gluconate is used specifically to counteract hydrofluoric acid burns. Observation will delay appropriate treatment and is associated with poor outcomes. Compartment pressure measurements are unnecessary.

REFERENCES: Failla JM, Linden MD: The acute pathologic changes of paint-injection injury and correlation to surgical treatment: A report of two cases. *J Hand Surg [Am]* 1997;22:156-159.
Schoo MJ, Scott FA, Boswick JA Jr: High-pressure injection injuries of the hand. *J Trauma* 1980;20:229-238.

Answers: Hand and Wrist

A-17: A 28-year-old woman has had progressive pain and loss of motion in her nondominant wrist for the past 6 months. Plain radiographs are shown in Figures 1A and 1B. Treatment should consist of

1. proximal row carpectomy.
2. total wrist arthrodesis.
3. lunate excision and silicone prosthesis replacement.
4. radial shortening osteotomy.
5. capitohamate fusion.

PREFERRED RESPONSE: 4

DISCUSSION: Based on the radiographic findings of lunate collapse without loss of carpal height nor a fixed carpal malalignment, the patient has stage IIIA Kienböck disease according to Lichtman's classification. Although much controversy remains regarding optimal treatment for Kienböck disease, radial shortening osteotomy decreases the radiolunate load and has shown excellent clinical results in patients with stage III or IIIA disease who have a negative ulnar variance. Proximal row carpectomy and total wrist arthrodesis are both salvage procedures that are applicable in stage IIIB or IV disease. The use of a silicone lunate prosthesis is no longer advised because of a high rate of particulate synovitis. Capitohamate fusion alone has not been shown to unload the lunate, although it is sometimes combined with capitate shortening, which decreases the load across the radiolunate articulation.

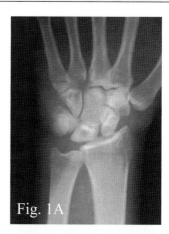

Fig. 1A

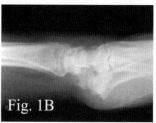

Fig. 1B

REFERENCES: Quenzer DE, Dobyns JH, Linscheid RL, Trail IA, Vidal MA: Radial recession osteotomy for Kienböck's disease. *J Hand Surg [Am]* 1997;22:386-395.
Trumble T, Glisson RR, Seaber AV, Urbaniak JR: A biomechanical comparison of the methods for treating Kienböck's disease. *J Hand Surg [Am]* 1986;11:88-93.

A-18: When evaluating fractures of the distal radius, which of the following factors most likely indicates an associated injury of the triangular fibrocartilage complex and potential instability of the distal radio-ulnar joint?

1. Avulsion of the ulnar styloid
2. Greater than 5 mm of radial shortening
3. Greater than 10° of dorsal angulation
4. An open fracture
5. A fracture involving the sigmoid notch

PREFERRED RESPONSE: 2

DISCUSSION: The primary findings that best predict distal radioulnar joint instability and triangular fibrocartilage complex injuries are greater than 5 mm of radial shortening or greater than 25° of dorsal angulation. Other findings that may be associated with triangular fibrocartilage complex injuries are basilar ulnar styloid fractures, ulnar dome fractures, and injuries to the sigmoid notch.

REFERENCE: Koval KJ (ed): *Orthopaedic Knowledge Update 7*. Rosemont, IL, American Academy of Orthopaedic Surgeons, 2002, pp 339-358.

A-19: A 23-year-old man undergoes surgery for the condition shown in Figure 2. At surgery, a nerve is seen to be contused but in continuity. Postoperatively, the muscles at the elbow and below which this nerve innervates show no motor function. Which of the following muscles will first show recovery of function?

1. Flexor carpi ulnaris (FCU)
2. Extensor pollicis longus (EPL)
3. Brachioradialis (BR)
4. Extensor carpi radialis brevis (ECRB)
5. Flexor digitorum profundus (FDP) to the little finger

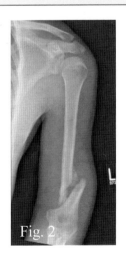

Fig. 2

PREFERRED RESPONSE: 3

DISCUSSION: Distal humerus fractures (Holstein-Lewis injuries) are notorious for radial nerve palsies. The order of innervation/reinnervation is the BR, extensor carpi radialis longus, and ECRB, followed by the supinator and the thumb and digital extensors. Brachioradialis function can be elicited by having the patient flex the elbow against resistance and the muscle belly can be palpated firing on the anterior proximal forearm/elbow. The FCU and FDP to the little finger are innervated by the ulnar nerve.

REFERENCES: Jawa A, McCarty P, Doornberg J, Harris M, Ring D: Extra-articular distal-third diaphyseal fractures of the humerus: A comparison of functional bracing and plate fixation. *J Bone Joint Surg Am* 2006;88:2343-2347.

Hoppenfeld S: *Surgical Exposures in Orthopaedics: The Anatomic Approach*, ed 2., Philadelphia, PA, 1994, JB Lippincott, p 73.

Total Joint Arthroplasty/ Joint Salvage

Section Editor

Thomas Parker Vail, MD

Q-1: Which of the following findings is a prerequisite for a high tibial valgus osteotomy for medial compartment gonarthrosis?

1. Inflammatory arthritis
2. Ligamentous instability
3. Lateral tibial subluxation
4. Preoperative arc of motion of at least 90°
5. Narrowing of the lateral compartment cartilaginous joint space

Q-2: What is the main benefit of using metal-backed tibial components in total knee arthroplasty?

1. Improve the conformity of the articular surfaces
2. Reduce the maximum compressive stresses on the underlying cancellous bone
3. Increase the tensile forces on the other condyle when one is loaded
4. Decrease the thickness of the polyethylene tray
5. Decrease the compressive forces on the polyethylene tray

Q-3: A 32-year-old woman with systemic lupus erythematosus treated with methotrexate and oral corticosteroids reports right groin pain with ambulation and night pain. Examination reveals pain with internal and external rotation and flexion that is limited to 105° because of discomfort. Laboratory studies show a serum WBC of 9.0/mm³ and an erythrocyte sedimentation rate of 35 mm/h. Figures 1A and 1B show AP and lateral radiographs of the right hip. Further evaluation should include

1. examination under fluoroscopy.
2. MRI.
3. a bone scan.
4. arthrography.
5. aspiration and arthrography.

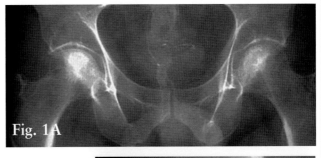
Fig. 1A

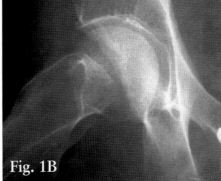
Fig. 1B

Q-4: Which of the following factors can contribute to patellar subluxation following routine total knee arthroplasty?

1. External rotation of the femoral component
2. Internal rotation of the tibial component
3. Symmetric patellar resection
4. Lateral placement of the tibial component
5. Neutral alignment of the mechanical axis

Q-5: During total knee arthroplasty using a posterior cruciate-retaining design, excessive tightness in flexion is noted, while the extension gap is felt to be balanced. Which of the following actions will effectively balance the knee?

1. Resect more distal femur.
2. Resect more anterior tibia.
3. Use a larger femoral component.
4. Use a smaller polyethylene insert.
5. Recess the posterior cruciate ligament.

Q-6: Figures 2A and 2B show the current radiographs of a 58-year-old man who underwent total knee arthroplasty with a cruciate ligament–sparing prosthesis 7 years ago. Examination reveals boggy synovitis and moderate pain, particularly anteriorly. Management should consist of

1. follow-up radiographs.
2. alendronate, with follow-up examinations every 6 months.
3. revision to a posterior stabilized prosthesis.
4. exchange of the tibial insert through a limited incision.
5. surgical exploration with revision or exchange based on the findings.

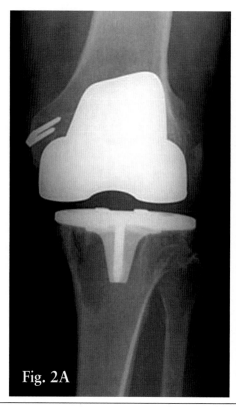

Fig. 2A

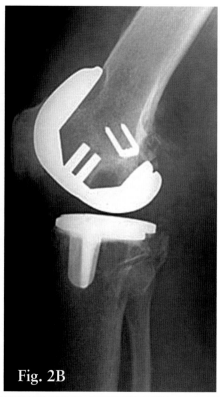

Fig. 2B

Q-7: What is the correct order of the elastic modulus of the following materials from greatest to least?

1. Stainless steel, cobalt-chromium, titanium, polymethylmethacrylate (PMMA), alumina ceramic
2. Cobalt-chromium, stainless steel, titanium, alumina ceramic, PMMA
3. Alumina ceramic, titanium, cobalt-chromium, stainless steel, PMMA
4. Alumina ceramic, cobalt-chromium, stainless steel, titanium, PMMA
5. Titanium, cobalt-chromium, alumina ceramic, stainless steel, PMMA

Q-8: Figure 3 shows the radiograph of a 75-year-old woman who reports the sudden onset of disabling medial knee pain. What is the most likely diagnosis?

1. Osteoarthritis
2. Osteonecrosis
3. Meniscal tear
4. Metastatic lesion
5. Synovial osteochondromatosis

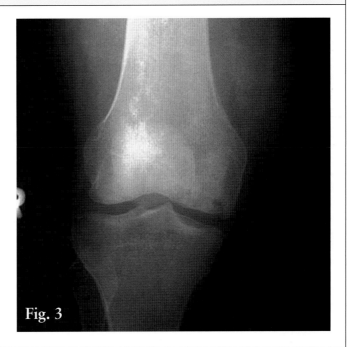

Fig. 3

Q-9: When using highly cross-linked ultra-high molecular weight polyethylene as an articulating surface for total knee arthroplasty, what property of the material raises concern?

1. Decreased volumetric wear
2. Decreased ductility
3. Increased mobility of the ultra-high molecular weight polyethylene chains in the material
4. Increased fatigue resistance
5. Increased fracture toughness

Q-10: An otherwise healthy 57-year-old man has persistent, severe hip pain after undergoing total hip arthroplasty 3 months ago. What is the next most appropriate step in management?

1. Serial radiographs to assess progressive radiolucency from osteolysis or mechanical loosening

2. Assessment of C-reactive protein, erythroctye sedimentation rate, and CBC, followed by aspiration

3. Technetium and/or indium-labeled leukocyte scintigraphy

4. A trial of broad-spectrum cefalosporin antibiotics to assess for a change in pain intensity

5. Injection with lidocaine and methylprednisolone acetate

Q-11: Which of the following treatments of polyethylene results in the highest amount of oxidative degradation?

1. Ethylene oxide sterilization

2. Gamma irradiation in air

3. Gamma irradiation in an inert environment

4. Gamma irradiation followed by cross-linking

5. Gas plasma sterilization

Q-12: Consider the theoretic articulation shown in Figure 4 as femoral and tibial components of a total knee prosthesis in which the components fit like a "roller in trough." Which of the following best describes the articulation?

1. Constrained to anteroposterior translation, unconstrained to medial-lateral translation, high contact stress on edge (ie, varus-valgus) loading

2. Constrained to anteroposterior translation, unconstrained to medial-lateral translation, low contact stress on edge (ie, varus-valgus) loading

3. Unconstrained to anteroposterior translation, constrained to medial-lateral translation, high contact stress on edge (ie, varus-valgus) loading

4. Unconstrained to anteroposterior translation, constrained to medial-lateral translation, low contact stress on edge (ie, varus-valgus) loading

5. Constraint is dependent on the status of the posterior cruciate ligament

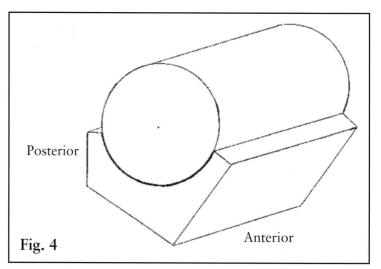

Fig. 4

Q-13: Wear particles of ultra-high molecular weight polyethylene that are generated by total hip implants are predominantly of what diameter?

1. Less than 1 micron

2. 10 to 50 microns

3. 100 to 200 microns

4. 500 to 750 microns

5. Greater than 1,000 microns

Q-14: Which of the following best describes the resultant forces on an increased offset stem when compared with a standard offset stem?

1. Increased joint reaction force, increased torsional load

2. Increased joint reaction force, decreased torsional load

3. Decreased joint reaction force, increased torsional load

4. Decreased joint reaction force, decreased torsional load

5. No change in joint reaction force or torsional load

Q-15: During total knee arthroplasty, what component position aids in proper tracking and stability of the patellar component?

1. Femoral component in external rotation

2. Tibial component in internal rotation

3. Medialization of the tibial tray

4. Lateralization of the patellar component

5. Medialization of the femoral component

Q-16: A 60-year-old woman reports anterior knee pain 2 years after undergoing primary total knee arthroplasty for rheumatoid arthritis. A Merchant view of the patella is shown in Figure 5. What is the most likely cause of her pain?

1. Elevation of the joint line
2. Lateral placement of the femoral component
3. Medial placement of the patellar component
4. Internal rotation of the femoral component
5. External rotation of the tibial component

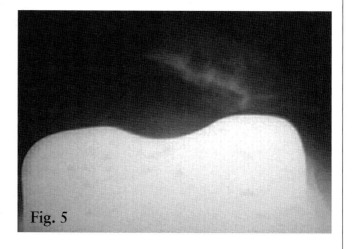

Fig. 5

Q-17: The anterior portal of a hip arthroscopy places what structure at greatest risk for injury?

1. Ascending branch of the lateral circumflex femoral artery
2. Ascending branch of the medial circumflex femoral artery
3. Femoral nerve
4. Lateral femoral cutaneous nerve
5. Superior gluteal nerve

Q-18: A 32-year-old man has posttraumatic arthritis after undergoing open reduction and internal fixation of a left acetabular fracture. A total hip arthroplasty is performed, and the radiograph is shown in Figure 6. What is the most common mode of failure leading to revision in this group of patients?

1. Infection
2. Heterotopic ossification
3. Dislocation
4. Periprosthetic fracture
5. Acetabular component loosening

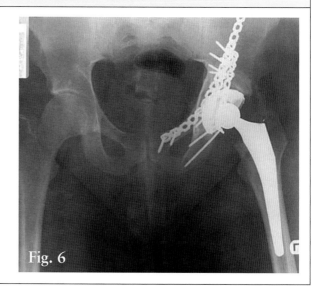

Fig. 6

Q-19: A 42-year-old man sustained the periprosthetic fracture shown in Figures 7A and 7B. The femoral component is well fixed. What is the next most appropriate step in management?

1. Closed reduction and bracing

2. Retrograde femoral intramedullary nailing

3. Open reduction and internal fixation of the fracture, leaving the femoral stem in place

4. Open reduction and internal fixation of the fracture and insertion of a proximally porous-coated stem

5. Open reduction and internal fixation of fracture fragments and insertion of a fully porous-coated femoral stem with diaphyseal fixation distal to the fracture

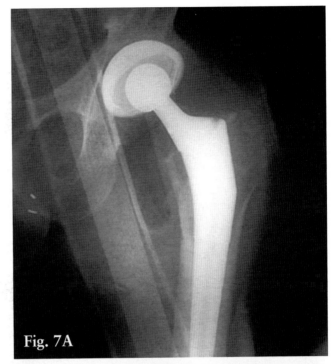

Fig. 7A

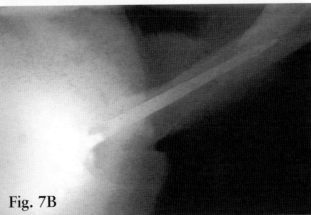

Fig. 7B

Q-20: A homebound 75-year-old woman with diabetes mellitus has had progressive left knee pain and swelling for the past 6 weeks. She is febrile with a temperature of 103°F (39.5°C). History reveals that she underwent arthroplasty 5 years ago. Examination shows passive range of motion of 0° to 100° with no active extension. Knee aspiration reveals purulent fluid with a Gram stain showing gram-negative rods. A radiograph is shown in Figure 8. In addition to IV antibiotics, which of the following management options offers the best chance of a successful outcome?

1. Incision and drainage with repair of the extensor mechanism

2. Removal of components and delayed revision knee arthroplasty with an allograft extensor mechanism

3. Removal of components and immediate exchange revision total knee arthroplasty

4. Removal of components and delayed knee arthrodesis

5. Removal of components and delayed revision knee arthroplasty with extensor mechanism repair

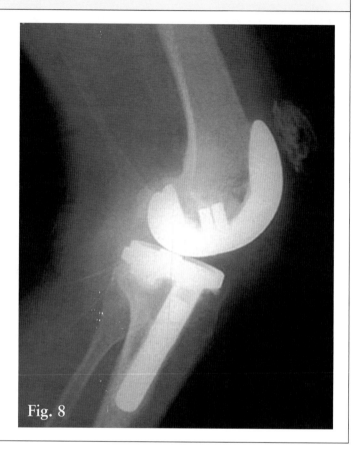

Fig. 8

Q-21: Varus intertrochanteric osteotomy for coxa valga commonly produces which of the following results?

1. Decreased abductor lever arm

2. Increased hip joint reaction force

3. Increased center edge angle

4. Abductor lag and lurch

5. Lengthening of the leg

Q-22: During a posterior cruciate ligament-sacrificing total knee arthroplasty with anterior referencing, 8 mm of distal femur is resected. It is noted that the flexion gap is tight and the extension gap appears stable. What is the next most appropriate step in management?

1. Cut more proximal tibia.
2. Cut more distal femur.
3. Cut both the proximal tibia and distal femur.
4. Decrease the size of the femoral component.
5. Decrease the tibial polyethylene insert thickness.

Q-23: A 58-year-old man has anterior knee pain after undergoing total knee arthroplasty for osteoarthritis 2 years ago. He denies any history of trauma. A Merchant view is shown in Figure 9. What is the most likely cause of his pain?

1. External rotation of the femoral component
2. Overstuffing of the patellofemoral joint
3. Less than 12 mm of bony patella remaining after resection
4. Lateral retinacular release
5. Use of a cemented patellar component

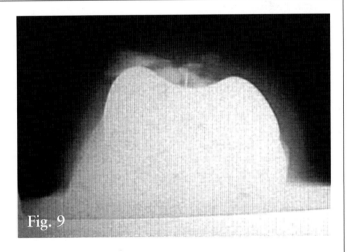

Fig. 9

Q-24: Etanercept is a recombinant genetically engineered fusion protein used to treat rheumatoid arthritis. What is its mode of action?

1. Monoclonal antibody that binds TNF-α
2. Blocks the binding of IL-1 to receptors
3. Soluble receptor that binds TNF-α
4. Soluble factor that binds rheumatoid factor
5. Directly inhibits pyrimidine synthesis

Q-25: A 68-year-old woman underwent a successful total right hip arthroplasty with a metal-on-metal articulation and cementless porous-coated components. Three months later, she underwent identical surgery on the left hip. Three months after surgery on the left hip, she reports groin pain on ambulation. Examination reveals significant groin discomfort with passive hip motion, particularly at the extremes of motion. Radiographs are shown in Figures 10A and 10B. Laboratory studies show an erythrocyte sedimentation rate of 35 mm/h and a C-reactive protein of 0.9. Aspiration yields scant growth of *Staphylococcus epidermidis* in the broth only, with no evidence of loosening on arthrography. A second aspiration yields scant growth of *S epidermidis* in the broth only. What is the most likely cause of the patient's pain?

1. Allergic metal synovitis

2. Aseptic loosening of the acetabular component

3. Septic loosening of the acetabulum

4. Deconditioning following hip arthroplasty

5. Iliopsoas tendinitis

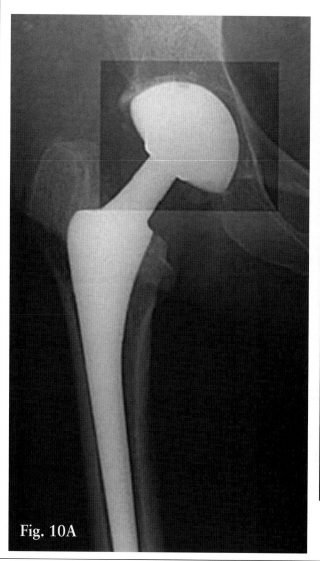

Fig. 10A

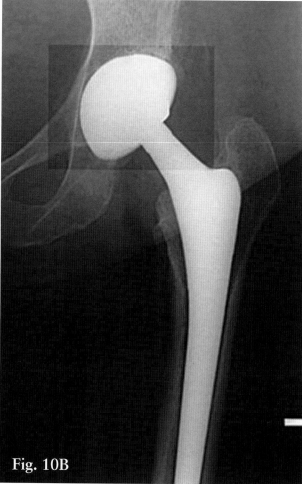

Fig. 10B

Q-26: Which of the following findings best describes the effects of increasing conformity of a fixed tibial bearing component and femoral component in total knee arthroplasty?

1. Increased peak contact stress, decreased component edge loading
2. Increased peak contact stress, increased component wear rates
3. Decreased peak contact stress, increased component wear rates
4. Decreased peak contact stress, decreased component wear rates
5. Decreased peak contact stress, decreased component edge loading

Q-27: Figure 11 shows the radiographs of a 56-year-old woman who has pain and varus knee deformity after undergoing total knee arthroplasty 8 years ago. Aspiration and studies for infection are negative. During revision surgery, management of the tibial bone loss is best achieved by

1. a custom tibial implant.
2. a hinged prosthesis.
3. reconstruction with structural allograft.
4. reconstruction with iliac crest bone graft.
5. filling the defect with cement.

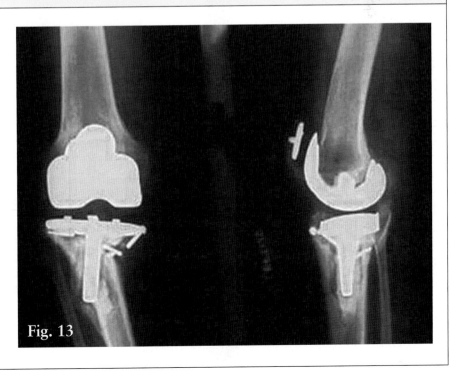

Fig. 13

Q-28: A 62-year-old man who underwent total knee arthroplasty 6 months ago now reports pain after falling on the anterior portion of the knee. Examination reveals weakness of knee extension but no extensor lag. Flexion that had once measured 115° is now limited to 70° because of pain. A radiograph is shown in Figure 12. Management should now consist of

1. immediate repair of the ruptured patellar tendon insertion.
2. knee joint aspiration and injection of a local anesthetic to facilitate examination.
3. joint aspiration for culture, broad-spectrum antibiotics, and immobilization.
4. immobilization until comfortable, followed by protected range of motion and strengthening.
5. immediate fracture repair.

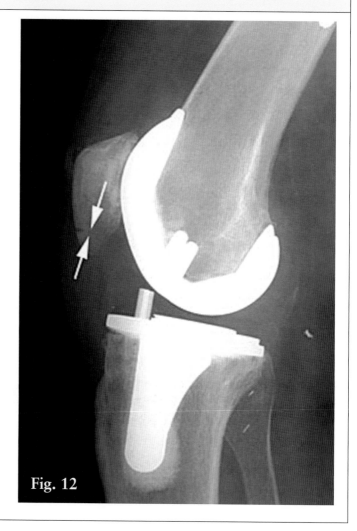

Fig. 12

Q-29: During primary total knee arthroplasty, what is the maximum distance the joint line can be raised or lowered before poor motion, joint instability, and increased chance of revision occur?

1. 4 mm
2. 8 mm
3. 12 mm
4. 16 mm
5. 20 mm

Q-30: Failure of high tibial osteotomy (HTO) is most closely associated with which of the following factors?

1. Patient age of less than 50 years at the time of surgery

2. Stable fixaton of the osteotomy

3. Development of deep venous thrombosis postoperatively

4. Type of osteotomy performed (ie, opening wedge versus dome osteotomy)

5. Presence of a lateral tibial thrust preoperatively

Q-31: Figure 13 shows the radiograph of a 47-year-old woman who has severe right hip pain and a limp. Management should consist of

1. acetabular osteotomy.

2. femoral and acetabular osteotomy.

3. total hip arthroplasty using standard trochanter osteotomy and cementless components.

4. total hip arthroplasty using femoral shortening osteotomy and cementless components.

5. total hip arthroplasty using femoral shortening osteotomy, a cemented socket, and a cementless femoral component.

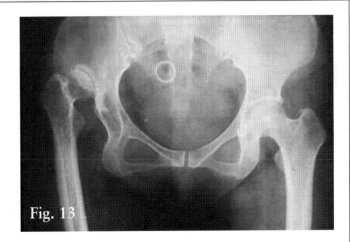

Fig. 13

Q-32: A 72-year-old woman with rheumatoid arthritis who underwent primary total knee arthroplasty 2 years ago has had diffuse knee pain that developed shortly after the surgery. The patient has difficulty with stair descent and arising from chairs. Evaluation for infection is negative. AP and lateral radiographs are shown in Figure 14. Management should now consist of

1. anti-inflammatory drugs.

2. a knee brace.

3. physical therapy for quadriceps strengthening.

4. revision to a thicker polyethylene insert.

5. revision to a posterior stabilized implant.

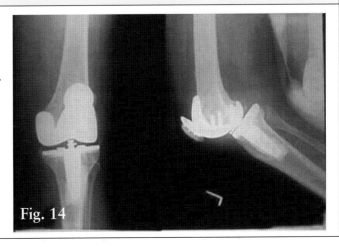

Fig. 14

Q-33: During the implantation of a cementless acetabular component in total hip arthroplasty, placement of a screw in the anterior superior quadrant puts which of the following structures at risk for damage?

1. Sciatic nerve

2. Internal iliac vessels

3. External iliac vessels

4. Femoral vessels

5. Obturator vessels

Q-34: Figure 15 shows the AP radiograph of an 18-year-old woman with progressive and severe right hip pain. Nonsteroidal anti-inflammatory drugs no longer control her pain. What is the next most appropriate step in management?

1. Total hip arthroplasty

2. Single innominate (Salter) osteotomy

3. Chiari osteotomy

4. Periacetabular osteotomy

5. Varus intertrochanteric osteotomy

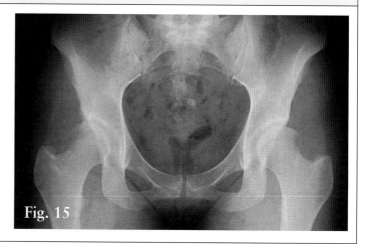

Fig. 15

Q-35: A 52-year-old man has had groin and deep buttock pain for the past 2 months. Examination reveals that hip range of motion is mildly restricted, and he has pain with both weight bearing and at rest. An MRI scan is shown in Figure 16. Management should consist of

1. protected weight bearing and anti-inflammatory drugs.

2. core decompression of the femoral head.

3. vascularized free fibular grafting to the femoral head.

4. bipolar hemiarthroplasty of the hip.

5. total hip arthroplasty.

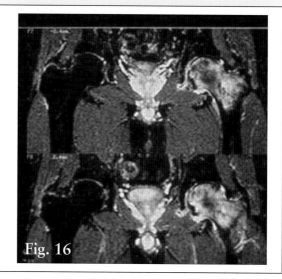

Fig. 16

Q-36: Figure 17 shows the radiograph of an 80-year-old woman who has right groin pain. She underwent a total hip arthroplasty 15 years ago and has no history of hip dislocation; however, she now reports that the pain results in functional impairment. Preoperative findings reveal that the component used has been discontinued, the locking mechanism is poor, and there is no replacement polyethylene available from the company. During surgery, the acetabular component is found to be well fixed, it is in satisfactory position, and adequate access can be obtained through the screw holes in the component to débride the osteolytic cavities. What is the best course of action for revision?

1. Remove the component and replace it with a "jumbo" cup with bone graft or substitute.

2. Remove the component and replace it with a bipolar component with bone graft or substitute.

3. Remove the component and replace it with a support ring with graft or graft substitute and cement a cup into the support ring.

4. Score the component for improved cement interdigitation and cement a cup into the retained socket with bone graft or substitute.

5. Use a structural acetabular graft to reconstruct the acetabulum and cement a cup into the structural graft.

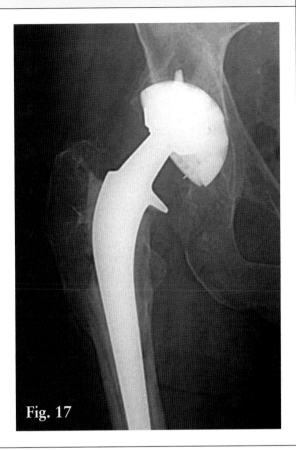

Fig. 17

Q-37: Figures 18A and 18B show the AP and lateral radiographs of a 67-year-old woman who has severe left knee pain when ambulating. History reveals that she underwent primary total knee arthroplasty 7 years ago. The patient reports increasing deformity over the past several years and uses a knee brace and a cane. Examination reveals that she walks with a varus thrust and has an uncorrectable varus deformity with valgus force. What is the primary reason for implant failure?

1. Osteolysis
2. Polyethylene wear
3. Tibial component fixation failure
4. Modular tibial component failure
5. Posterior cruciate ligament retention

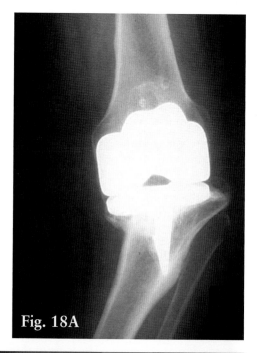

Fig. 18A

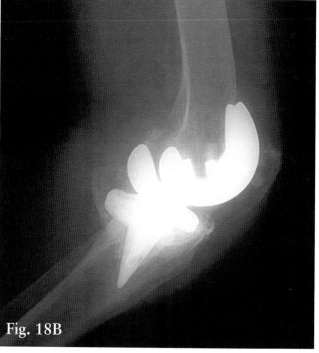

Fig. 18B

Q-38: Which of the following statements best characterizes polymethylmethacrylate (PMMA) when it is used to secure joint components in bone and to distribute the forces evenly across the bone-implant interface?

1. PMMA is stronger in tension than compression.
2. Porosity reduction increases the fatigue strength of PMMA.
3. Hypotension that occasionally results after PMMA is placed in the femoral canal is independent of a patient's intraoperative blood volume.
4. Inclusion of antibiotics does not alter the strength of PMMA.
5. PMMA bonds chemically to bone and the implant surface.

Q-39: A 35-year-old male laborer with isolated posttraumatic degenerative arthritis of the right hip undergoes the procedure shown in Figure 19. What is the most appropriate position of the right lower extremity?

1. 0° of flexion, 10° of abduction, 0° of rotation
2. 15° of flexion, 20° of abduction, 15° of external rotation
3. 20° of flexion, 10° of abduction, and 5° of external rotation
4. 30° of flexion, 5° of adduction, and 5° of external rotation
5. 45° of flexion, 10° of adduction, 0° of rotation

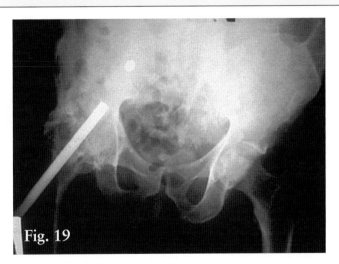
Fig. 19

Q-40: Which of the following bearing materials is most resistant to scratching from third-body debris?

1. Alumina
2. Stainless steel
3. Forged cobalt-chromium
4. Ion bombarded and forged cobalt-chromium
5. Oxidized titanium

Q-41: A 48-year-old woman has knee pain that is worse with weight bearing. She reports no night pain or pain at rest. History reveals that she underwent total knee arthroplasty with cementless components 2 years ago. Examination reveals tenderness along the medial joint line. Figures 20A through 20C show radiographs and a bone scan. What is the most likely cause of the patient's pain?

1. Deep infection
2. Malalignment
3. Fibrous ingrowth of the femoral component
4. Fibrous ingrowth of the tibial component
5. Patellar component loosening

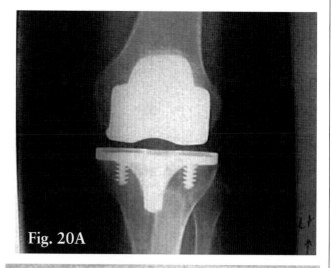

Fig. 20A

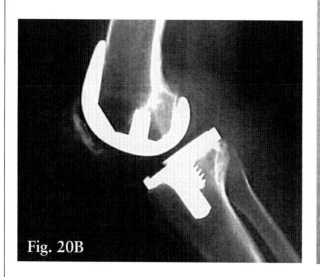

Fig. 20B

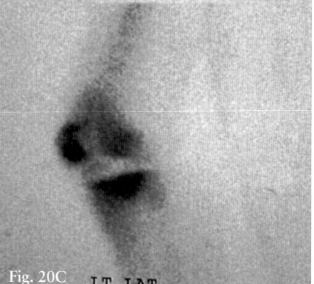

Fig. 20C   LT LAT

Q-42: A 65-year-old woman has nausea, vomiting, and abdominal distention after undergoing total knee arthroplasty 48 hours ago. An abdominal radiograph is shown in Figure 21. Associated risk factors for this disorder include

1. hypokalemia.
2. administration of warfarin.
3. administration of antibiotics.
4. general anesthesia.
5. early mobilization and physical therapy.

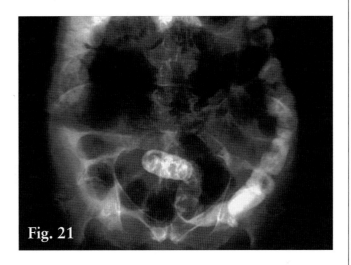

Fig. 21

Q-43: Which of the following methods is considered effective in decreasing the dislocation rate following a total hip arthroplasty using a posterior approach to the hip?

1. Use of a shorter neck length

2. Use of a smaller diameter head with a skirted neck extension

3. Reconstruction of the external rotators and capsular attachments during closure

4. Placement of the acetabular component in 60° of abduction as opposed to 45° of abduction

5. Placement of the acetabular component in neutral (0°) anteversion as opposed to 15° to 20° of anteversion

A-1: Which of the following findings is a prerequisite for a high tibial valgus osteotomy for medial compartment gonarthrosis?

1. Inflammatory arthritis
2. Ligamentous instability
3. Lateral tibial subluxation
4. Preoperative arc of motion of at least 90°
5. Narrowing of the lateral compartment cartilaginous joint space

PREFERRED RESPONSE: 4

DISCUSSION: The indications for high tibial valgus osteotomy include a physiologically young age, arthritis confined to the medial compartment, 10 to 15° of varus alignment on weight-bearing radiographs, a preoperative arc of motion of at least 90°, flexion contracture of less than 15°, and a motivated, compliant patient. Contraindications include lateral compartment narrowing of the articular cartilage, lateral tibial subluxation of greater than 1 cm, medial compartment bone loss, ligamentous instability, and inflammatory arthritis.

REFERENCES: Naudie D, Bourne RB, Rorabeck CH, Bourne TT: The Insall Award: Survivorship of the high tibial valgus osteotomy: A 10- to 22-year followup study. *Clin Orthop Relat Res* 1999;367:18-27. Pellicci PM, Tria AJ Jr, Garvin KL (eds): *Orthopaedic Knowledge Update: Hip and Knee Reconstruction 2.* Rosemont, IL, American Academy of Orthopaedic Surgeons, 2000, pp 255-264.

A-2: What is the main benefit of using metal-backed tibial components in total knee arthroplasty?

1. Improve the conformity of the articular surfaces
2. Reduce the maximum compressive stresses on the underlying cancellous bone
3. Increase the tensile forces on the other condyle when one is loaded
4. Decrease the thickness of the polyethylene tray
5. Decrease the compressive forces on the polyethylene tray

PREFERRED RESPONSE: 2

DISCUSSION: In a normal knee, the hard subchondral bone helps to distribute loads across the joint surface. A metal-backed tibial component in total knee arthroplasty decreases the compressive stresses on the underlying, softer cancellous bone by distributing the load over a larger surface area, particularly when one condyle is loaded. Although metallic base plates also increase the tensile forces on the other condyle when one is loaded and may decrease the thickness of the polyethylene tray, these are not benefits. Compressive forces on the polyethylene tray are increased with metal backing. The conformity of the articular surfaces is not affected by metal backing of the tibial component.

REFERENCE: Pellicci PM, Tria AJ Jr, Garvin KL (eds): *Orthopaedic Knowledge Update: Hip and Knee Reconstruction 2.* Rosemont, IL, American Academy of Orthopaedic Surgeons, 2000, pp 265-274.

Answers: Total Joint Arthroplasty/Joint Salvage

A-3: A 32-year-old woman with systemic lupus erythematosus treated with methotrexate and oral corticosteroids reports right groin pain with ambulation and night pain. Examination reveals pain with internal and external rotation and flexion that is limited to 105° because of discomfort. Laboratory studies show a serum WBC of 9.0/mm³ and an erythrocyte sedimentation rate of 35 mm/h. Figures 1A and 1B show AP and lateral radiographs of the right hip. Further evaluation should include

1. examination under fluoroscopy.

2. MRI.

3. a bone scan.

4. arthrography.

5. aspiration and arthrography.

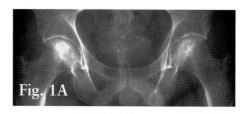

Fig. 1A

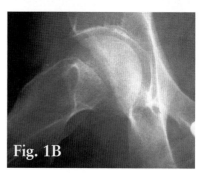

Fig. 1B

PREFERRED RESPONSE: 2

DISCUSSION: The radiographs show Ficat and Arlet stage 2 osteonecrosis. The femoral head remains round, and there are sclerotic changes in the superolateral quadrant. Patients with systemic lupus erythematosus are at risk for osteonecrosis because of prednisone use and the underlying metabolic changes associated with the condition (hypofibrinolysis and thrombophilia). MRI is the best diagnostic method for detecting osteonecrosis, with a greater than 98% sensitivity and specificity. For this patient, an MRI can assess the contralateral hip for any involvement and can quantify the extent of the lesion.

REFERENCES: Mont MA, Jones LC, Sotereanos DG, Amstutz HC, Hungerford DS: Understanding and treating osteonecrosis of the femoral head. *Instr Course Lect* 2000;49:169-185.
Koval KJ (ed): *Orthopaedic Knowledge Update 7*. Rosemont, IL, American Academy of Orthopaedic Surgeons, 2002, pp 417-451.

A-4: Which of the following factors can contribute to patellar subluxation following routine total knee arthroplasty?

1. External rotation of the femoral component
2. Internal rotation of the tibial component
3. Symmetric patellar resection
4. Lateral placement of the tibial component
5. Neutral alignment of the mechanical axis

PREFERRED RESPONSE: 2

DISCUSSION: Excessive resection of the lateral facet of the patella can lead to subluxation. Rotational alignment of the components can have a significant impact on patellar tracking. Internal rotation of the femoral component leads to more lateral alignment of the patella within the trochlear groove. Internal rotation and medial placement of the tibial component results in lateralization of the tibial tubercle with an increase in the Q angle. Excessive valgus alignment of the mechanical axis, or insufficient correction of preoperative valgus, has a similar effect on the Q angle, and both can result in a higher rate of tracking problems.

REFERENCE: Ayers DC, Dennis DA, Johanson NA, Pelligrini VD: Common complications of total knee arthroplasty. *J Bone Joint Surg Am* 1997;79:278-311.

A-5: During total knee arthroplasty using a posterior cruciate-retaining design, excessive tightness in flexion is noted, while the extension gap is felt to be balanced. Which of the following actions will effectively balance the knee?

1. Resect more distal femur.
2. Resect more anterior tibia.
3. Use a larger femoral component.
4. Use a smaller polyethylene insert.
5. Recess the posterior cruciate ligament.

PREFERRED RESPONSE: 5

DISCUSSION: Excessive flexion gap tightness can be addressed with a variety of techniques; including: (a) recess and release the posterior cruciate ligament; (b) resect a posterior slope in the tibia; (c) avoid an oversized femoral component that moves the posterior condyles more distally; (d) resect more posterior femoral condyle and use a smaller femoral component placed more anteriorly; and (e) release the tight posterior capsule and balance the collateral ligaments.

REFERENCE: Ayers DC, Dennis DA, Johanson NA, Pelligrini VD: Common complications of total knee arthroplasty. *J Bone Joint Surg Am* 1997;79:278-311.

Answers: Total Joint
Arthroplasty/Joint Salvage

A-6: Figures 2A and 2B show the current radiographs of a 58-year-old man who underwent total knee arthroplasty with a cruciate ligament–sparing prosthesis 7 years ago. Examination reveals boggy synovitis and moderate pain, particularly anteriorly. Management should consist of

1. follow-up radiographs.

2. alendronate, with follow-up examinations every 6 months.

3. revision to a posterior stabilized prosthesis.

4. exchange of the tibial insert through a limited incision.

5. surgical exploration with revision or exchange based on the findings.

PREFERRED RESPONSE: 5

DISCUSSION: The patient has symptoms of synovitis that are most likely the result of the release of particles from the tibial polyethylene. While observation may be warranted in a completely asymtomatic knee, some intervention is indicated for this patient as there is clear radiographic evidence of lysis in both the tibia and femur. The decision about the extent of the revision should be made at the time of surgery. A limited incision technique is not indicated. Grafting (or using graft substitute) the defect is the most appropriate approach for treating the osteolytic lesions. While a posterior stabilized prosthesis might be the solution, surgical findings might dictate otherwise.

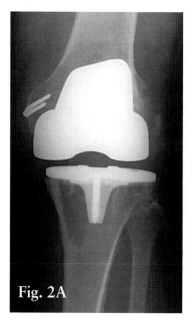
Fig. 2A

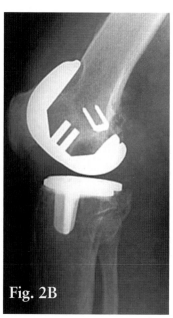
Fig. 2B

REFERENCE: Brassard MF, Insall JN, Scuderi GR: Complications of total knee arthroplasty, in Insall JN, Scott WN (eds): *Surgery of the Knee*, ed 3. Philadelphia, PA, Churchill Livingstone, 2001, vol 2, pp 1801-1844.

A-7: What is the correct order of the elastic modulus of the following materials from greatest to least?

1. Stainless steel, cobalt-chromium, titanium, polymethylmethacrylate (PMMA), alumina ceramic
2. Cobalt-chromium, stainless steel, titanium, alumina ceramic, PMMA
3. Alumina ceramic, titanium, cobalt-chromium, stainless steel, PMMA
4. Alumina ceramic, cobalt-chromium, stainless steel, titanium, PMMA
5. Titanium, cobalt-chromium, alumina ceramic, stainless steel, PMMA

PREFERRED RESPONSE: 4

DISCUSSION: In Young's modulus of elasticity, E is a measure of the stiffness of a material and its ability to resist deformation. In the elastic region of the stress-stain curve, E = stress/strain. The moduli of elasticity for these materials are alumina ceramic = 380 Gigapascals (GPa), cobalt-chromium = 210 GPa, stainless steel = 190 GPa, titanium = 116 GPa, and PMMA = 1.1 to 4.1 GPa.

REFERENCES: Buckwalter JA, Einhorn TA, Simon SR (eds): *Orthopaedic Basic Science*, ed 2. Rosemont, IL, American Academy of Orthopaedic Surgeons, 2000, pp 182-215.

A-8: Figure 3 shows the radiograph of a 75-year-old woman who reports the sudden onset of disabling medial knee pain. What is the most likely diagnosis?

1. Osteoarthritis
2. Osteonecrosis
3. Meniscal tear
4. Metastatic lesion
5. Synovial osteochondromatosis

PREFERRED RESPONSE: 2

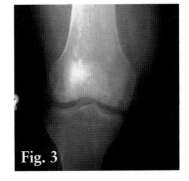

Fig. 3

DISCUSSION: Idiopathic osteonecrosis of the medial femoral condyle occurs predominantly in women older than age 60 years. It is characterized by pain centered in the medial anterior aspect of the knee, and onset is sudden. Flattening, sclerosis, and the radiolucent crescent sign are radiographic indicators of osteonecrosis. The radiographs show no narrowing of the joint space or osteophyte formation to indicate osteoarthritis, and there are no loose bodies to indicate synovial osteochondromatosis. A meniscal tear is not consistent with the radiographic findings shown here. Meniscal tears can coexist with osteonecrosis, but the pain is not eliminated merely by partial meniscectomy. Metastatic lesions to the distal femoral epiphysis are exceedingly rare.

REFERENCES: Urbaniak JR, Jones JP Jr (eds): *Osteonecrosis: Etiology, Diagnosis, and Treatment.* Rosemont, IL, American Academy of Orthopaedic Surgeons, 1997, pp 413-418.
Insall JN, Windsor RE, Scott WN, Kelly MA, Aglietti P (eds): *Surgery of the Knee*, ed 2. New York, NY, Churchill Livingstone, 1993, pp 609-634.

Answers: Total Joint
Arthroplasty/Joint Salvage

A-9: When using highly cross-linked ultra-high molecular weight polyethylene as an articulating surface for total knee arthroplasty, what property of the material raises concern?

1. Decreased volumetric wear

2. Decreased ductility

3. Increased mobility of the ultra-high molecular weight polyethylene chains in the material

4. Increased fatigue resistance

5. Increased fracture toughness

PREFERRED RESPONSE: 2

DISCUSSION: The decreased mobility of the polymer chains from cross-linking leads to decreased volumetric wear but also to decreases in ductility and fatigue resistance. Stresses at the knee are higher and varied in the point of application, leading to the concern for fatigue resistance and fracture.

REFERENCE: Koval KJ (ed): *Orthopaedic Knowledge Update 7*. Rosemont, IL, American Academy of Orthopaedic Surgeons, 2002, pp 193-199.

A-10: An otherwise healthy 57-year-old man has persistent, severe hip pain after undergoing total hip arthroplasty 3 months ago. What is the next most appropriate step in management?

1. Serial radiographs to assess progressive radiolucency from osteolysis or mechanical loosening

2. Assessment of C-reactive protein, erythroctye sedimentation rate, and CBC, followed by aspiration

3. Technetium and/or indium-labeled leukocyte scintigraphy

4. A trial of broad-spectrum cefalosporin antibiotics to assess for a change in pain intensity

5. Injection with lidocaine and methylprednisolone acetate

PREFERRED RESPONSE: 2

DISCUSSION: Any patient who is severely symptomatic this quickly after surgery must be evaluated for infection. Loosening is also a possible cause, but infection must be ruled out. Bone scans are not helpful at this early postoperative stage. Normal laboratory values argue strongly against infection, but when abnormal, need to be supplemented with a hip aspiration. Aspiration remains the most selective and sensitive measure, especially when linked to a WBC count of the synovial tissues in the joint. There is no indication for an antibiotic trial because it may make future culture sensitivity more difficult.

REFERENCES: Drancourt M, Stein A, Argenson JN, et al: Oral rifampin plus ofloxacin for treatment of staphylococcus-infected orthopedic implants. *Antimicrob Agents Chemother* 1993;37:1214-1218.
Duncan CP, Beauchamp C: A temporary antibiotic-loaded joint replacement system for the management of complex infections involving the hip. *Orthop Clin North Am* 1993;24:751-759.
Oyen WJ, Claessens RA, van Horn JR, et al: Scintigraphic detection of bone and joint infections with indium-111-labeled nonspecifonal human immunoglobulin G. *J Nucl Med* 1990;31:403-412.

A-11: Which of the following treatments of polyethylene results in the highest amount of oxidative degradation?

1. Ethylene oxide sterilization

2. Gamma irradiation in air

3. Gamma irradiation in an inert environment

4. Gamma irradiation followed by cross-linking

5. Gas plasma sterilization

PREFERRED RESPONSE: 2

DISCUSSION: Oxidative degradation of polyethylene occurs as a function of time in an air environment. In an environment such as argon, nitrogen, or a vacuum, the process is reduced. Ethylene oxide is an alternative for sterilization in which the cross-link degradation is minimized because of the absence of oxidative interactions. Gamma sterilization or use of ethylene oxide gas is the industry standard; however, oxygen concentrations are now reduced to a minimal level to retard the oxidation phenomenon.

REFERENCES: Sanford WM, Saum KA: Accelerated oxidative aging testing of UHMWPE. *Trans Orthop Res Soc* 1995;20:119.

Sun DC, Schmidig G, Stark C, et al: On the origins of a subsurface oxidation maximum and its relationship to the performance of UHMWPE implants. *Trans Soc Biomater* 1995;18:362.

Callaghan JJ, Dennis DA, Paprosky WA, Rosenberg AG (eds): *Orthopaedic Knowledge Update: Hip and Knee Reconstruction*. Rosemont, IL, American Academy of Orthopaedic Surgeons, 1995, pp 35-41.

McKellop HA: Bearing surfaces in total hip replacement: State of the art and future developments. *Instr Course Lect* 2001;50:165-179.

A-12: Consider the theoretic articulation shown in Figure 4 as femoral and tibial components of a total knee prosthesis in which the components fit like a "roller in trough." Which of the following best describes the articulation?

1. Constrained to anteroposterior translation, unconstrained to medial-lateral translation, high contact stress on edge (ie, varus-valgus) loading

2. Constrained to anteroposterior translation, unconstrained to medial-lateral translation, low contact stress on edge (ie, varus-valgus) loading

3. Unconstrained to anteroposterior translation, constrained to medial-lateral translation, high contact stress on edge (ie, varus-valgus) loading

4. Unconstrained to anteroposterior translation, constrained to medial-lateral translation, low contact stress on edge (ie, varus-valgus) loading

5. Constraint is dependent on the status of the posterior cruciate ligament

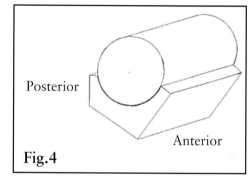

Posterior

Anterior

Fig.4

PREFERRED RESPONSE: 1

DISCUSSION: The theoretic total knee components will resist anteroposterior motion by making the femoral component "climb the walls" of the tibial component. As drawn, there is no constraint to medial-lateral translation. The cylinder is not rounded on the edges, so varus-valgus motion will impart load from the cylinder to the trough over a small area, thus having a high contact stress.

REFERENCE: Alicea J: Scoring systems and their validation for the arthritic knee, in Insall JN, Scott WN (eds): *Surgery of the Knee*, ed 3. Philadelphia, PA, Churchill Livingstone, 2001, vol 2, pp 1507-1515.

A-13: Wear particles of ultra-high molecular weight polyethylene that are generated by total hip implants are predominantly of what diameter?

1. Less than 1 micron
2. 10 to 50 microns
3. 100 to 200 microns
4. 500 to 750 microns
5. Greater than 1,000 microns

PREFERRED RESPONSE: 1

DISCUSSION: Multiple studies have shown that the size of an ultra-high molecular weight polyethylene particle generated by total hip implants is typically less than 1 micron. This finding is significant in that particles of that size are readily phagocytized by macrophages.

REFERENCES: Campbell P, Ma S, Yeom B, McKellop H, Schmalzried TP, Amstutz HC: Isolation of predominantly submicron-sized UHMWPE wear particles from periprosthetic tissues. *J Biomed Mater Res* 1995;29:127-131.
Shanbhag AS, Jacobs JJ, Glant TT, Gilbert JL, Black J, Galante JO: Composition and morphology of wear debris in failed uncemented total hip replacement. *J Bone Joint Surg Br* 1994;76:60-67.
Maloney WJ, Smith RL, Schmalzried TP, Chiba J, Huene D, Rubash H: Isolation and characterization of wear particles generated in patients who have had failure of a hip arthroplasty without cement. *J Bone Joint Surg Am* 1995;77:1301-1310.

A-14: Which of the following best describes the resultant forces on an increased offset stem when compared with a standard offset stem?

1. Increased joint reaction force, increased torsional load
2. Increased joint reaction force, decreased torsional load
3. Decreased joint reaction force, increased torsional load
4. Decreased joint reaction force, decreased torsional load
5. No change in joint reaction force or torsional load

PREFERRED RESPONSE: 3

DISCUSSION: The increased emphasis on restoring offset in total hip arthroplasty has implications for the forces applied to the components and the fixation interfaces. Static analysis has shown that with an increased affect, joint reaction force on the articulation is decreased. When the resultant load on the hip is "out of plane" (ie, directed anterior to posterior), there is increased torsion where the stem is turned into more retroversion.

REFERENCES: Buckwalter JA, Einhorn TA, Simon SR (eds): *Orthopaedic Basic Science*, ed 2. Rosemont, IL, American Academy of Orthopaedic Surgeons, 2000, pp 134-180.
Hurwitz DE, Andriaacchi TP: Biomechanics of the hip, in Callaghan J, Rosenberg AG, Rubash HE (eds): *The Adult Hip*. Philadelphia, PA, Lippincott-Raven, 1998.
Pauwels F: *Biomechanics of the Normal and Diseased Hip*. New York, NY, Springer-Verlag, 1976.

Answers: Total Joint Arthroplasty/Joint Salvage

A-15: During total knee arthroplasty, what component position aids in proper tracking and stability of the patellar component?

1. Femoral component in external rotation
2. Tibial component in internal rotation
3. Medialization of the tibial tray
4. Lateralization of the patellar component
5. Medialization of the femoral component

PREFERRED RESPONSE: 1

DISCUSSION: The femoral component should be implanted with enough external rotation to facilitate patellar tracking. Proper tracking requires a normal Q angle and is affected by axial and rotational alignment of the femur and tibia. An excessive Q angle can result from internal rotation of either component, medialization of the tibial tray, or lateralization of the patellar component.

REFERENCES: Beaty JH (ed): *Orthopaedic Knowledge Update 6.* Rosemont, IL, American Academy of Orthopaedic Surgeons, 1999, pp 559-582.
Lonner JH, Lotke PA: Aseptic complications after total knee arthroplasty. *J Am Acad Orthop Surg* 1999;7:311-324.

A-16: A 60-year-old woman reports anterior knee pain 2 years after undergoing primary total knee arthroplasty for rheumatoid arthritis. A Merchant view of the patella is shown in Figure 5. What is the most likely cause of her pain?

1. Elevation of the joint line
2. Lateral placement of the femoral component
3. Medial placement of the patellar component
4. Internal rotation of the femoral component
5. External rotation of the tibial component

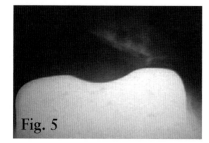

Fig. 5

PREFERRED RESPONSE: 4

DISCUSSION: Patellar complications commonly occur after primary total knee arthroplasty; therefore, proper component positioning is critical in obtaining a successful result. This patient has lateral tilting and subluxation of the patellar component. Internal rotation of the femoral component has the most deleterious effect on patellar tracking. Lateral placement of the femoral component, medial placement of the patellar component, and external rotation of the tibial component have beneficial effects on patellar tracking. Elevation of the joint line, if not excessive, should not impact patellar tracking.

REFERENCES: Rand JA: Patellar resurfacing in total knee arthroplasty. *Clin Orthop Relat Res* 1990;260:110-117.
Healy WL, Wasliewski SA, Takei R, Oberlander M: Patellofemoral complications following total knee arthroplasty: Correlation with implant design and patient risk factors. *J Arthroplasty* 1995;10:197-201.

A-17: The anterior portal of a hip arthroscopy places what structure at greatest risk for injury?

1. Ascending branch of the lateral circumflex femoral artery

2. Ascending branch of the medial circumflex femoral artery

3. Femoral nerve

4. Lateral femoral cutaneous nerve

5. Superior gluteal nerve

PREFERRED RESPONSE: 4

DISCUSSION: The average location of the anterior portal is 6.3 cm distal to the anterior superior iliac spine. The lateral femoral cutaneous nerve typically has divided into three or more branches at the level of the anterior portal. The portal usually passes within several millimeters of the most medial branch. Injury to the nerve can lead to meralgia paresthetica. The femoral nerve lies an average minimum distance of 3.2 cm from the anterior portal. The ascending branch of the lateral circumflex artery lies approximately 3.7 cm inferior to the anterior portal. Neither the ascending branch of the medial circumflex artery nor the superior gluteal nerve are at risk.

REFERENCES: Byrd JWT: *Operative Hip Arthroscopy*. New York, NY, Thieme Medical Publishers, 1998, pp 83-91.

Arendt EA (ed): *Orthopaedic Knowledge Update: Sports Medicine 2*. Rosemont, IL, American Academy of Orthopaedic Surgeons, 1999, pp 281-289.

A-18: A 32-year-old man has posttraumatic arthritis after undergoing open reduction and internal fixation of a left acetabular fracture. A total hip arthroplasty is performed, and the radiograph is shown in Figure 6. What is the most common mode of failure leading to revision in this group of patients?

1. Infection

2. Heterotopic ossification

3. Dislocation

4. Periprosthetic fracture

5. Acetabular component loosening

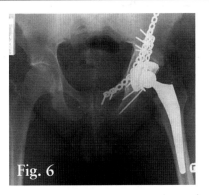
Fig. 6

PREFERRED RESPONSE: 5

DISCUSSION: Acetabular component loosening has been reported as the most common mode of failure following total hip arthroplasty in patients with a previous acetabular fracture. Following acetabular fracture and subsequent open reduction and internal fixation, the bone quality and vascularity are compromised, thus reducing the success rate of acetabular component cementless fixation.

REFERENCES: Jimenez ML, Tile M, Schenk RS: Total hip replacement after acetabular fracture. *Orthop Clin* 1997;28:435-446.

Romness DW, Lewallen DG: Total hip arthroplasty after fracture of the acetabulum: Long-term results. *J Bone Joint Surg Br* 1990;72:761-764.

A-19: A 42-year-old man sustained the periprosthetic fracture shown in Figures 7A and 7B. The femoral component is well fixed. What is the next most appropriate step in management?

1. Closed reduction and bracing

2. Retrograde femoral intramedullary nailing

3. Open reduction and internal fixation of the fracture, leaving the femoral stem in place

4. Open reduction and internal fixation of the fracture and insertion of a proximally porous-coated stem

5. Open reduction and internal fixation of fracture fragments and insertion of a fully porous-coated femoral stem with diaphyseal fixation distal to the fracture

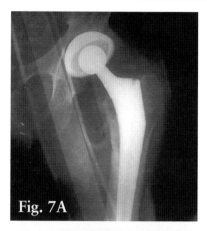

Fig. 7A

PREFERRED RESPONSE: 3

DISCUSSION: The patient has a periprosthetic fracture below the femoral stem. The component is porous coated and well fixed. Open reduction and internal fixation, leaving the stem in place, can be performed when bone quality is good. Plating with or without allograft struts and supplemental cerclage fixation generally is acceptable. If the component is loose, revision to a longer device is recommended with appropriate stabilization of the fracture using the aforementioned methods. If bone

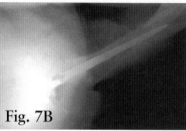

Fig. 7B

loss has occurred, allograft supplementation or a tumor prosthesis may be indicated. Fractures located well below the stem tip can be treated without regard for the prosthesis. Closed reduction and bracing is not associated with good results for periprosthetic femoral fractures. Retrograde intramedullary nailing is not appropriate for this fracture.

REFERENCES: Duncan CP, Masri BA: Fractures of the femur after hip replacement. *Instr Course Lect* 1995;44:293-304.

Bono JV, McCarthy JC, Thornhill TS, Bierbaum BE, Turner RH (eds): *Revision Total Hip Arthroplasty.* New York, NY, Springer Verlag, 1999, pp 530-592.

A-20: A homebound 75-year-old woman with diabetes mellitus has had progressive left knee pain and swelling for the past 6 weeks. She is febrile with a temperature of 103°F (39.5°C). History reveals that she underwent arthroplasty 5 years ago. Examination shows passive range of motion of 0° to 100° with no active extension. Knee aspiration reveals purulent fluid with a Gram stain showing gram-negative rods. A radiograph is shown in Figure 8. In addition to IV antibiotics, which of the following management options offers the best chance of a successful outcome?

1. Incision and drainage with repair of the extensor mechanism

2. Removal of components and delayed revision knee arthroplasty with an allograft extensor mechanism

3. Removal of components and immediate exchange revision total knee arthroplasty

4. Removal of components and delayed knee arthrodesis

5. Removal of components and delayed revision knee arthroplasty with extensor mechanism repair

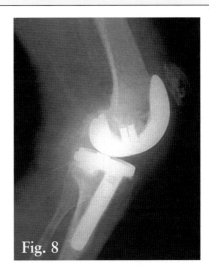

Fig. 8

PREFERRED RESPONSE: 4

DISCUSSION: The patient has an infected total knee arthroplasty and an interrupted extensor mechanism. A late infection of a total knee arthroplasty in a patient with diabetes mellitus and a virulent organism requires removal of the components, débridement, antibiotic spacers, and surveillance to ensure eradication of the infection. Reconstruction of an incompetent extensor mechanism in an infected knee is extremely unlikely to be successful. Arthrodesis is the procedure of choice if a revision total knee arthroplasty is not likely to succeed. Resection arthroplasty is recommended only as a long-term solution if the patient is medically unable to undergo further surgery.

REFERENCES: Koval KJ (ed): *Orthopaedic Knowledge Update 7*. Rosemont, IL, American Academy of Orthopaedic Surgery, 2002, pp 513-536.
Hanssen AD, Rand JA: Evaluation and treatment of infection at the site of a total hip or knee arthroplasty. *Instr Course Lect* 1999;48:111-122.

A-21: Varus intertrochanteric osteotomy for coxa valga commonly produces which of the following results?

1. Decreased abductor lever arm

2. Increased hip joint reaction force

3. Increased center edge angle

4. Abductor lag and lurch

5. Lengthening of the leg

PREFERRED RESPONSE: 4

DISCUSSION: The greater trochanter is raised as a by-product of varus osteotomy, and a temporary abductor lag and lurch is common for 6 months following surgery. In the absence of hip joint subluxation, varus intertrochanteric osteotomy has no effect on the center edge angle of Wiberg. Varus osteotomy typically increases femoral offset, thereby improving the abductor lever arm and reducing the hip joint reaction force. Even without taking a wedge, varus osteotomy always produces some degree of shortening.

REFERENCE: Millis MB, Murphy SB, Poss R: Osteotomies about the hip for the prevention and treatment of osteoarthrosis. *Instr Course Lect* 1996;45:209-226.

A-22: During a posterior cruciate ligament-sacrificing total knee arthroplasty with anterior referencing, 8 mm of distal femur is resected. It is noted that the flexion gap is tight and the extension gap appears stable. What is the next most appropriate step in management?

1. Cut more proximal tibia.

2. Cut more distal femur.

3. Cut both the proximal tibia and distal femur.

4. Decrease the size of the femoral component.

5. Decrease the tibial polyethylene insert thickness.

PREFERRED RESPONSE: 4

DISCUSSION: If the flexion gap is tight and the extension gap is correct, it is preferable to change only the flexion gap and leave the extension gap unchanged; therefore, the treatment of choice is to decrease the size of the femoral component. The smaller component will be smaller in both medial-lateral as well as anterior-posterior dimensions. A smaller anterior-posterior size will allow more space for the flexion gap without significantly affecting the extension gap. Decreasing the size of the tibial polyethylene insert thickness or cutting more proximal tibia will affect both the flexion and extension gaps. Cutting more distal femur will increase the extension gap and not change the flexion gap, making the described situation worse. Cutting both the proximal tibia and distal femur will increase both the flexion and extension gaps.

REFERENCE: Pellicci PM, Tria AJ Jr, Garvin KL (eds): *Orthopaedic Knowledge Update: Hip and Knee Reconstruction 2*. Rosemont, IL, American Academy of Orthopaedic Surgeons, 2000, pp 281-286, 339-365.

A-23: A 58-year-old man has anterior knee pain after undergoing total knee arthroplasty for osteoarthritis 2 years ago. He denies any history of trauma. A Merchant view is shown in Figure 9. What is the most likely cause of his pain?

1. External rotation of the femoral component
2. Overstuffing of the patellofemoral joint
3. Less than 12 mm of bony patella remaining after resection
4. Lateral retinacular release
5. Use of a cemented patellar component

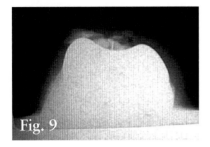

Fig. 9

PREFERRED RESPONSE: 3

DISCUSSION: The patient has a patellar stress fracture after resurfacing in a total knee arthroplasty. Several studies have shown that over-resection of the patella to less than 12 to 15 mm increases anterior patellar surface strains to a point where the risk of fracture is increased. Increasing the patellar thickness, positioning of the femoral component, lateral releases, and component types have not been clearly associated with increased fracture risk.

REFERENCES: Reuben JD, McDonald CL, Woodard PL, Hennington LJ: Effect of patella thickness on patella strain following total knee arthroplasty. *J Arthroplasty* 1991;6:251-258.
Hsu HC, Luo ZP, Rand JA, An KN: Influence of patellar thickness on patellar tracking and patellofemoral contact characteristics after total knee arthroplasty. *J Arthroplasty* 1996;11:69-80.
Greenfield MA, Insall JN, Case GC, Kelly MA: Instrumentation of the patellar osteotomy in total knee arthroplasty: The relationship of patellar thickness and lateral retinacular release. *Am J Knee Surg* 1996;9:129-131.

A-24: Etanercept is a recombinant genetically engineered fusion protein used to treat rheumatoid arthritis. What is its mode of action?

1. Monoclonal antibody that binds TNF-α
2. Blocks the binding of IL-1 to receptors
3. Soluble receptor that binds TNF-α
4. Soluble factor that binds rheumatoid factor
5. Directly inhibits pyrimidine synthesis

PREFERRED RESPONSE: 3

DISCUSSION: Etanercept is a molecule consisting of the Fc portion of IgG fused to the extracellular domain of the p76 human THF-α receptor. It is soluble and binds TNF-α. Infliximab is the monoclonal antibody that binds TNF-α. IL-1 receptor antagonists are still in development. Leflunomide is a drug that inhibits pyrimidine synthesis and is similar to methotrexate as an antimetabolite.

REFERENCE: Koval KJ (ed): *Orthopaedic Knowlegde Update 7*. Rosemont, IL, American Academy of Orthopaedic Surgeons, 2002, pp 193-199.

Answers: Total Joint
Arthroplasty/Joint Salvage

A-25: A 68-year-old woman underwent a successful total right hip arthroplasty with a metal-on-metal articulation and cementless porous-coated components. Three months later, she underwent identical surgery on the left hip. Three months after surgery on the left hip, she reports groin pain on ambulation. Examination reveals significant groin discomfort with passive hip motion, particularly at the extremes of motion. Radiographs are shown in Figures 10A and 10B. Laboratory studies show an erythrocyte sedimentation rate of 35 mm/h and a C-reactive protein of 0.9. Aspiration yields scant growth of *Staphylococcus epidermidis* in the broth only, with no evidence of loosening on arthrography. A second aspiration yields scant growth of *S epidermidis* in the broth only. What is the most likely cause of the patient's pain?

1. Allergic metal synovitis

2. Aseptic loosening of the acetabular component

3. Septic loosening of the acetabulum

4. Deconditioning following hip arthroplasty

5. Iliopsoas tendinitis

PREFERRED RESPONSE: 3

DISCUSSION: The difference in the clinical results combined with the laboratory findings points to infection. While there is a significant risk of false-positive findings with aspiration, the fact that two successive aspirations grew the same organism strongly suggests infection. The radiograph shows that there is more radiolucency around the left acetabular component than the right component.

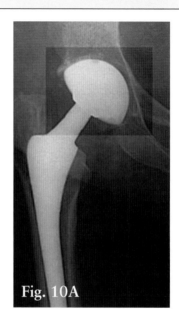
Fig. 10A

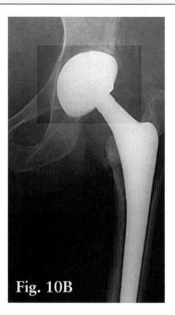
Fig. 10B

REFERENCES: White RE: Evaluation of the painful total hip arthroplasty, in Callaghan JJ, Rosenberg AG, Rubash HE (eds): *The Adult Hip.* Philadelphia, PA, Lippincott-Raven, 1998, vol 2, pp 1377-1385. Barrack RL, Harris WH: The value of aspiration of the hip joint before revision total hip arthroplasty. *J Bone Joint Surg Am* 1993;75:66-76.

A-26: Which of the following findings best describes the effects of increasing conformity of a fixed tibial bearing component and femoral component in total knee arthroplasty?

1. Increased peak contact stress, decreased component edge loading
2. Increased peak contact stress, increased component wear rates
3. Decreased peak contact stress, increased component wear rates
4. Decreased peak contact stress, decreased component wear rates
5. Decreased peak contact stress, decreased component edge loading

PREFERRED RESPONSE: 4

DISCUSSION: In the design of tibial and femoral components, a compromise must be made between contact stresses and constraint. Increased conformity increases constraint, limits motion, and potentially increases stress on the knee-cement interface. By increasing conformity, the surface area over which force is applied is increased, resulting in decreased peak contact stresses and decreased component wear rates.

REFERENCES: Pellicci PM, Tria AJ Jr, Garvin KL (eds): *Orthopaedic Knowledge Update: Hip and Knee Reconstruction 2*. Rosemont, IL, American Academy of Orthopaedic Surgeons, 2000, pp 265-274.
Bartel DL, Rawlinson JJ, Burstein AH, Ranawat CS, Flynn WF Jr: Stresses in polyethylene components of contemporary total knee replacements. *Clin Orthop Relat Res* 1995;317:76-82.

A-27: Figure 11 shows the radiographs of a 56-year-old woman who has pain and varus knee deformity after undergoing total knee arthroplasty 8 years ago. Aspiration and studies for infection are negative. During revision surgery, management of the tibial bone loss is best achieved by

1. a custom tibial implant.
2. a hinged prosthesis.
3. reconstruction with structural allograft.
4. reconstruction with iliac crest bone graft.
5. filling the defect with cement.

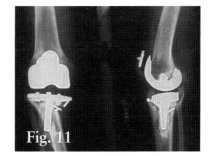

Fig. 11

PREFERRED RESPONSE: 3

DISCUSSION: Massive bone loss encountered in revision total knee arthroplasty remains a significant challenge. Recent reports have shown high success rates using structural allograft to reconstruct massive bone defects. Custom and hinged prostheses in this setting are no longer favored. The defect shown is segmental and is too large to be filled with cement or iliac crest bone graft.

REFERENCES: Mow CS, Wiedel JD: Structural allografting in revision total knee arthroplasty. *J Arthroplasty* 1996;11:235-241.
Engh GA, Herzwurm PJ, Parks NL: Treatment of major defects of bone with bulk allografts and stemmed components during total knee arthroplasty. *J Bone Joint Surg Am* 1997;79:1030-1039.
Clatworthy MG, Ballance J, Brick GW, Chandler HP, Gross AE: The use of structural allograft for uncontained defects in revision total knee arthroplasty: A minimum five-year review. *J Bone Joint Surg Am* 2001;83:404-411.

Answers: Total Joint
Arthroplasty/Joint Salvage

A-28: A 62-year-old man who underwent total knee arthroplasty 6 months ago now reports pain after falling on the anterior portion of the knee. Examination reveals weakness of knee extension but no extensor lag. Flexion that had once measured 115° is now limited to 70° because of pain. A radiograph is shown in Figure 12. Management should now consist of

1. immediate repair of the ruptured patellar tendon insertion.
2. knee joint aspiration and injection of a local anesthetic to facilitate examination.
3. joint aspiration for culture, broad-spectrum antibiotics, and immobilization.
4. immobilization until comfortable, followed by protected range of motion and strengthening.
5. immediate fracture repair.

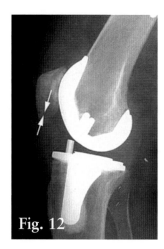

Fig. 12

PREFERRED RESPONSE: 4

DISCUSSION: The patient has a type IIIB patellar fracture (inferior pole fracture with an intact patellar tendon). Nonsurgical management is the treatment of choice if there is little displacement and the extensor mechanism is intact.

REFERENCES: Brown TE, Diduch DR: Fractures of the patella, in Insall JN, Scott WN (eds): *Surgery of the Knee*, ed 3. Philadelphia, PA, Churchill Livingstone, 2001, vol 2, pp 1290-1312.
Pellicci PM, Tria AJ Jr, Garvin KL (eds): *Orthopaedic Knowledge Update: Hip and Knee Reconstruction 2*. Rosemont, IL, American Academy of Orthopaedic Surgeons, 2000, pp 323-337.

A-29: During primary total knee arthroplasty, what is the maximum distance the joint line can be raised or lowered before poor motion, joint instability, and increased chance of revision occur?

1. 4 mm
2. 8 mm
3. 12 mm
4. 16 mm
5. 20 mm

PREFERRED RESPONSE: 2

DISCUSSION: Positioning of the femoral and tibial components is a common cause of early failure of total knee arthroplasty. Two modes of possible position are raising or lowering the joint line from its anatomic level. Raising or lowering the joint line beyond an established threshold can cause limited range of motion, poor patellar function, and possible instability. It has been determined that a threshold of approximately 8 mm provides consistently good results after knee arthroplasty.

REFERENCE: Pellicci PM, Tria AJ Jr, Garvin KL (eds): *Orthopaedic Knowledge Update: Hip and Knee Reconstruction 2*. Rosemont, IL, American Academy of Orthopaedic Surgeons, 2000, pp 339-365.

A-30: Failure of high tibial osteotomy (HTO) is most closely associated with which of the following factors?

1. Patient age of less than 50 years at the time of surgery

2. Stable fixaton of the osteotomy

3. Development of deep venous thrombosis postoperatively

4. Type of osteotomy performed (ie, opening wedge versus dome osteotomy)

5. Presence of a lateral tibial thrust preoperatively

PREFERRED RESPONSE: 5

DISCUSSION: Long-term survivorship studies have attempted to clarify patient factors related to good outcomes in HTO. One particular study showed that a patient age of less than 50 years was related to good outcomes in those who had good preoperative knee flexion. The same study found no relation between HTO failure and the presence of postoperative infection or deep venous thrombosis. The presence of a lateral tibial thrust is a contraindication to performing this surgery. As expected, good patient selection is critical to obtaining good long-term results with HTO.

REFERENCES: Naudie D, Borne RB, Rorabeck CH, Bourne TJ: Survivorship of the high tibial valgus osteotomy: A 10- to 22-year followup study. *Clin Orthop Relat Res* 1999;367:18-27.

Rinonapoli E, Mancini GB, Corvaglia A, Musiello S: Tibial osteotomy for varus gonarthrosis: A 10- to 21-year followup study. *Clin Orthop Relat Res* 1998;353:185-193.

Coventry MB, Ilstrup DM, Wallrichs SL: Proximal tibial osteotomy: A critical long-term study of eighty-seven cases. *J Bone Joint Surg Am* 1993;75:196-201.

A-31: Figure 13 shows the radiograph of a 47-year-old woman who has severe right hip pain and a limp. Management should consist of

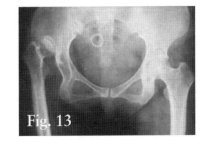

Fig. 13

1. acetabular osteotomy.

2. femoral and acetabular osteotomy.

3. total hip arthroplasty using standard trochanter osteotomy and cementless components.

4. total hip arthroplasty using femoral shortening osteotomy and cementless components.

5. total hip arthroplasty using femoral shortening osteotomy, a cemented socket, and a cementless femoral component.

PREFERRED RESPONSE: 4

DISCUSSION: Femoral shortening osteotomy for a Crowe type IV hip dislocation has been shown to provide superior results with minimal complications. Cementless fixation of the stem allows for modular implants that greatly simplify the reconstruction.

REFERENCE: Jaroszynski G, Woodgate IG, Saleh KJ, Gross AE: Total hip replacement for the dislocated hip. *Instr Course Lect* 2001;50:307-316.

A-32: A 72-year-old woman with rheumatoid arthritis who underwent primary total knee arthroplasty 2 years ago has had diffuse knee pain that developed shortly after the surgery. The patient has difficulty with stair descent and arising from chairs. Evaluation for infection is negative. AP and lateral radiographs are shown in Figure 14. Management should now consist of

1. anti-inflammatory drugs.
2. a knee brace.
3. physical therapy for quadriceps strengthening.
4. revision to a thicker polyethylene insert.
5. revision to a posterior stabilized implant.

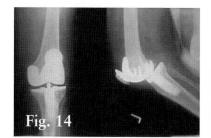
Fig. 14

PREFERRED RESPONSE: 5

DISCUSSION: The radiographs show posterior flexion instability that is the result of flexion-extension gap imbalance and/or posterior cruciate ligament incompetence after a posterior cruciate-retaining total knee arthroplasty. The radiographs also show anterior femoral displacement on the tibia. Pagnano and associates reported on a series of patients with painful total knee arthroplasties who had been previously diagnosed as having pain of unknown etiology, showing that the pain was secondary to flexion instability. Pain relief was achieved by revision to a posterior stabilized implant.

REFERENCES: Pagnano MW, Hanssen AD, Lewallen DG, Stuart MJ: Flexion instability after primary posterior cruciate retaining total knee arthroplasty. *Clin Orthop Relat Res* 1998;356:39-46.
Fehring TK, Valadie AL: Knee instability after total knee arthroplasty. *Clin Orthop Relat Res* 1994;299:157-162.
Fehring TK, Odum S, Griffin WL, Mason B, Nadaud M: Early failures of total knee arthroplasty. *Clin Orthop Relat Res* 2001;392:315-318.

A-33: During the implantation of a cementless acetabular component in total hip arthroplasty, placement of a screw in the anterior superior quadrant puts which of the following structures at risk for damage?

1. Sciatic nerve
2. Internal iliac vessels
3. External iliac vessels
4. Femoral vessels
5. Obturator vessels

PREFERRED RESPONSE: 3

DISCUSSION: A knowledge of the safe quadrants for screw placement for acetabular component implantation is essential when performing total hip arthroplasty. The external iliac vessels are on the inner wall of the pelvis, corresponding to the anterior superior quadrant of the acetabulum.

REFERENCES: Keating EM, Ritter MA, Faris PM: Structures at risk from medially placed acetabular screws. *J Bone Joint Surg Am* 1990;72:509-511.
Wasielewski RC, Cooperstein L, Kruger MP, Rubash HE: Acetabular anatomy and the transacetabular fixation of screws in total hip arthroplasty. *J Bone Joint Surg Am* 1990;72:501-508.

A-34: Figure 15 shows the AP radiograph of an 18-year-old woman with progressive and severe right hip pain. Nonsteroidal anti-inflammatory drugs no longer control her pain. What is the next most appropriate step in management?

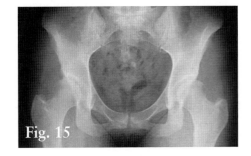
Fig. 15

1. Total hip arthroplasty

2. Single innominate (Salter) osteotomy

3. Chiari osteotomy

4. Periacetabular osteotomy

5. Varus intertrochanteric osteotomy

PREFERRED RESPONSE: 4

DISCUSSION: A concentric hip with acetabular dysplasia in a symptomatic patient is best treated by periacetabular osteotomy. The Salter osteotomy is less optimal because the method has limited correction, is uniaxial, cannot be tailored to the deformity, and lateralizes the entire hip joint, thereby increasing the joint reactive forces. Because the hyaline cartilage of the joint is histologically normal, rotating the hyaline cartilage into an optimal position is preferable to augmenting the acetabulum with a shelf or by Chiari osteotomy. Varus intertrochanteric osteotomy has no significant role in the treatment of acetabular dysplasia. Total hip arthroplasty may be required in the future but should not be the first choice.

REFERENCE: Millis MB, Murphy SB, Poss R: Osteotomies about the hip for the prevention and treatment of osteoarthritis. *Instr Course Lect* 1996;45:209-226.

A-35: A 52-year-old man has had groin and deep buttock pain for the past 2 months. Examination reveals that hip range of motion is mildly restricted, and he has pain with both weight bearing and at rest. An MRI scan is shown in Figure 16. Management should consist of

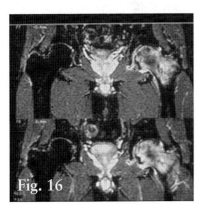
Fig. 16

1. protected weight bearing and anti-inflammatory drugs.

2. core decompression of the femoral head.

3. vascularized free fibular grafting to the femoral head.

4. bipolar hemiarthroplasty of the hip.

5. total hip arthroplasty.

PREFERRED RESPONSE: 1

DISCUSSION: The MRI findings show highly increased signal through the entire femoral head and neck that is diagnostic of transient osteoporosis of the femoral head. This recently described entity is often seen in middle-aged men and should be treated nonsurgically with protected weight bearing and anti-inflammatory drugs. The natural history is that of self-resolution.

REFERENCES: Guerra JJ, Steinberg ME: Distinguishing transient osteoporosis from avascular necrosis of the hip. *J Bone Joint Surg Am* 1995;77:616-624.

Urbanski SR, de Lange EE, Eschenroeder HC Jr: Magnetic resonance imaging of transient osteoporosis of the hip. A case report. *J Bone Joint Surg Am* 1991;73:451-455.

A-36: Figure 17 shows the radiograph of an 80-year-old woman who has right groin pain. She underwent a total hip arthroplasty 15 years ago and has no history of hip dislocation; however, she now reports that the pain results in functional impairment. Preoperative findings reveal that the component used has been discontinued, the locking mechanism is poor, and there is no replacement polyethylene available from the company. During surgery, the acetabular component is found to be well fixed, it is in satisfactory position, and adequate access can be obtained through the screw holes in the component to débride the osteolytic cavities. What is the best course of action for revision?

1. Remove the component and replace it with a "jumbo" cup with bone graft or substitute.

2. Remove the component and replace it with a bipolar component with bone graft or substitute.

3. Remove the component and replace it with a support ring with graft or graft substitute and cement a cup into the support ring.

4. Score the component for improved cement interdigitation and cement a cup into the retained socket with bone graft or substitute.

5. Use a structural acetabular graft to reconstruct the acetabulum and cement a cup into the structural graft.

PREFERRED RESPONSE: 4

DISCUSSION: The clinical result in this patient has been good, with no dislocations, suggesting that the components are in reasonably good position. The radiograph and examination

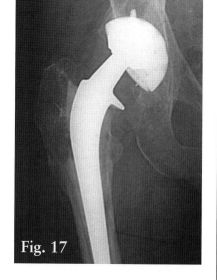

Fig. 17

at the time of surgery suggest that the acetabular component is well fixed. The surrounding bone of the acetabulum is osteopenic and there would most likely be considerable bone loss if the acetabular component is removed. Access to the osteolytic lesions is possible. Cementing an acetabular component into the retained socket will cause the least amount of bone loss, shorten the procedure, and most likely result in a functional hip.

REFERENCES: Maloney WJ: Socket retention: Staying in place. *Orthopedics* 2000;23:965-966.
Blaha JD: Well-fixed acetabular component retention or replacement: The whys and the wherefores. *J Arthroplasty* 2002;17:157-161.

A-37: Figures 18A and 18B show the AP and lateral radiographs of a 67-year-old woman who has severe left knee pain when ambulating. History reveals that she underwent primary total knee arthroplasty 7 years ago. The patient reports increasing deformity over the past several years and uses a knee brace and a cane. Examination reveals that she walks with a varus thrust and has an uncorrectable varus deformity with valgus force. What is the primary reason for implant failure?

1. Osteolysis
2. Polyethylene wear
3. Tibial component fixation failure
4. Modular tibial component failure
5. Posterior cruciate ligament retention

PREFERRED RESPONSE: 3

DISCUSSION: Both cemented and cementless total knee arthroplasties depend on adequate fixation of the tibial component to promote long-term survivorship. An effective stem and adequate peripheral fixation of the tibial component to the cancellous-cortical portion of the proximal tibia are necessary for cementless fixation. Peripheral screws and pegs can serve as adjunctive fixation to decrease micromotion and shear forces and allow bone ingrowth to occur. Careful preparation of the proximal tibial surface can minimize fixation failure. Cemented fixation of the tibial stem should be performed in addition to the plateau. Osteolysis, polyethylene wear, and failure at the insert/tray locking mechanism have not occurred. Posterior cruciate ligament retention has not caused the tibial component fixation failure.

REFERENCE: Pellicci PM, Tria AJ Jr, Garvin KL (eds): *Orthopaedic Knowledge Update: Hip and Knee Reconstruction 2.* Rosemont, IL, American Academy of Orthopaedic Surgeons, 2000, pp 275-279.

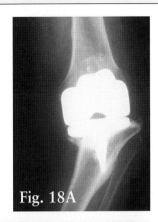

Fig. 18A

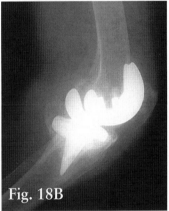

Fig. 18B

A-38: Which of the following statements best characterizes polymethylmethacrylate (PMMA) when it is used to secure joint components in bone and to distribute the forces evenly across the bone-implant interface?

1. PMMA is stronger in tension than compression.

2. Porosity reduction increases the fatigue strength of PMMA.

3. Hypotension that occasionally results after PMMA is placed in the femoral canal is independent of a patient's intraoperative blood volume.

4. Inclusion of antibiotics does not alter the strength of PMMA.

5. PMMA bonds chemically to bone and the implant surface.

PREFERRED RESPONSE: 2

DISCUSSION: PMMA has no adhesive properties and can be more accurately described as grout than glue. It does not chemically bond to bone or implants; however, mechanical bonding is accomplished with porous or coated components and with cancellous bone. PMMA is approximately three times stronger in compression than in tension. Peak blood levels of monomer are usually seen approximately 3 minutes after the cement is placed. The monomer is cleared by the lungs. Associated hypotension is more closely related to diminished blood volume than to circulating monomer levels. High porosity decreases the tensile and fatigue properties of cement. Manually mixed cement may have porosity as high as 27%. Porosity may be reduced to less than 1% through vacuum mixing or centrifugation of the cement. When adding antibiotics to cement, the compressive and tensile forces are not appreciably decreased, but the overall fatigue strength may be reduced.

REFERENCES: <edb>Canale ST (ed): *Campbell's Operative Orthopaedics*, ed 9. St Louis, MO, Mosby, 1998, pp 221-224.
Callaghan JJ, Dennis DA, Paprosky WG, Rosenberg AG (eds): *Orthopaedic Knowledge Update: Hip and Knee Reconstruction*. Rosemont, IL, American Academy of Orthopaedic Surgeons, 1995, pp 27-33.

A-39: A 35-year-old male laborer with isolated posttraumatic degenerative arthritis of the right hip undergoes the procedure shown in Figure 19. What is the most appropriate position of the right lower extremity?

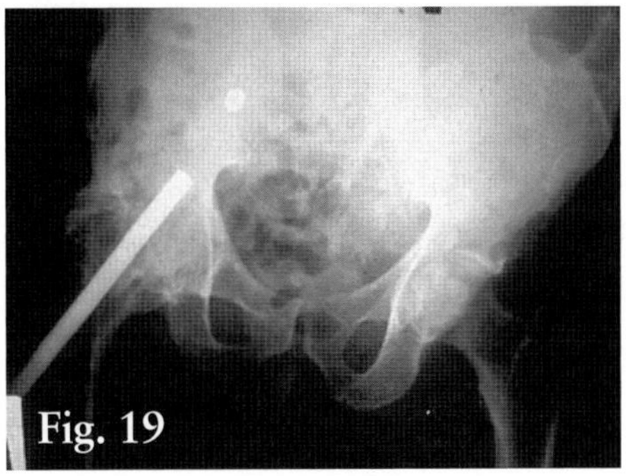

1. 0° of flexion, 10° of abduction, 0° of rotation
2. 15° of flexion, 20° of abduction, 15° of external rotation
3. 20° of flexion, 10° of abduction, and 5° of external rotation
4. 30° of flexion, 5° of adduction, and 5° of external rotation
5. 45° of flexion, 10° of adduction, 0° of rotation

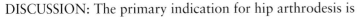
Fig. 19

PREFERRED RESPONSE: 4

DISCUSSION: The primary indication for hip arthrodesis is isolated unilateral hip disease in a young, active patient. Avoiding abductor damage and preserving proximal femoral anatomy are imperative to allow conversion to a future total hip arthroplasty. Optimal positioning is 30° of flexion to allow swing-through. Neutral abduction and adduction and slight external rotation allow the most efficient gait while allowing sufficient support in stance. A small degree of adduction is acceptable for a successful hip arthrodesis.

REFERENCES: Callaghan JJ, Brand RA, Pedersen DR: Hip arthrodesis: A long term follow-up. *J Bone Joint Surg Am* 1985;67:1328-1335.
Koval KJ (ed): *Orthopaedic Knowledge Update 7*. Rosemont, IL, American Academy of Orthopaedic Surgeons, 2002, pp 417-451.

A-40: Which of the following bearing materials is most resistant to scratching from third-body debris?

1. Alumina
2. Stainless steel
3. Forged cobalt-chromium
4. Ion bombarded and forged cobalt-chromium
5. Oxidized titanium

PREFERRED RESPONSE: 1

DISCUSSION: Alumina is the hardest of all the materials listed. Clinical retrieval demonstrates resistance to scratching from third-body debris.

REFERENCE: Cooper JR, Dowson D, Fisher J, Jobbins B: Ceramic bearing surfaces in total articular joints: Resistance to third body damage from bone cement particles. *J Med Eng Technol* 1991;15:63-67.

A-41: A 48-year-old woman has knee pain that is worse with weight bearing. She reports no night pain or pain at rest. History reveals that she underwent total knee arthroplasty with cementless components 2 years ago. Examination reveals tenderness along the medial joint line. Figures 20A through 20C show radiographs and a bone scan. What is the most likely cause of the patient's pain?

1. Deep infection
2. Malalignment
3. Fibrous ingrowth of the femoral component
4. Fibrous ingrowth of the tibial component
5. Patellar component loosening

PREFERRED RESPONSE: 4

DISCUSSION: The radiographs show a halo-like sclerotic margin around the tibial stem and lucency under the baseplate. The bone scan shows markedly increased uptake under the tibial component, particularly on the medial side (not diffusely through the knee as seen with infection). These studies indicate lack of bone ingrowth fixation of the cementless porous-coated tibial component. The recent report of Fehring and associates has identified failure of ingrowth of a porous-coated implant as a dominant mode of early failure of total knee arthroplasties.

REFERENCES: Fehring TK, Odum S, Griffin WL, Mason B, Nadaud M: Early failures of total knee arthroplasty. *Clin Orthop Relat Res* 2001;392:315-318.
Fehring TK: Revision TJA corrects flexion extension gap imbalance. *Orthop Today* 2002;22:44.

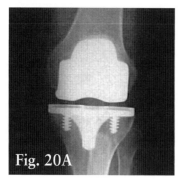
Fig. 20A

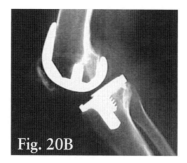
Fig. 20B

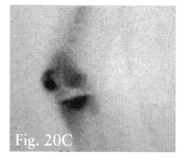
Fig. 20C

A-42: A 65-year-old woman has nausea, vomiting, and abdominal distention after undergoing total knee arthroplasty 48 hours ago. An abdominal radiograph is shown in Figure 21. Associated risk factors for this disorder include

1. hypokalemia.
2. administration of warfarin.
3. administration of antibiotics.
4. general anesthesia.
5. early mobilization and physical therapy.

PREFERRED RESPONSE: 1

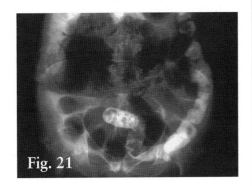

Fig. 21

DISCUSSION: The prevalence of postoperative ileus associated with total joint arthroplasty has been reported to be as high as 3%. Metabolic abnormalities such as hypokalemia are believed to contribute to the onset of ileus and Ogilvie syndrome (acute pseudo-obstruction of the colon). Prolonged bed rest also has been associated with the development of ileus and Ogilvie syndrome. Untreated Ogilvie syndrome can result in cecal perforation. Ileus usually is not accompanied by mechanical obstruction. Antibiotic administration and the type of anesthesia used have not been correlated with development of ileus. Administration of warfarin has been associated with elevated prothrombin time/partial thromboplastin time and international normalized ratio levels when ileus is managed with a nasogastric tube and suction. Metabolic imbalances must be corrected to reverse the ileus process.

REFERENCES: Iorio R, Healy WL, Appleby D: The association of excessive warfarin anticoagulation and postoperative ileus after total joint replacement surgery. *J Arthroplasty* 2000;15:220-223.
Clarke HD, Berry DJ, Larson DR: Acute pseudo-obstruction of the colon as a postoperative complication of hip arthroplasty. *J Bone Joint Surg Am* 1997;79:1642-1647.

A-43: Which of the following methods is considered effective in decreasing the dislocation rate following a total hip arthroplasty using a posterior approach to the hip?

1. Use of a shorter neck length

2. Use of a smaller diameter head with a skirted neck extension

3. Reconstruction of the external rotators and capsular attachments during closure

4. Placement of the acetabular component in 60° of abduction as opposed to 45° of abduction

5. Placement of the acetabular component in neutral (0°) anteversion as opposed to 15° to 20° of anteversion

PREFERRED RESPONSE: 3

DISCUSSION: A total hip arthroplasty using the posterior approach has resulted in hip dislocation under certain circumstances. Reconstruction of the external rotator/capsular complex is recognized as a stability-enhancing mechanism for the posterior approach. Although the correct position for an acetabular component has not been definitively determined, many surgeons prefer to place the acetabular component in 15° to 20° of anteversion and approximately 45° of abduction. Relative retroversion is a risk factor for posterior dislocation. High abduction angles result in edge loading of the polyethylene and possible early failure, as well as an increased risk of dislocation. Smaller diameter heads and skirted neck extensions used together decrease the range of motion that is allowed before impingement occurs, and this can result in dislocation. Shorter neck lengths generally result in soft-tissue envelope laxity. If laxity occurs, increased offset, neck length, or both can improve stability.

REFERENCES: Pellicci PM, Bostrom M, Poss R: Posterior approach to total hip replacement using enhanced posterior soft tissue repair. *Clin Orthop Relat Res* 1998;355:224-228.
Morrey BF: Difficult complications after hip joint replacement: Dislocation. *Clin Orthop Relat Res* 1997;344:179-187.

Foot and Ankle

Section Editor

Brian G. Donley, MD

Q-1: The main advantage of surgical repair of an acute Achilles tendon rupture, when compared with nonsurgical management, is reduced

1. stiffness of the ankle joint.
2. risk of deep venous thrombosis.
3. risk of rerupture.
4. cost of care.
5. tendon healing time.

Q-2: Figures 1A and 1B show a clinical photograph and radiograph of a patient who has difficulty wearing shoes and has persistent symptoms medially and laterally at the first and fifth metatarsophalangeal joints. Because shoe modifications have failed to provide relief, management should now consist of

1. bunion repair only.
2. bunionette repair only with lateral condylectomy.
3. repair of both with lateral condylectomy.
4. repair of both with a proximal fifth metatarsal osteotomy.
5. repair of both with a fifth metatarsal head excision.

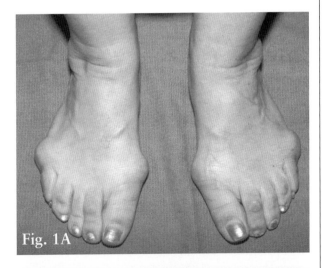

Fig. 1A

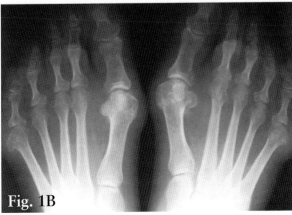

Fig. 1B

Q-3: A patient requires excision of a symptomatic os trigonum employing a posterolateral approach. What intermuscular interval is used?

1. Peroneus longus and peroneus brevis
2. Tibialis posterior and flexor hallucis longus
3. Flexor digitorum longus and flexor hallucis longus
4. Flexor hallucis longus and peroneus brevis
5. Tibialis posterior and flexor digitorum longus

Q-4: What is the most appropriate orthotic management for the lesion shown in Figure 2?

1. Metatarsal pad
2. Morton extension orthosis
3. Medial longitudinal arch support
4. Budin splint
5. Viscoelastic heel lift

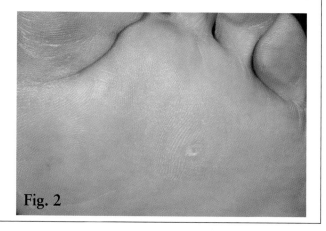
Fig. 2

Q-5: A Canale view best visualizes which of the following structures?

1. Posterior facet of the subtalar joint
2. Lisfranc joint
3. Talar neck
4. Sustentaculum tali
5. Lateral column of the foot

Q-6: Which of the following procedures is used for acute repair of dislocated peroneal tendons?

1. Deepening the fibular groove with an osteotome
2. Borrowing fascia to create new retinacula
3. Repairing the periosteal tendon sheath attachment
4. Creating a fibular bone-block extension
5. Rerouting the tendons through the fibula

Q-7: Talar compression syndrome in ballet dancers typically involves injury to which of the following structures?

1. Sustentaculum tali
2. Lateral process of the talus
3. Posterior process of the calcaneus
4. Os tibialis externum
5. Os trigonum

Q-8: The abductor digiti quinti muscle of the foot is most frequently innervated by what peripheral nerve?

1. Medial plantar
2. Deep peroneal
3. Saphenous
4. Sural
5. Lateral plantar

Q-9: In ankle arthroscopy, the anteromedial portal is located between what structures?

1. Medial malleolus and saphenous vein
2. Saphenous vein and anterior tibial tendon
3. Anterior tibial tendon and extensor hallucis longus
4. Anterior tibial tendon and anterior tibial neurovascular bundle
5. Extensor hallucis longus tendon and anterior tibial neurovascular bundle

Q-10: The dorsal-medial aspect of the great toe receives sensory innervation from which nerve?

1. Deep peroneal
2. Saphenous
3. Posterior tibial
4. Superficial peroneal
5. Medial plantar

Q-11: A 60-year-old man reports that he has had shoe pressure pain over his right great toe for several years but has minimal discomfort when barefoot or in sandals. A clinical photograph and radiographs are shown in Figures 3A through 3C. Management should consist of

1. cheilectomy.
2. extra-depth shoes.
3. steroid injection.
4. arthrodesis.
5. joint replacement arthroplasty.

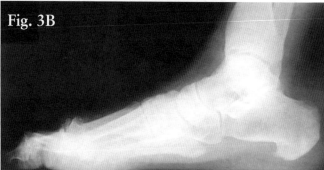

Fig. 3A

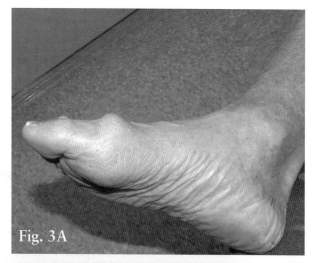

Fig. 3B

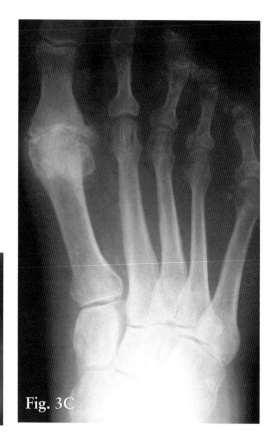

Fig. 3C

Q-12: Which of the following ligaments is intracapsular?

1. Lisfranc
2. Deltoid
3. Calcaneofibular
4. Anterior talofibular
5. Inferior tibiofibular

Q-13: Sensation on the plantar aspect of the great toe is derived from which of the following nerves?

1. Sural
2. Lateral plantar
3. Medial plantar
4. Lesser saphenous
5. Greater saphenous

Q-14: A 35-year-old woman who runs long distance has had posterior calf tenderness for the past 3 months. A clinical photograph is shown in Figure 4A, and MRI scans are shown in Figures 4B and 4C. Management at this point should consist of

1. a non-weight-bearing cast for 4 weeks.
2. eccentric calf stretching and physical therapy.
3. a cortisone injection.
4. tendon débridement.
5. tendon débridement and augmentation.

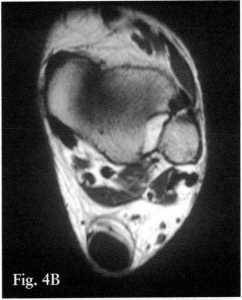

Fig. 4B

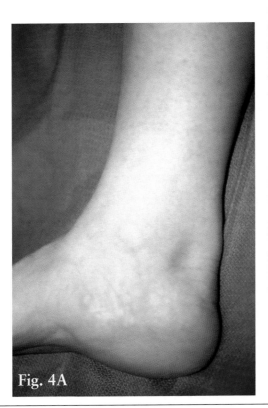

Fig. 4A

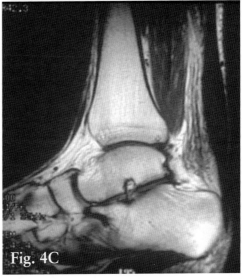

Fig. 4C

Q-15: Which of the following nerves is most likely responsible for symptoms associated with plantar fasciitis?

1. Medial plantar
2. Medial calcaneal
3. First branch of lateral plantar
4. Lateral plantar
5. Lateral calcaneal

Q-16: The so-called high ankle sprain from an external rotation mechanism of injury typically involves injury to which of the following structures?

1. Posterior talofibular ligament
2. Deltoid ligament
3. Anterior inferior tibiofibular ligament
4. Calcaneofibular ligament
5. Extensor retinaculum

Q-17: The modified Broström lateral ankle ligamentous reconstruction uses which of the following structures to provide supplementary stabilization?

1. One half of the peroneus brevis tendon
2. The entire peroneus brevis tendon
3. Peroneus longus tendon
4. Plantaris
5. Inferior extensor retinaculum

Q-18: When performing ankle arthroscopy through the anterolateral portal, what anatomic structure is at greatest risk?

1. Anterior tibialis tendon
2. Anterior tibial artery
3. Sural nerve
4. Deep peroneal nerve
5. Superficial peroneal nerve

Q-19: Turf toe typically involves injury to which of the following structures of the great toe?

1. Nail bed
2. Extensor tendon
3. Flexor tendon
4. Capsule of the first metatarsophalangeal joint
5. Distal phalanx of the first toe

A-1: The main advantage of surgical repair of an acute Achilles tendon rupture, when compared with nonsurgical management, is reduced

1. stiffness of the ankle joint.
2. risk of deep venous thrombosis.
3. risk of rerupture.
4. cost of care.
5. tendon healing time.

PREFERRED RESPONSE: 3

DISCUSSION: The literature supports similar clinical outcomes after surgical and nonsurgical methods. The chief difference lies in the complications between the groups. Surgical patients experience more wound problems but a significantly lower rerupture rate. Although suturing the tendon allows earlier mobility, the tendon healing time is unchanged. Nonsurgical methods are less expensive to provide.

REFERENCES: Maffulli N: Rupture of the Achilles tendon. *J Bone Joint Surg Am* 1999;81:1019-1036.
Cetti R, Christensen SE, Ejsted R, Jensen NM, Jorgensen U: Operative versus nonoperative treatment of Achilles tendon rupture: A prospective randomized study and review of the literature. *Am J Sports Med* 1993;21:791-799.
Nistor L: Surgical and non-surgical treatment of Achilles tendon rupture. *J Bone Joint Surg Am* 1981;63:394-399.

A-2: Figures 1A and 1B show a clinical photograph and radiograph of a patient who has difficulty wearing shoes and has persistent symptoms medially and laterally at the first and fifth metatarsophalangeal joints. Because shoe modifications have failed to provide relief, management should now consist of

1. bunion repair only.
2. bunionette repair only with lateral condylectomy.
3. repair of both with lateral condylectomy.
4. repair of both with a proximal fifth metatarsal osteotomy.
5. repair of both with a fifth metatarsal head excision.

PREFERRED RESPONSE: 3

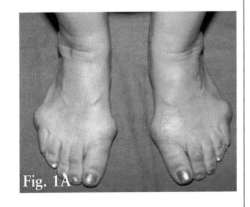

Fig. 1A

(continued on next page)

(A-2 continued)

DISCUSSION: A significant bunionette deformity that fails to respond to conservative management is best addressed surgically, in this case with the bunion deformity. The radiograph reveals a prominent lateral condyle at the fifth metatarsal head without a significant increase in the intermetatarsal angle. Simple exostectomy is preferred with less risk of complications. Complete excision would risk transfer lesions to the medial metatarsals.

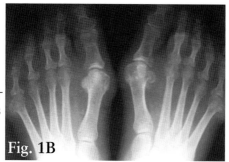

Fig. 1B

REFERENCES: Mann RA, Coughlin MJ: Adult hallux valgus, in Coughlin MJ, Mann RA (eds): *Surgery of the Foot and Ankle*, ed 7. St Louis, MO, Mosby, 1999, pp 415-435.

Mizel MS, Miller RA, Scioli MW (eds): *Orthopaedic Knowledge Update: Foot and Ankle 2*. Rosemont, IL, American Academy of Orthopaedic Surgeons, 1998, pp 163-173.

A-3: A patient requires excision of a symptomatic os trigonum employing a posterolateral approach. What intermuscular interval is used?

1. Peroneus longus and peroneus brevis
2. Tibialis posterior and flexor hallucis longus
3. Flexor digitorum longus and flexor hallucis longus
4. Flexor hallucis longus and peroneus brevis
5. Tibialis posterior and flexor digitorum longus

PREFERRED RESPONSE: 4

DISCUSSION: The posterolateral approach to the ankle uses an intramuscular plane (which is also internervous) between the peroneus brevis (superficial peroneal nerve) and the flexor hallucis longus (tibial nerve). The flexor hallucis longus courses directly medial to the os trigonum and is at risk for injury.

REFERENCE: Hoppenfeld S, deBoer P: *Surgical Exposures in Orthopaedics: The Anatomic Approach.* Philadelphia, PA, JB Lippincott, 1984, pp 487-492.

A-4: What is the most appropriate orthotic management for the lesion shown in Figure 2?

1. Metatarsal pad
2. Morton extension orthosis
3. Medial longitudinal arch support
4. Budin splint
5. Viscoelastic heel lift

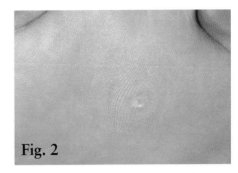

Fig. 2

PREFERRED RESPONSE: 1

DISCUSSION: The figure shows an intractable plantar keratosis (IPK). The keratoma usually forms beneath a bony prominence. This can occur under the sesamoids, most commonly the tibial sesamoid, or under the fibular condyle of a prominent metatarsal head. The initial treatment of an IPK consists of paring down the callused lesion and placing a metatarsal pad proximal to the lesion to provide posting to unload the bony prominence.

REFERENCE: Rudicel SA: Intractable plantar keratoses, in Gould J (ed): *Operative Foot Surgery.* Philadelphia, PA, WB Saunders, 1994, p 70.

A-5: A Canale view best visualizes which of the following structures?

1. Posterior facet of the subtalar joint
2. Lisfranc joint
3. Talar neck
4. Sustentaculum tali
5. Lateral column of the foot

PREFERRED RESPONSE: 3

DISCUSSION: The Canale view, which visualizes the talar neck, is taken with the ankle in maximum plantar flexion and the foot pronated 15°. The radiograph is directed at a 75° angle from the horizontal plane in the anteroposterior plane. The Broden view, which is different from the Canale view, is best for imaging the posterior facet of the subtalar joint.

REFERENCES: Canale ST, Kelly FB Jr: Fractures of the neck of the talus: Long-term evaluation of seventy-one cases. *J Bone Joint Surg Am* 1978;60:143-156.
Bruden B: Roentgen examination of the subtaloid joint in fractures of the calcaneus. *Acta Radiol* 1949;31:85-91.

A-6: Which of the following procedures is used for acute repair of dislocated peroneal tendons?

1. Deepening the fibular groove with an osteotome
2. Borrowing fascia to create new retinacula
3. Repairing the periosteal tendon sheath attachment
4. Creating a fibular bone-block extension
5. Rerouting the tendons through the fibula

PREFERRED RESPONSE: 3

DISCUSSION: Acute dislocation of the peroneal tendons involves avulsion of the periosteal attachment of the peroneal sheath and the superior retinaculum. Repair of these structures and cast immobilization for several weeks provides excellent functional stability of the tendons and avoids chronic subluxation. The other methods are used in chronic tendon dislocation.

REFERENCES: Eckert WR, Davis EA Jr: Acute rupture of the peroneal retinaculum. *J Bone Joint Surg Am* 1976;58:670-672.
Arrowsmith SR, Fleming LL, Allman FL: Traumatic dislocations of the peroneal tendons. *Am J Sports Med* 1983;11:142-146.

A-7: Talar compression syndrome in ballet dancers typically involves injury to which of the following structures?

1. Sustentaculum tali
2. Lateral process of the talus
3. Posterior process of the calcaneus
4. Os tibialis externum
5. Os trigonum

PREFERRED RESPONSE: 5

DISCUSSION: Talar compression syndrome is also known as os trigonum syndrome or posterior ankle impingement syndrome and occurs in activities involving extreme ankle plantar flexion. It involves pinching of the posterior talus (os trigonum or posterior process of the talus) between the calcaneus and tibia. The flexor hallucis longus also may be impinged. The other structures are not commonly injured in this syndrome.

REFERENCES: Brodsky AE, Khalil MA: Talar compression syndrome. *Am J Sports Med* 1986;14:472-476.
Wredmark T, Carlstedt CA, Bauer H, Saartok T: Os trigonum syndrome: A clinical entity in ballet dancers. *Foot Ankle* 1991;11:404-406.
Marotta JJ, Micheli LJ: Os trigonum impingement in dancers. *Am J Sports Med* 1992;20:533-536.

A-8: The abductor digiti quinti muscle of the foot is most frequently innervated by what peripheral nerve?

1. Medial plantar
2. Deep peroneal
3. Saphenous
4. Sural
5. Lateral plantar

PREFERRED RESPONSE: 5

DISCUSSION: Distal to the laciniate ligament the tibial nerve divides into four or five branches. The nerve to the abductor digiti quinti arises as a branch off the lateral plantar nerve or may come directly off the tibial nerve. It passes beneath the deep fascial edge of the abductor hallucis muscle where it can become compressed. It continues laterally, deep to the origin of the plantar fascia and flexor digitorum brevis muscle, and terminates in the proximal portion of the abductor digiti quinti.

REFERENCES: Chapman MW: *Operative Orthopaedics*. Philadelphia, PA, JB Lippincott, 1993, p 2327. Baxter DE, Thigpen CM: Heel pain: Operative results. *Foot Ankle* 1984;5:16-25.

A-9: In ankle arthroscopy, the anteromedial portal is located between what structures?

1. Medial malleolus and saphenous vein
2. Saphenous vein and anterior tibial tendon
3. Anterior tibial tendon and extensor hallucis longus
4. Anterior tibial tendon and anterior tibial neurovascular bundle
5. Extensor hallucis longus tendon and anterior tibial neurovascular bundle

PREFERRED RESPONSE: 2

DISCUSSION: The anteromedial portal is placed just medial to the anterior tibial tendon and lateral to the saphenous vein at the level of the ankle joint. The anterolateral portal is located just lateral to the tendon of the peroneus tertius.

REFERENCE: Ferkel RS: Arthroscopy of the ankle and foot, in Mann RA, Coughlin MJ (eds): *Surgery of the Foot and Ankle*, ed 6. St Louis, MO, Mosby, 1993, vol 2, p 1279.

A-10: The dorsal-medial aspect of the great toe receives sensory innervation from which nerve?

1. Deep peroneal
2. Saphenous
3. Posterior tibial
4. Superficial peroneal
5. Medial plantar

PREFERRED RESPONSE: 4

DISCUSSION: The medial or internal division of the superficial peroneal nerve consistently provides sensory innervation to the dorsal-medial aspect of the great toe.

REFERENCE: Sarrafian SK: *Anatomy of the Foot and Ankle*. Philadelphia, PA, JB Lippincott, 1993, p 368.

A-11: A 60-year-old man reports that he has had shoe pressure pain over his right great toe for several years but has minimal discomfort when barefoot or in sandals. A clinical photograph and radiographs are shown in Figures 3A through 3C. Management should consist of

1. cheilectomy.
2. extra-depth shoes.
3. steroid injection.
4. arthrodesis.
5. joint replacement arthroplasty.

PREFERRED RESPONSE: 2

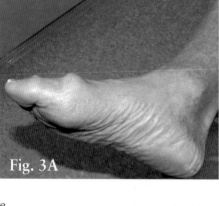

Fig. 3A

DISCUSSION: Some patients have minimal symptoms associated with hallux rigidus despite significant radiographic evidence of osteoarthritis. This patient's symptoms are primarily related to shoe pressure from the exostosis and can be managed with extra-depth shoe wear.

REFERENCES: Smith RW, Katchis SD, Ayson LC: Outcomes in hallux rigidus patients treated nonoperatively: A long-term follow-up study. *Foot Ankle Int* 2000;21:906-913.
Shereff MJ, Baumhauer JF: Hallux rigidus and osteoarthrosis of the first metatarsophalangeal joint. *J Bone Joint Surg Am* 1998;80:898-908.

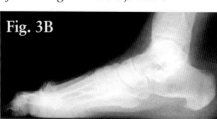

Fig. 3B

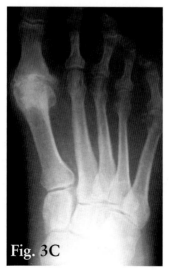

Fig. 3C

A-12: Which of the following ligaments is intracapsular?

1. Lisfranc
2. Deltoid
3. Calcaneofibular
4. Anterior talofibular
5. Inferior tibiofibular

PREFERRED RESPONSE: 4

DISCUSSION: The anterior talofibular ligament lies within the lateral capsule of the ankle, similar to the anterior glenohumeral ligaments of the shoulder. The other four ligaments mentioned are extracapsular.

REFERENCE: Brostroem L: Sprained ankles: I. Anatomic lesions in recent sprains. *Acta Chir Scand* 1964;128:483-495.

A-13: Sensation on the plantar aspect of the great toe is derived from which of the following nerves?

1. Sural
2. Lateral plantar
3. Medial plantar
4. Lesser saphenous
5. Greater saphenous

PREFERRED RESPONSE: 3

DISCUSSION: The medial and lateral plantar nerves supply all the musculature of the sole of the foot. The medial plantar nerve supplies most of the terminal sensory branches, including the proper digital nerves to the great toe and the common digital nerves to the next three interspaces. The three and one-half toes supplied by the medial plantar nerve are analogous to the median nerve innervation in the hand.

REFERENCE: Gross RH: Fractures and dislocations of the foot, in Rockwood CA Jr, Wilkins KE, Beaty JH (eds): *Fractures in Children*, ed 4. Philadelphia, PA, Lippincott-Raven, 1996, p 1383.

A-14: A 35-year-old woman who runs long distance has had posterior calf tenderness for the past 3 months. A clinical photograph is shown in Figure 4A, and MRI scans are shown in Figures 4B and 4C. Management at this point should consist of

1. a non-weight-bearing cast for 4 weeks.
2. eccentric calf stretching and physical therapy.
3. a cortisone injection.
4. tendon débridement.
5. tendon débridement and augmentation.

PREFERRED RESPONSE: 2

DISCUSSION: The initial treatment for peritendinitis should consist of calf stretching in an eccentric mode and physical therapy. In a recent study, this treatment has been found superior to surgical débridement in nonextensive peritendinitis and pantendinitis. A non-weight-bearing cast, while useful in reducing inflammation, will result in calf atrophy and poorly organized collagen repair. Cortisone is contraindicated because of the danger of tendon damage. Tendon débridement at this stage is not indicated.

REFERENCES: Alfredson H, Pietila T, Jansson P, Lorentzon R: Heavy-load eccentric calf muscle training for the treatment of chronic Achilles tendinosis. *Am J Sports Med* 1998;26:360-366.
Angermann P, Hougaard D: Chronic Achilles tendinopathy in athletic individuals: Results of nonsurgical treatment. *Foot Ankle Int* 1999;20:304-306.

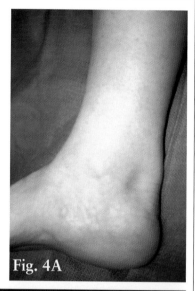
Fig. 4A

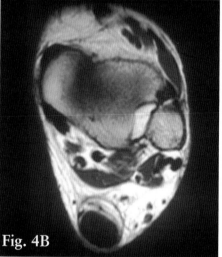
Fig. 4B

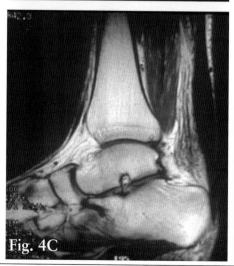
Fig. 4C

Answers: Foot and Ankle

A-15: Which of the following nerves is most likely responsible for symptoms associated with plantar fasciitis?

1. Medial plantar
2. Medial calcaneal
3. First branch of lateral plantar
4. Lateral plantar
5. Lateral calcaneal

PREFERRED RESPONSE: 5

DISCUSSION: The first branch of the lateral calcaneal nerve innervates the abductor digiti minimi. It is reported to be trapped at the interval between the abductor hallucis and the quadratus plantae muscles.

REFERENCE: Baxter DE, Pfeffer GB, Thigpen M: Chronic heel pain: Treatment rationale. *Orthop Clin North Am* 1989;20:563-569.

A-16: The so-called high ankle sprain from an external rotation mechanism of injury typically involves injury to which of the following structures?

1. Posterior talofibular ligament
2. Deltoid ligament
3. Anterior inferior tibiofibular ligament
4. Calcaneofibular ligament
5. Extensor retinaculum

PREFERRED RESPONSE: 3

DISCUSSION: Ankle sprains most commonly involve injury to the lateral collateral ligaments of the ankle (anterior talofibular, posterior talofibular, and calcaneofibular) from an inversion mechanism of injury. A different entity has been more recently described that involves an external rotation mechanism of injury that widens the ankle mortise and disrupts the anterior inferior tibiofibular ligament. Deltoid ligament and extensor retinaculum injuries do occur, although infrequently, and involve eversion and extreme plantar flexion mechanisms, respectively.

REFERENCES: Last RJ: *Anatomy: Regional and Applied,* ed 6. London, England, Churchill Livingstone, 1978, p 182.
Kaye RA: Stabilization of ankle syndesmosis injuries with a syndesmosis screw. *Foot Ankle* 1989;9:290-293.
Baxter DE: *The Foot and Ankle in Sports.* St Louis, MO, Mosby-Year Book, 1995, p 30.
Pfeffer GB (ed): *Chronic Ankle Pain in the Athlete.* Rosemont, IL, American Academy of Orthopaedic Surgeons, 2000, p 11.

Answers: Foot and Ankle

A-17: The modified Broström lateral ankle ligamentous reconstruction uses which of the following structures to provide supplementary stabilization?

1. One half of the peroneus brevis tendon
2. The entire peroneus brevis tendon
3. Peroneus longus tendon
4. Plantaris
5. Inferior extensor retinaculum

PREFERRED RESPONSE: 5

DISCUSSION: The modified Broström lateral ankle ligament stabilization procedure uses the remnants of the anterior talofibular and the calcaneofibular ligaments, supplemented by the inferior extensor retinaculum and the transferred talocalcaneal ligament to stabilize the lateral ankle. Chrisman and associates described the use of one half of the peroneus brevis. Watson-Jones and Evans used the entire peroneus brevis. The peroneus longus has been taken by mistake. The plantaris has been used in triligamentous reconstruction.

REFERENCES: Gould N, Seligson D, Gassman J: Early and late repair of lateral ligament of the ankle. *Foot Ankle* 1980;1:84-89.

Hamilton WG, Thompson FM, Snow SW: The modified Brostrom procedure for lateral ankle instability. *Foot Ankle* 1993;14:1-7.

Chrisman OD, Snook GA: Reconstruction of lateral ligament tears of the ankle: An experimental study and clinical evaluation of seven patients treated by a new modification of the Elmslie procedure. *J Bone Joint Surg Am* 1969;51:904-912.

Evans DL: Recurrent instability of the ankle: My method of surgical treatment. *Proc R Soc Med* 1953;46:343.

Watson-Jones R: *Fractures and Joint Injuries,* ed 3. Baltimore, MD, Williams and Wilkins, 1946, p 234.

Liu SH, Baker CL: Comparison of lateral ankle ligamentous reconstruction procedures. *Am J Sports Med* 1994;22:313-317.

Broström L: Sprained ankles: VI. Surgical treatment of "chronic" ligament ruptures. *Acta Chir Scand* 1966;132:551-565.

A-18: When performing ankle arthroscopy through the anterolateral portal, what anatomic structure is at greatest risk?

1. Anterior tibialis tendon
2. Anterior tibial artery
3. Sural nerve
4. Deep peroneal nerve
5. Superficial peroneal nerve

PREFERRED RESPONSE: 5

DISCUSSION: The superficial branch of the peroneal nerve travels subcutaneously anterior to the lateral malleolus at the ankle. It can be easily damaged by deep penetration of the knife blade when making this portal or when passing shavers in and out of the portal. Anesthesia or dysesthesia from laceration or neuroma formation can cause significant postoperative morbidity. The anterior tibialis tendon, anterior tibial artery, and the deep peroneal nerve are located much more anterior and central on the ankle. The sural nerve is posterior lateral to the ankle and is not at risk from this portal.

REFERENCES: Ferkel RD, Heath DD, Guhl JF: Neurological complications of ankle arthroscopy. *Arthroscopy* 1996;12:200-208.
Cooper PS, Murray TF Jr: Arthroscopy of the foot and ankle in the athlete. *Clin Sports Med* 1996;15:805-824.

A-19: Turf toe typically involves injury to which of the following structures of the great toe?

1. Nail bed
2. Extensor tendon
3. Flexor tendon
4. Capsule of the first metatarsophalangeal joint
5. Distal phalanx of the first toe

PREFERRED RESPONSE: 4

DISCUSSION: The term turf toe includes a range of injuries of the capsuloligamentous complex of the first metatarsophalangeal joint with or without osteochondral fracture of the first metatarsal head or one of the sesamoids. The mechanism of injury is hyperextension.

REFERENCES: Clanton TO, Butler JE, Eggert A: Injuries to the metatarsophalangeal joints in athletes. *Foot Ankle* 1986;7:162-176.
Sammarco GJ: How I manage turf toe. *Phys Sports Med* 1988;16:113-118.